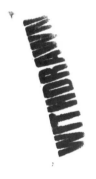

Ethics and Newborn Genetic Screening

Ethics and Newborn Genetic Screening

New Technologies, New Challenges

Edited by

Mary Ann Baily, *Research Scholar*

and

Thomas H. Murray, *President and CEO*

The Hastings Center
Garrison, New York

The Johns Hopkins University Press
Baltimore

© 2009 The Johns Hopkins University Press
All rights reserved. Published 2009
Printed in the United States of America on acid-free paper
9 8 7 6 5 4 3 2 1

Copyright in this volume excludes the specific work by Scott D. Grosse, Michele A.
Lloyd-Puryear, and Marie Y. Mann, which was performed as work of the U.S.
government.

The Johns Hopkins University Press
2715 North Charles Street
Baltimore, Maryland 21218-4363
www.press.jhu.edu

Library of Congress Cataloging-in-Publication Data

Ethics and newborn genetic screening : new technologies, new challenges / edited
by Mary Ann Baily and Thomas H. Murray.
    p. ; cm.
  Includes bibliographical references and index.
  ISBN-13: 978-0-8018-9151-9 (hardcover : alk. paper)
  ISBN-10: 0-8018-9151-5 (hardcover : alk. paper)
    1. Genetic disorders—Diagnosis—Moral and ethical aspects. 2. Newborn
infants—Diseases—Diagnosis—Moral and ethical aspects. 3. Genetic
screening—Moral and ethical aspects. I. Baily, Mary Ann. II. Murray,
Thomas H., 1946–
    [DNLM: 1. Genetic Diseases, Inborn—diagnosis. 2. Neonatal Screening—
ethics. 3. Genetic Screening—ethics. 4. Health Policy. 5. Infant, Newborn.
WS 200 E84 2009]
    RJ255.6.D55.E84   2009
    618.92'0042—dc22   2008033831

A catalog record for this book is available from the British Library.

*Special discounts are available for bulk purchases of this book. For more information, please
contact Special Sales at 410-516-6936 or specialsales@press.jhu.edu.*

The Johns Hopkins University Press uses environmentally friendly book materials,
including recycled text paper that is composed of at least 30 percent post-consumer
waste, whenever possible. All of our book papers are acid-free, and our jackets and
covers are printed on paper with recycled content.

Contents

Contributors

Andrea Bonnicksen, Ph.D., Professor, Department of Political Science, Northern Illinois University, DeKalb, Illinois

Jeffrey R. Botkin, M.D., M.P.H., Professor of Pediatrics and Medical Ethics, Associate Vice President for Research, University of Utah, Salt Lake City, Utah

Ned Calonge, M.D., M.P.H., Chief Medical Officer, Department of Public Health and Environment, Denver, Colorado

Toby Citrin, J.D., Director, Center for Public Health and Community Genomics, University of Michigan School of Public Health, Ann Arbor, Michigan

Ellen Wright Clayton, M.D., M.S., J.D., Rosalind E. Franklin Professor of Genetics and Health Policy, Co-Director, Center for Biomedical Ethics and Society, Vanderbilt University, Nashville, Tennessee

Jannine De Mars Cody, Ph.D., President, The Chromosome 18 Registry and Research Society, and Associate Professor, Chromosome 18 Clinical Research Center, Department of Pediatrics, University of Texas Health Science Center, San Antonio, Texas

Anne Marie Comeau, Ph.D., Deputy Director, New England Newborn Screening Program, and Associate Professor, Department of Pediatrics, University of Massachusetts Medical School, Jamaica Plain, Massachusetts

James R. Eckman, M.D., Professor of Hematology, Oncology, and Medicine, Winship Cancer Institute; Professor of Medicine, Emory University School of Medicine; and Director, Georgia Sickle Cell Comprehensive Care Center at Grady, Atlanta, Georgia

Scott D. Grosse, Ph.D., National Center on Birth Defects and Developmental Disabilities, Centers for Disease Control and Prevention, Atlanta, Georgia

Bruce Jennings, M.A., Director, Center for Humans and Nature, New York, New York; and Lecturer, Yale School of Public Health, New Haven, Connecticut

Donna E. Levin, J.D., General Counsel, Massachusetts Department of Public Health, Boston, Massachusetts

Michele A. Lloyd-Puryear, M.D., Ph.D., Maternal and Child Health Bureau, Health Resources and Services Administration, U.S. Department of Health and Human Services, Rockville, Maryland

Marie Y. Mann, M.D., M.P.H., Maternal and Child Health Bureau, Health Resources and Services Administration, U.S. Department of Health and Human Services, Rockville, Maryland

Karen J. Maschke, Ph.D., Research Scholar and Editor, *IRB: Ethics and Human Research*, The Hastings Center, Garrison, New York

Stephen M. Modell, M.D., M.S., Dissemination Activities Director, Center for Public Health and Community Genomics, University of Michigan School of Public Health, Ann Arbor, Michigan

Virginia A. Moyer, M.D., M.P.H., Professor of Pediatrics, Baylor College of Medicine and Texas Children's Hospital, Houston, Texas

Lainie Friedman Ross, M.D., Ph.D., Carolyn and Matthew Bucksbaum Professor of Clinical Ethics; Associate Director, MacLean Center for Clinical Medical Ethics; and Professor, Departments of Pediatrics, Medicine, and Surgery, University of Chicago, Chicago, Illinois

Joseph Telfair, Dr.P.H., M.S.W., M.P.H., Professor, Public Health Research and Practice, and Director of Graduate Studies, Department of Public Health Education, School of Health and Human Performance, University of North Carolina at Greensboro, Greensboro, North Carolina

Steven M. Teutsch, M.D., M.P.H., Executive Director, U.S. Outcomes Research, Merck & Co., Inc., West Point, Pennsylvania

Bradford L. Therrell, Ph.D., Director, National Newborn Screening and Genetics Resource Center, Austin, Texas; and Professor, Department of Pediatrics, University of Texas Health Science Center at San Antonio, San Antonio, Texas

Benjamin S. Wilfond, M.D., Professor, Department of Pediatrics, University of Washington, and Director, Treuman Katz Center for Pediatric Bioethics, Seattle Children's Hospital, Seattle, Washington

Preface

This book is the product of a multiyear Hastings Center effort to study new screening technologies and new knowledge about the origin and treatment of genetic conditions. The project focused on the impact of these changes on newborn screening, an ongoing public health program that tests virtually all newborns for genetic disorders. Titled "Ethical Decision-Making for Newborn Genetic Screening," the project was funded by grant 5R HG002579 from the National Human Genome Research Institute, in the National Institutes of Health.

The long-term objective of the research was to provide guidance to the professionals, policymakers, and members of the public who must make decisions about newborn screening in this new environment. The project's aims included:

1 Carrying out an in-depth analysis of a set of closely related ethical and social issues that are critical to newborn screening decisions. These issues relate to fairness in the distribution of the costs and benefits of newborn screening; information, consent, and privacy; consultation and decision making; and race, ethnicity, and socioeconomic status.
2 Using this analysis as the basis for a framework for the determination and assessment of newborn screening policy that adequately responds to these issues.
3 Disseminating the results in formats appropriate to the needs of specific groups of decision makers.

To accomplish this, the Hastings Center assembled an interdisciplinary group with expertise and experience in a range of fields, including the technology of screening, its clinical utility and application, ethics, public health, economics, law, public policy, and consumer advocacy. (See table P.1 for the list of project members.) The group met four times over several years to explore key issues in the areas identified, using five genetic disorders as examples to help focus the discussions: phenylketonuria (PKU), sickle cell disease (SCD), cystic fibrosis (CF), medium-chain acyl-CoA dehydrogenase deficiency (MCAD), and severe combined immunodeficiency (SCID). (These disorders are described in the Appendix.) At the meetings, project members and other invited guests presented and debated the findings of their own experience and research on the issues.

Most of the chapters in this book originated as background papers prepared by project members and outside consultants and presented to the group. Chapter 2 is developed from a background paper for the project, but also draws heavily from work carried out by the author under a previous contract funded by the Health Resources and Services Administration. Chapter 8 was not written as part of the project process but provides an important outside perspective on the American College of Medical Genetics report that is playing a key role in the expansion of newborn screening test panels currently under way. The authors of the background papers benefited from the interchanges among project participants; however, the papers and the chapters developed from them reflect the authors' own views, not those of the entire group of project members.

Chapter 1 provides an overview of the issues, and chapter 16, the final chapter, presents conclusions and recommendations for the future. These chapters are the work of the book's editors (the principal investigator and project manager). The analysis in these two chapters has been heavily influenced by the deliberations of the group; nevertheless, we emphasize that, except where expressly stated otherwise, the analysis, conclusions, and recommendations are those of the editors alone. The period from 2002 to 2007 was marked by considerable turmoil and controversy in newborn screening policy. The project members were able to agree on an overarching conclusion about the requirements for ethical policy, but they disagreed strongly on the extent to which the actual policy process and outcome conformed to the requirements during this period. As a result, we did not attempt to achieve consensus among the project members on the contents of these chapters.

The chapters address the questions raised from a variety of perspectives. In chapter 2, "Fair Distribution of Newborn Screening Costs and Benefits," Mary Ann Baily explains the rationale for making newborn screening a public health program and analyzes the meaning of fairness, arguing that assessment of the fairness of a policy requires attention to the policy decision process as well as the policy outcomes. She uses this conceptual framework to discuss

TABLE P.1
Project Members

Adrienne Asch, Ph.D., M.S. The Center for Ethics at Yeshiva University New York, NY	Fernando Guerra, M.D. Department of Health of the San Antonio Metropolitan Health District San Antonio, TX
Mary Ann Baily, Ph.D. The Hastings Center Garrison, NY	Bruce Jennings, M.A. Center for Humans and Nature New York, NY
Andrea Bonnicksen, Ph.D. Northern Illinois University DeKalb, IL	Michele A. Lloyd-Puryear, M.D., Ph.D. Maternal and Child Health Bureau, Health Resources and Services Administration Rockville, MD
Jeffrey R. Botkin, M.D., M.P.H. University of Utah Salt Lake City, UT	Karen J. Maschke, Ph.D. The Hastings Center Garrison, NY
Ellen Wright Clayton, M.D., M.S., J.D. Vanderbilt University Nashville, TN	Thomas H. Murray, Ph.D. The Hastings Center Garrison, NY
Jannine De Mars Cody, Ph.D. University of Texas Health Science Center San Antonio, TX	Kenneth Pass, Ph.D. New York State Department of Health New York, NY
Anne Marie Comeau, Ph.D. New England Newborn Screening Program Jamaica Plain, MA	Lainie Friedman Ross, M.D., Ph.D. MacLean Center for Clinical Medical Ethics at University of Chicago Chicago, IL
George Cunningham, M.D., M.P.H. California Department of Health Services Richmond, CA	Charmaine Royal, M.S., Ph.D. Duke University Durham, NC
Jessica Davis, M.D. New York Hospital–Cornell Medical Center New York, NY	Bradford L. Therrell, Ph.D. National Newborn Screening and Genetics Resource Center Austin, TX
Paul Fernhoff, M.D. Emory University School of Medicine Atlanta, GA	Ann Umemoto, M.P.H., M.P.A. March of Dimes White Plains, NY
Alan Fleischman, M.D. March of Dimes White Plains, NY	Doris Wethers, M.D. Columbia University College of Physicians and Surgeons New York, NY
Nancy Green, M.D. Columbia Medical Center New York, NY	Benjamin S. Wilfond, M.D. University of Washington School of Medicine Seattle, WA
Scott D. Grosse, Ph.D. National Center on Birth Defects and Developmental Disabilities Centers for Disease Control and Prevention Atlanta, GA	

Note: Organizational affiliations are for identification purposes only; affiliations are current as of 2007.

the existing structure of newborn screening programs and the decision making that produces it. The discussion of program structure includes test panel composition, financing, provision of follow-up services, and research and evaluation using newborn screening bloodspots. The discussion of decision making considers the roles of the federal government, state governments, health care professionals, parent advocacy groups, test manufacturers, and economic evaluation tools such as cost-benefit analysis and cost-effectiveness analysis in the policy process.

Chapter 3 focuses specifically on the use of cost-effectiveness as a criterion for newborn screening policy decisions. In a world of limited resources, every dollar spent on one method of preventing or treating disease is a dollar that is not available for other worthwhile goals (i.e., there is an opportunity cost to newborn screening programs). Scott Grosse describes cost-effectiveness analysis (CEA) and explores its use—or, more accurately, nonuse—in newborn screening policy in the United States and the United Kingdom. His detailed critique of CEAs of newborn screening for specific disorders reveals dramatic variation in the values used for key parameters. This highlights the inadequacy of the information policymakers have available to them and may explain why CEA does not play a bigger role in newborn screening decisions.

Jannine Cody presents "An Advocate's Perspective on Newborn Screening Policy" in chapter 4. Drawing on her experience as a parent and advocate, she argues that the historical criteria used to judge whether a condition should be added to newborn screening need to be reevaluated in the light of changed circumstances: treatment, she argues, should no longer be thought of as complete prevention or cure but as symptom reduction; the balance of power in medicine has changed as patients become more assertive and informed; and the increasing focus on health care consumers results in more attention—uneven to be sure—to particular disorders. Her critique of the Wilson and Jungner criteria deserves a careful reading by public health policymakers, as does her claim that multiplex tests have changed the argument from which conditions to *include* to which conditions to *exclude*.

In chapter 5, Lainie Ross uses the disorder Duchenne muscular dystrophy (DMD) to consider a set of ethical and policy questions about the screening of newborns (and older infants) for conditions that do not meet the Wilson and Jungner criteria. What are the risks and benefits of expanding newborn screening to include DMD? If newborn screening were to expand to include DMD, should it require informed consent? Should newborn screening for DMD be limited to boys? Why or why not? What is the ideal timing for screening (prenatal, newborn, or later in infancy), and what factors influence this determination? She concludes that screening for DMD is a valid moral option, but should not be included in the test panels of mandatory public newborn screening programs. Rather, it should be offered only on a voluntary basis, with full informed consent and after the newborn period, to families of both boys and girls.

In chapter 6, Ellen Wright Clayton uses the experience of the Tennessee Genetics Advisory Committee to draw lessons about efforts to expand newborn screening programs. Her narrative of enthusiastic but incompletely informed legislators, parents advocating for enlarged panels of tests, along with clinicians and companies likely to benefit from such an expansion, is a cautionary tale. She identifies the mandatory, nonvoluntary nature of most state newborn screening programs as a reason to resist adding conditions for which the outcome is highly uncertain or no good prevention or treatment is available.

Bruce Jennings and Andrea Bonnicksen, in chapter 7, go more deeply into the role of state newborn screening advisory committees in introducing public participation into newborn screening decision making. They note that the ideal advisory body brings to its work legitimacy, credibility, and a commitment to the common good. They examine newborn screening advisory committees to ask whether those expectations are reasonable and whether they are ever met in practice. They ask further how these advisory bodies see themselves and what can be done to improve the democratic functioning of such committees. They conclude with recommendations for bringing practice closer to the ideal of citizen involvement.

In chapter 8, Toby Citrin and Stephen Modell build on the Communities of Color and Genetics Policy project, which underscored the importance of racial and ethnic identities in research, clinical care, and public health programs in genetics. They describe why it is important to develop educational programs that take race and ethnicity into account, as well as how and why to engage populations of various racial/ethnic backgrounds in shaping newborn screening policy. Finally, they describe how community organizations can effectively participate in these vital activities.

Newborn screening is carried out by individual states; what role does and should the federal government play? Chapter 9 provides a historical perspective on federal support for state newborn screening programs, focusing on a variety of areas, including research, policy development, service delivery, quality assessment and improvement, and education and training. Michele Lloyd-Puryear, Bradford Therrell, Marie Mann, James Eckman, and Joseph Telfair use four specific examples to illustrate the federal role in providing strategic support for newborn screening: research on PKU; implementation of screening for SCD; policy development by the Newborn Screening Task Force and other federal advisory committees; and evaluation and quality assurance through the newborn screening consultation and review team.

Chapter 10 makes a strong plea for evidence-based decision making in the development of policies to expand newborn screening test panels. It is written by Virginia Moyer, Ned Calonge, Steven Teutsch, and Jeffrey Botkin, on behalf of the United States Preventive Services Task Force, an independent panel of experts in primary care and prevention that systematically reviews the evidence of effectiveness and develops recommendations for clinical preventive services. (The task force was first convened by the U.S. Public Health Service in 1984, and since 1998 has been sponsored by the U.S. Agency for Healthcare Research and Quality. Its recommendations are considered the "gold standard" for preventive services [www.ahrq.gov/clinic/uspstfab.htm]. For information on the task force's methods, see Harris et al. 2001.) The authors are highly critical of the methods used by the ACMG expert group to fashion recommendations for a uniform newborn screening panel. They argue that the recommendations are helping to produce an expansion of testing that cannot be justified on rational screening principles or on the basis of equity. They also argue that state and federal policymakers should ask probing questions before mandating that all newborns be screened for disorders for which evidence of utility is lacking or incomplete.

Jeffrey Botkin also highlights the need to improve the evidence base for newborn screening policy. In chapter 11, he briefly reviews the evidence base for several conditions and then develops a proposal for a structured sequence of research protocols to evaluate potential applications for newborn screening before their formal implementation in public health programs. He argues that such a framework for research will require collaboration between states and the federal government, and notes that such collaboration seems to be emerging through recent federal legislation and funding.

Research with newborn screening samples can be beneficial to the screening programs and to society, but the later research use of stored bloodspots that were collected for screening raises significant ethical, regulatory, and policy issues. In chapter 12, Karen Maschke describes these issues, examines existing policy recommendations, and identifies the unresolved ethical and policy challenges that newborn screening programs face as they continue to collect and store newborn screening samples.

In chapter 13, Botkin tackles directly the newborn screening Catch-22 that is implicit in the previous chapters. There is a great need for scientific evidence concerning the clinical usefulness and cost-effectiveness of tests for almost all disorders for which newborn screening is being done or contemplated. Further, there is a strong tradition in research ethics that says informed consent or, in the case of children, parental permission is required for research to be morally justified. Yet, as a public health program, newborn screening in most states is simply done with, at most, parental notification. Botkin argues that, with proper safeguards, population-based research on newborn screening can be justified without a strict requirement for parental permission.

Anne Marie Comeau and Donna Levin address the same issue in chapter 14 by examining two different models for population-based research run in concert with state-authorized newborn screening services in Massachusetts. In the first, parents were offered optional testing for CF and 19 metabolic disorders as part of a statewide newborn screening research protocol. The newborn screening program made the results of optional testing available to each participant through the health care provider. The second research protocol used newborn screening bloodspots to test all newborns for maternal HIV antibody, with all specimens de-identified before testing. HIV status could not be reported to participants because the HIV test results for specific individuals were never generated; however, individuals could determine their HIV status confidentially by seeking testing at one of many free and anonymous test sites located throughout the state. The authors discuss the advantages and disadvantages of each protocol in the light of their experience in Massachusetts and relative to alternative approaches.

Carrier testing and newborn screening programs for certain conditions (such as SCD and CF) tend to be considered independently in policy discussions in the United States. In fact, the presence of each program influences how the other program operates and how the information produced is interpreted. Using CF as an example, Benjamin Wilfond describes these interactions in chapter 15 and argues that both public and private policymakers must recognize the interactions and take them into account in their decisions. The overall policy goal should be to provide information that allows individuals to manage the impact of genetic conditions on their families in ways that respond to diverse family needs and preferences, in a manner that is both cost-effective and respectful of basic ethical values.

Chapter 16 presents the overall conclusion of the Hastings Center's project, drawn from the analyses presented throughout the book: to be ethical, newborn screening policy should be evidence-based; should take into account the opportunity cost of the newborn screening program; should distribute the costs and benefits of the program fairly; and should appropriately respect human rights. In this final chapter, the editors explain this conclusion, discuss its implications for policy, and make some specific recommendations for the future.

The editors of this volume thank, first, the contributing authors. We appreciate their cooperation in the lengthy process of completing the manuscript, and their excellent work speaks for itself in these pages. We also thank the participants in our project, "Ethical Decision-Making for Newborn Genetic Screening." The knowledge and commitment they brought to the deliberations at project meetings and the peer review they provided to the authors were invaluable contributions to this work.

We are grateful to the March of Dimes, and especially to Nancy Green and Ann Umemoto, for collaborating with us in the design and execution of the project, and we are grateful to the National Human Genome Research Institute for funding it.

Many members of the Hastings Center staff provided help to the project and to the preparation of this book. Mary Ann Hasbrouck managed the logistics of the four project meetings, with the help of other administrative staff, especially Vicki Peyton and Jodi Fernandes. Research assistants Denise Wong, Alyssa Lyon, Alison Jost, and Jacob Moses provided valuable support to the project. Jacob deserves special thanks for mastering the requirements of the Johns Hopkins University Press and ensuring that our manuscript complied with them. Gregory Guzauskas, student of public health and summer intern, drafted the Appendix describing the key features of phenylketonuria, sickle cell disease, medium-chain acyl-CoA dehydrogenase deficiency, cystic fibrosis, and severe combined immunodeficiency disorder.

Finally, Tom Murray would like to thank his family for their forbearance while he worked on the project and on this volume, especially Cynthia Murray.

REFERENCE

Harris, R. P., Helfand, M., Woolf, S. H., Lohr, K. N., Mulrow, C. D., Teutsch, S. M., and Atkins, D., for the Methods Work Group Third U.S. Preventive Services Task Force. 2001. Current methods of the U.S. Preventive Services Task Force: a review of the process. *Am J Prev Med* 20 (Suppl 3): 21–35.

Ethics and Newborn Genetic Screening

CHAPTER 1

Overview

MARY ANN BAILY, PH.D.
THOMAS H. MURRAY, PH.D.

Newborn screening programs are public health programs that screen infants shortly after birth to identify conditions for which early intervention can prevent mortality, morbidity, and disability. They began in the 1960s, after Dr. Robert Guthrie developed a simple blood test for phenylketonuria (PKU), a genetic metabolic disorder that, if untreated, leads to mental retardation and other symptoms. Treatment for PKU consists of a special dietary regimen and, if begun very early in life (ideally, within 7 to 10 days after birth), it can reduce or eliminate the major symptoms associated with the condition (National Institutes of Health 2000). (See the Appendix for more information about PKU.) To use the Guthrie test to screen newborns for PKU, clinicians took a small blood sample from a newborn's heel and deposited it on a special filter paper card that could be easily transported to a testing facility. Massachusetts developed the first screening program, which was voluntary. Over time, other states introduced PKU testing and made it mandatory, partly in response to intensive grassroots lobbying by children's advocates.

Some states also began expanding newborn screening to include tests for other disorders. The federal government contributed to the development of newborn screening by funding research on the effectiveness of the PKU test, funding quality control of testing laboratories, providing maternal and child health block grants to state health departments, and, beginning in 1976, providing funding explicitly for screening for genetic diseases and eventually for other supportive genetic services. Nevertheless, despite this federal involvement, newborn screening has remained primarily a state public health activity.

At this time, all states have newborn screening systems to provide initial screening and follow-up services such as diagnostic services, short- and long-term treatment and management, parent education, and program evaluation. State governments make the difficult decisions about which conditions to test for, what supportive services to make available to parents and newborns, how to pay for testing and supportive services, whether to make screening voluntary or mandatory, what information to provide to parents, and how to safeguard confidentiality in the storage and use of screening samples and test results. The result is an array of programs that vary across the country along many dimensions. For example, all 50 states and the District of Columbia test for PKU, sickle cell disease, congenital hypothyroidism, and galactosemia, but beyond these, the selection of additional tests varies. States have also made different decisions about the content of treatment protocols, the systems available for follow-up, and the extent to which the cost of the system falls on the families of the newborns screened.

Table 1.1 lists the conditions tested for in each state as of December 2007. The conditions vary significantly in incidence; impact on mortality and quality of life; availability, complexity, effectiveness, and cost of treatment; and extent of association with a particular race or ethnicity. To provide perspective on this variation and avoid the implicit identification of newborn screening solely with PKU, we provide information about four additional disorders—sickle cell disease (SCD), cystic fibrosis (CF), medium-chain acyl-CoA dehydrogenase deficiency (MCAD), and severe combined immunodeficiency disorder (SCID)—in the Appendix. Screening for SCD has been included in the majority of state newborn screening programs for many years, CF and MCAD screening were introduced more recently in a number of states, and efforts are currently under way to develop a test for SCID that is suitable for a newborn screening program.

The December 2007 distribution of tests by state is a snapshot of a rapidly evolving reality, as dramatic advances in scientific knowledge and screening technology change the environment in which newborn screening policy decisions are made. For example, tandem mass spectrometry is making it possible to easily detect many more metabolic conditions in newborns with the blood samples already being collected. This laboratory technology uses two machines called mass spectrometers in sequence to perform a bloodspot analysis. The result is a profile of the levels of certain metabolites in the newborn's blood; abnormal levels of one or more of these can signal the presence of a disorder such as PKU or MCAD. In the near future, better understanding of the disease-gene relationship and the use of DNA-based testing technologies such as gene chips and microarrays will provide more ways to use a single blood sample to test for many genetic conditions instead of a few, at minimal additional cost.

Meanwhile, new medical knowledge is increasing the number of disorders for which there are significant early interventions. Health care professionals and support groups for families affected by genetic conditions are advocating for incorporation of the new tests into screening programs, in the hope of improved health outcomes. Companies that stand to profit from new tests and technologies are marketing them aggressively. The results are already being seen in a significant expansion of the number of conditions tested for, despite well-founded doubts about both the process used to decide which conditions to include in newborn screening and the value of the screening for at least some of these conditions.

There is also pressure to modify the goal of the programs. In a World Health Organization report, J. M. G. Wilson and G. Jungner (1968) laid out criteria for appraising the validity of population screening programs (table 1.2). These criteria had a major influence on screening policies worldwide. In newborn screening, they were the basis for a consensus that the goal of screening should be to improve the health of the child and that screening of newborns is appropriate only for conditions with effective, medically accepted treatments that must begin in infancy. The new technologies have resulted in pressure to depart from this consensus by including tests for conditions for which there is no immediate medical treatment or no treatment at all, including adult-onset conditions, trait-carrier identification, and genetic predispositions to disease. There is also pressure to broaden the focus to the entire family; for example, some argue that screening newborns for an untreatable genetic disorder may be justified because parents can use the information that the results imply about parental carrier status to make later reproductive decisions.

These and other technical and social changes on the horizon will greatly increase the complexity of setting up and maintaining screening systems that are both effective and ethically acceptable. Creating an integrated system in

TABLE 1.1
National Newborn Screening Status Report, December 2007

State	Hearing HEAR	Endocrine CH	Endocrine CAH	Hemoglobin Hb S/S	Hemoglobin Hb S/A	Hemoglobin Hb S/C	Other BIO	Other GALT	Other CF	Additional Conditions Included in Screening Panel (universally required unless otherwise indicated)
Alabama	A	•	•	•	•	•	•	•		
Alaska	•	•	•	•	•	•	•	•	•	
Arizona	A	•	•	•	•	•	•	•	C	
Arkansas	•	•	C	•	•	•	C	•	C	
California	B	•	•	•	•	•	C	•	•	HHH; PRO; EMA
Colorado	•	•	•	•	•	•	•	•	•	
Connecticut	•	•	•	•	•	•	•	•	B	HHH; HIV†; NKH
District of Columbia	•	•	•	•	•	•	•	•	•	G6PD
Delaware	•	•	•	•	•	•	•	•	•	
Florida	•	•	•	•	•	•	•	•	•	
Georgia	A	•	•	•	•	•	•	•	•	
Hawaii	•	•	•	•	•	•	•	•	•	
Idaho	A	•	•	•	•	•	•	•	•	
Illinois	•	•	•	•	•	•	•	•	•	NKH; 5-OXO; HIV†
Indiana	•	•	•	•	•	•	•	•	•	
Iowa	•	•	•	•	•	•	C	•	C	
Kansas	A	•	C	•	•	•	C	•	C	
Kentucky	•	•	•	•	•	•	•	•	C	
Louisiana	•	•	•	•	•	•	•	•	•	
Maine	A	•	•	•	•	•	•	•	•	HHH; CPS (D)
Maryland	•	•	•	•	•	•	•	•	•	EMA
Massachusetts	A	•	•	•	•	•	•	•	A	TOXO; HHH (A); CPS (D)
Michigan	A	•	•	•	•	•	•	•	•	

Core* Conditions

State		Notes
Minnesota		5-OXO; CPS; HHH
Mississippi		
Missouri	C	
Montana	C	
Nebraska	A	5-OXO; HHH; NKH (A)
Nevada	A	
New Hampshire	A	TOXO
New Jersey		
New Mexico		
New York		HIV; HHH; Krabbe disease
North Carolina		
North Dakota	A	HHH; NKH
Ohio		
Oklahoma		
Oregon	A	
Pennsylvania		5-OXO; CPS; G6PD; HHH; NKH (B)
Rhode Island		
South Carolina	A	
South Dakota	A	5-OXO; EMA; HHH; NKH
Tennessee	A	HHH; NKH
Texas	B	
Utah		
Vermont		
Virginia		
Washington	A	
West Virginia		
Wisconsin	A	
Wyoming		

See table key on page 10.

(continued)

TABLE 1.1 *(continued)*

	Fatty Acid Disorders					Organic Acid Disorders										Amino Acid Disorders				
State	CUD	LCHAD	MCAD	TFP	VLCAD	GA-I	HMG	IVA	3MCC	Cbl-A,B	BKT	MUT	PROP	MCD	ASA	CIT	HCY	MSUD	PKU	TYR-1
Alabama	•	•	•	•	•	•	•	•	•	•	•	•	•	•	D	•	•	•	•	•
Alaska	•	•	•	•	•	•	•	•	•	•	•	•	•	•	•	•	•	•	•	•
Arizona	•	•	•	•	•	•	•	•	•	•	•	•	•	•	•	•	•	•	•	•
Arkansas	C	C	C	C	C	C	C	C	C	C	C	C	C	C	C	C	C	C	•	C
California	•	C	C	C	C	C	C	C	C	C	C	C	C	C	C	C	C	C	•	C
Colorado	•	•	•	•	•	•	•	•	•	•	•	•	•	•	•	•	•	•	•	•
Connecticut	•	•	•	•	•	•	•	•	•	•	•	•	•	•	•	•	•	•	•	•
District of Columbia	•	•	•	•	•	•	•	•	•	•	•	•	•	•	•	•	•	•	•	•
Delaware	•	•	•	•	•	•	•	•	•	•	•	•	•	•	•	•	•	•	•	•
Florida	•	•	•	•	•	•	•	•	•	•	•	•	•	•	•	•	•	•	•	•
Georgia	•	•	•	•	•	•	•	•	•	•	•	•	•	•	•	•	•	•	•	•
Hawaii	•	•	•	•	•	•	•	•	•	•	•	•	•	•	•	•	•	•	•	•
Idaho	•	•	•	•	•	•	•	•	•	•	•	•	•	•	•	•	•	•	•	•
Illinois	•	•	•	•	•	•	•	•	•	•	•	•	•	•	•	•	•	•	•	•
Indiana	•	•	•	•	•	•	•	•	•	•	•	•	•	•	•	•	•	•	•	•
Iowa	•	•	•	•	•	•	•	•	•	•	•	•	•	•	•	•	•	•	•	•
Kansas	C	C	C	C	C	C	C	C	C	C	C	C	C	C	C	C	C	C	•	C
Kentucky	•	C	C	•	C	C	C	C	C	C	C	C	C	C	C	C	C	C	•	C
Louisiana	•	•	•	•	•	•	•	•	•	•	•	•	•	•	•	•	•	•	•	•
Maine	D	•	•	D	•	•	•	•	•	•	•	•	•	D	•	•	•	•	•	•
Maryland	•	•	•	•	•	•	•	•	•	•	•	•	•	•	•	•	•	•	•	•
Massachusetts	D	A	•	D	A	A	A	A	A	A	A	A	A	D	A	A	•	•	•	•
Michigan	•	•	•	•	•	•	•	•	•	•	•	•	•	•	A	A	•	•	•	A
Minnesota	•	•	•	•	•	•	•	•	•	•	•	•	•	•	•	•	•	•	•	•

State	1	2	3	4	5	6	7	8	9	10	11	12	13	14	15	16	17	18
Mississippi	•	•	•	•	•	•	•	•	•	•	•	•	•	•	•	•	•	•
Missouri	•	C	C	•	C	C	C	C	C	C	C	C	C	C	C	C	C	•
Montana	C	C	C	C	C	C	C	C	C	C	C	C	C	C	C	C	C	C
Nebraska	A	A	A	A	A	A	A	A	A	A	A	A	A	A	A	A	A	A
Nevada	•	•	•	•	•	•	•	•	•	•	•	•	•	•	•	•	•	•
New Hampshire	•	•	•	•	•	•	•	•	•	•	•	•	•	•	•	•	•	•
New Jersey	A	A	A	•	A	•	B	•	B	•	B	•	B	•	B	•	B	B
New Mexico	•	•	•	•	•	•	•	•	•	•	•	•	•	•	•	•	•	•
New York	•	•	•	•	•	•	•	•	•	•	•	•	•	•	•	•	•	•
North Carolina	•	•	•	•	•	•	•	•	•	•	•	•	•	•	•	•	•	•
North Dakota	•	•	•	•	•	•	•	•	•	•	•	•	•	•	•	•	•	•
Ohio	•	•	•	•	•	•	•	•	•	•	•	•	•	•	•	•	•	•
Oklahoma	C	C	C	C	C	C	C	C	C	C	C	C	C	C	C	C	C	C
Oregon	D	D	•	D	•	•	D	•	D	•	D	•	•	D	•	D	•	•
Pennsylvania	B	B	B	B	B	B	B	B	B	B	B	B	B	B	B	B	B	B
Rhode Island	•	•	•	•	•	•	•	•	•	•	•	•	•	•	•	•	•	•
South Carolina	•	•	•	•	•	•	•	•	•	•	•	•	•	•	•	•	•	•
South Dakota	•	•	•	•	•	•	•	•	•	•	•	•	•	•	•	•	•	•
Tennessee	•	•	•	•	•	•	•	•	•	•	•	•	•	•	•	•	•	•
Texas	•	•	•	•	•	•	•	•	•	•	•	•	•	•	•	•	•	•
Utah	•	•	•	•	•	•	•	•	•	•	•	•	•	•	•	•	•	•
Vermont	•	•	•	•	•	•	•	•	•	•	•	•	•	•	•	•	•	•
Virginia	•	•	•	•	•	•	•	•	•	•	•	•	•	•	•	•	•	•
Washington	•	•	C	•	•	•	•	•	•	•	•	•	•	•	•	•	•	•
West Virginia	C	C	C	C	C	C	C	C	C	C	C	C	C	•	C	C	C	C
Wisconsin	•	•	C	•	•	•	•	•	•	•	•	•	•	•	•	•	•	C
Wyoming	•	•	•	•	•	•	•	•	•	•	•	•	•	•	•	•	•	•

See table key on page 10. *(continued)*

TABLE 1.1 (continued)

State	Fatty Acid Disorders								Organic Acid Disorders							Amino Acid Disorders							Other Metabolic		Hbg
	CACT	CPT-Ia	CPT-II	DE-RED	GA-II	MCKAT	M/SCHAD	SC AD	2M3HBA	2MBG	3MGA	Cbl-C,D	IBG	MAL	ARG	BIOPT-BS	BIOPT-RG	CIT-II	H-PHE	MET	TYR-II	TYR-III	GALE	GALK	Variant Hbg's
Alabama	•		•		•			•	•	•	•	•	•	•	•	D	D	•	•	•	•	•			D
Alaska	•	D	•		•			•	•	•	•	•	•	•	•	B	B	•	•	•	•	•	B	B	
Arizona	D	D	D		D				D		D	D						D	D		D	D			D
Arkansas	•		•		•			•	•	•	•	•	•	•	•	•	•	•	C	•	•	•			C
California	•	•	•		•		•	•	•	•	•	•	•	•	•	•	•	•	•	•	•	•	•	•	•
Colorado	•	•	•	•	•	•	•	•	•	•	•	•	•	•	•	•	A	•	•	•	•	•	•	•	•
Connecticut	•	•	•	•	•	•	•	•	•	•	•	•	•	•	•	A	A	•	•	•	•	•	•	•	•
District of Columbia	•	•	•	•	•	D	•	•	D	•	D	•	•	D	•	D	D	•	•	•	D	D	•	•	•
Delaware	•	•	•	•	•	D	•	•	•	•	•	•	•	•	•	B	B	•	•	•	•	•	•	•	•
Florida	•	•	•	•	•	•	•	•	•	•	•	•	D	D	A	D	D	•	•	•	•	•	•	•	•
Georgia	D	D	•	D	•	D	•	•	D	•	•	•	D	•	•	D	D	•	•	•	•	•	B	B	•
Hawaii	•	•	•	•	•	•	•	•	•	•	•	•	•	•	•	B	B	•	•	•	•	•	B	B	•
Idaho	D	D	•	D	•	D	•	•	•	•	•	•	•	•	•	D	D	•	•	•	•	•	•	•	•
Illinois	•	•	•	•	•	•	•	•	D	•	•	•	•	•	D	•	•	D	•	•	•	•			
Indiana	•	•	•	•	•	•	•	•	•	•	•	•	•	•	•	•	•	•	•	•	•	•			
Iowa	•	•	•	•	•	•	•	•	•	•	•	•	•	•	A	B	B	•	•	A	•	•			
Kansas	D	•	A	•	A	•	•	•	•	•	•	•	D	•	•	B	B	•	•	•	•	D			
Kentucky	•	D	A	D	•	•	•	•	•	•	•	•	•	•	A	B	B	•	•	D	•	D	•	•	•
Louisiana	•	•	•	•	•	•	•	•	•	•	•	•	•	•	A	B	B	•	•	•	•	•	•	•	•
Maine	D	D	•	•	•	•	•	•	D	D	D	•	D	•	•	B	B	•	•	D	•	D	•	•	•
Maryland	D	D	•	•	A	•	•	A	D	D	D	A	D	•	A	D	D	A	•	D	A	A	•	•	•
Massachusetts	D	D	A	•	A	•	•	A	D	•	D	A	D	•	A	D	D	A	•	D	A	D	•	•	•

State																								
Michigan	·	·	·	·	·	·	·	·	·	·	·	·	·	·	·	·	·	·	·	·	·	·	·	·
Minnesota	·	·	·	·	D	·	·	·	·	·	·	·	·	·	·	·	·	·	·	·	·	·	·	·
Mississippi	·	·	A	·	A	A	·	·	A	A	A	A	A	A	A	A	A	A	A	A	A	A	A	A
Missouri	D	D	D	D	D	D	D	D	D	D	D	D	D	D	D	D	D	D	D	D	D	C	D	D
Montana	C	C	C	C	C	C	C	C	C	C	C	C	C	C	C	C	C	C	C	C	C	C	C	C
Nebraska	A	A	A	A	A	A	A	A	A	A	A	A	A	A	A	A	A	A	A	A	A	A	A	A
Nevada	·	·	·	·	·	·	·	·	·	·	·	·	·	B	B	B	B	B	B	B	·	·	B	A
New Hampshire	D	D	·	·	·	·	D	D	D	D	D	D	D	D	D	D	D	D	D	·	·	·	·	·
New Jersey	A	A	A	A	A	A	A	A	A	A	A	A	A	A	A	A	A	A	A	A	A	A	A	A
New Mexico	A	A	A	A	A	A	A	D	A	D	D	B	A	B	B	A	A	A	A	A	B	D	D	D
New York	·	·	·	·	·	·	·	·	·	·	·	·	·	·	·	·	·	·	·	·	·	·	·	·
North Carolina	·	·	·	·	·	·	·	·	·	·	·	·	·	·	·	·	·	·	·	·	·	·	·	·
North Dakota	·	·	·	·	·	·	·	·	·	·	·	·	·	·	·	·	·	·	·	·	·	·	·	·
Ohio	C	C	C	C	C	C	C	C	C	C	C	C	C	C	C	C	C	C	C	C	C	C	C	C
Oklahoma	C	C	·	C	C	D	D	D	D	D	D	D	D	B	B	D	·	D	D	B	B	·	B	B
Oregon	D	D	D	B	B	B	B	B	B	B	B	B	B	B	B	B	B	B	B	B	B	·	·	·
Pennsylvania	B	B	B	B	B	·	·	·	·	·	·	·	·	·	·	·	·	·	·	·	·	·	·	·
Rhode Island	D	·	·	·	·	·	·	·	·	·	·	·	·	·	·	·	·	·	·	·	·	·	·	·
South Carolina	·	·	·	·	·	·	·	·	·	·	·	·	·	·	·	·	·	·	·	·	·	·	·	·
South Dakota	·	·	·	·	·	·	·	·	·	·	·	·	·	·	·	·	·	·	·	·	·	·	·	·
Tennessee	·	·	D	·	·	·	·	·	·	·	·	·	·	·	·	·	·	·	·	·	·	·	·	·
Texas	·	·	·	D	·	·	·	·	·	·	·	·	·	D	·	·	·	·	·	·	·	·	·	·
Utah	D	D	·	D	·	·	·	D	D	D	D	·	·	·	·	·	·	·	·	·	·	·	D	D
Vermont	D	D	D	D	D	D	D	D	D	D	D	D	D	D	D	D	·	·	·	·	·	·	D	D
Virginia	D	D	D	D	D	D	D	D	D	D	D	D	D	D	D	D	D	D	D	C	C	C	D	D
Washington	·	·	·	·	·	·	·	·	·	·	·	·	·	·	·	·	·	·	·	·	·	·	·	·
West Virginia	D	D	D	D	D	D	D	D	D	D	D	D	D	D	D	D	D	D	D	D	D	D	D	D
Wisconsin	·	·	·	·	·	·	·	·	·	·	·	·	·	·	·	·	A	A	A	·	·	·	·	·
Wyoming	A	A	A	A	A	A	A	A	A	A	A	A	A	A	A	A	A	A	A	B	A	A	·	·

(continued)

See table key on page 10.

TABLE 1.1 (*continued*)

Source: Adapted with permission from http://genes-r-us.uthscsa.edu/. Data updated December 17, 2007.

Note: Dot (•) indicates that screening for the condition is universally required by law or rule and fully implemented. A = universally offered but not yet required; B = offered to select populations, or by request; C = testing required but not yet implemented; D = likely to be detected (and reported) as a by-product of mass reaction monitoring screening (MS/MS, tandem mass spectrometry) targeted by law or rule.

Abbreviations:

2M3HBA	2-methyl 3-hydroxybutyric aciduria
2MBG	2-methylbutyryl-CoA dehydrogenase deficiency
3MCC	3-methylcrotonyl-CoA carboxylase deficiency
3MGA	3-methylglutaconic aciduria
5-OXO	5-oxoprolinuria (pyroglutamic aciduria)
ARG	argininemia (arginase deficiency)
ASA	argininosuccinate acidemia (argininosuccinic acidemia; argininosuccinic aciduria)
BIO	biotinidase deficiency (also abbreviated as BIOT)
BIOPT-BS	defects of biopterin cofactor biosynthesis
BIOPT-RG	defects of biopterin cofactor regeneration (also abbreviated as BIOT-REG)
BKT	β-ketothiolase (mitochondrial acetoacetyl-CoA thiolase; short-chain ketoacyl thiolase; T2) deficiency
CACT	carnitine acylcarnitine translocase deficiency
CAH	congenital adrenal hyperplasia
Cbl-A,B	methylmalonic acidemia (or aciduria) related to lack of vitamin B$_{12}$ cofactor cobalamin A or B
Cbl-C,D	methylmalonic acidemia (or aciduria) related to lack of vitamin B$_{12}$ cofactor cobalamin C or D
CF	cystic fibrosis
CH	congenital hypothyroidism
CIT-I	citrullinemia type I (argininosuccinate synthetase deficiency) (also abbreviated as CIT)
CIT-II	citrullinemia type II (citrin deficiency)
CPS	carbamoylphosphate (carbamylphosphate) synthetase deficiency
CPT-Ia	carnitine palmitoyltransferase I deficiency (also abbreviated as CPT-IA)
CPT-II	carnitine palmitoyltransferase II deficiency
CUD	carnitine uptake defect (carnitine transport defect)
DE-RED	dienoyl-CoA reductase deficiency
EMA	ethylmalonic encephalopathy
G6PD	glucose-6-phosphate dehydrogenase deficiency
GA-I	glutaric acidemia (or aciduria) type I (or 1) (also abbreviated as GA-1)
GA-II	glutaric acidemia (or aciduria) type II (or 2) (also abbreviated as GA-2)
GALE	galactose epimerase deficiency
GALK	galactokinase deficiency
GALT	transferase deficient galactosemia (classical galactosemia)
Hb S/A	S-β-thalassemia (also abbreviated as Hb S/β-Th, or Hb S/Th)
Hb S/C	sickle-hemoglobin C (sickle-C) disease
Hb S/S	sickle cell anemia
Hbg	hemoglobinopathy
HCY	homocystinuria (cystathionine β-synthase deficiency)
HEAR	hearing screening
HHH	hyperammonemia/ornithinemia/citrullinemia (ornithine transporter defect)
HIV	human immunodeficiency virus
HMG	3-hydroxy 3-methylglutaric aciduria (3-hydroxy 3-methylglutaryl-CoA [HMG-CoA] lyase deficiency)
H-PHE	benign hyperphenylalaninemia
IBG	isobutyryl-CoA dehydrogenase deficiency
IVA	isovaleric acidemia (isovaleryl-CoA dehydrogenase deficiency)
LCHAD	long-chain L-3-hydroxyacyl-CoA dehydrogenase (long-chain 3-hydroxyacyl-CoA dehydrogenase; long chain hydroxyacyl-CoA dehydrogenase deficiency)
MAL	malonic acidemia (malonyl-CoA decarboxylase deficiency)
MCAD	medium-chain acyl-CoA dehydrogenase deficiency
MCD	multiple carboxylase (holocarboxylase synthetase) deficiency
MCKAT	medium-chain ketoacyl-CoA thiolase deficiency
MET	hypermethioninemia
M/SCHAD	medium-/short-chain L-3-hydroxyacyl-CoA dehydrogenase deficiency
MSUD	maple syrup urine disease (branched-chain ketoacid dehydrogenase deficiency)
MUT	methylmalonic acidemia (or aciduria) related to methylmalonyl-CoA mutase deficiency
NKH	nonketotic hyperglycinemia
PKU	phenylketonuria/hyperphenylalaninemia
PRO	prolinemia
PROP	propionic acidemia (propionyl-CoA carboxylase deficiency)
SCAD	short-chain acyl-CoA dehydrogenase deficiency
TFP	trifunctional protein deficiency
TOXO	toxoplasmosis
TYR-I	tyrosinemia type I
TYR-II	tyrosinemia type II
TYR-III	tyrosinemia type III
VLCAD	very long-chain acyl-CoA dehydrogenase deficiency

* Terminology consistent with American College of Medical Genetics 2006.

† Newborn screened for HIV only if mother was not screened during pregnancy.

TABLE 1.2
Wilson and Jungner Criteria

1	The condition being screened for should be an important health problem.
2	The natural history of the condition should be well understood.
3	There should be a detectable early stage.
4	Treatment should be of more benefit at an early stage than at a later stage.
5	A suitable test should be devised for the early stage.
6	The test should be acceptable.
7	Intervals for repeating the test should be determined.
8	Adequate health service provision should be made for the extra clinical workload resulting from screening.
9	The risks, both physical and psychological, should be less than the benefits.
10	The costs should be balanced against the benefits.

Source: Adapted from Wilson and Jungner 1968.

which all parents receive appropriate information and their newborns receive appropriate, continuing care has always been a challenge in the U.S. context, given its many uncoordinated financing and delivery structures and its diverse population. With more tests, and tests with more complex and at times ambiguous implications, new ethical and policy challenges arise in selecting tests, providing adequate information and counseling to parents, protecting privacy, and achieving fairness in the financing of screening and supportive services.

The rapid change under way in health care delivery, financing, medical practice, information management, and public health agency structures and the growing diversity in socioeconomic class, race, and ethnicity are making it more difficult to manage the existing system, let alone deal with increasing complexity. In recognition of these challenges, people involved in newborn screening programs have responded in a variety of ways. The most notable effort was the Newborn Screening Task Force (2000), sponsored by the American Academy of Pediatrics and the Health Resources and Services Administration (HRSA), which brought together the major public and private organizations involved in newborn screening and issued a comprehensive report on the state of the field. Other activities include the work of the Council of Regional Networks for Genetic Services, which published a report in 2000 on the follow-up and management of children with disorders detected through newborn screening (Pass et al. 2000), and the work of the New York State Task Force on Life and the Law, which reviewed newborn screening standards in New York in its 2001 report on genetic testing. On genetic testing in general, the Secretary's Advisory Committee on Genetic Testing issued a report in 2000 that sets broad guidelines for oversight of testing, and a successor committee, the Secretary's Advisory Committee on Genetics, Health, and Society, continues to play a role in the study of genetic testing issues.

The report that has had perhaps the greatest impact on newborn screening programs in recent years is "Newborn Screening: Toward a Uniform Screening Panel and System," released in 2005 and published in 2006 (American College of Medical Genetics 2006). This report was produced by a group assembled by the American College of Medical Genetics (ACMG) with funding from HRSA. It presents a long list of conditions and recommends that states test all newborns for these conditions and report the results to parents. The list includes 29 conditions that meet the ACMG group's criteria for inclusion in a uniform panel and 25 secondary, "report only" conditions that do not meet the criteria but are automatically identified in screening for the 29 core conditions and in following up to a definitive diagnosis (see table 1.1). The Secretary's Advisory Committee on Heritable Disorders and Genetic Diseases in Newborns and Children endorsed this report and is engaging in activities to refine the methodology for adding conditions to the uniform panel and to provide guidance and technical assistance to states as they expand the scope of their programs. The March of Dimes and other parent and professional advocacy groups have actively promoted expansion of programs to conform to the ACMG report's recommendations, and a number of states began using the list to guide ambitious program expansions even before HRSA released the full report explaining the methods used to develop the list.

As newborn screening responds to all these changes, new ethical questions arise and old ones return in new form. The project that resulted in this book was designed to explore four closely related areas of recognized need for in-depth ethical and policy analysis: fairness in the distribution of costs and benefits; information, consent, and privacy; consultation and decision making; and race, ethnicity, and socioeconomic status.

Fairness in the Distribution of Costs and Benefits

In debates about newborn screening policymaking, conflict has often arisen over the place of cost. Some argue that cost should be irrelevant, because saving a child's life has infinite value (Howse and Katz 2000). Others argue that with resources scarce and compelling social needs abundant, priority setting cannot be avoided; the real question is how the available resources should be allocated so that everyone is treated fairly. Specifically, what does fairness in the distribution of the costs and benefits of newborn screening mean, and how should newborn screening programs be structured to achieve it?

The fairness issue is particularly salient in discussions of the composition of states' test panels. With the increase in the number of tests that are candidates for inclusion, decisions about what to test for have become more challenging. Does society have a moral obligation to the health of the next generation, and, if so, to what extent does it require using collective resources to identify and treat genetic conditions in newborns? Is it fair to have test panels that vary across states, so that a child with a genetic condition is identified and successfully treated in one state, while a child in another state with the same condition is not identified and dies? How should society balance the financial and emotional costs to the many families of children who have false positive screening results against the benefits to the few children with true positive results who are identified and successfully treated? Are the methods of cost-effectiveness, cost-utility, and cost-benefit analysis, often used in the economic evaluation of health programs, compatible with the answers to basic questions about fairness?

Important fairness questions also arise in the financing of newborn screening tests and supportive services. Current programs rely on a mix of parental payments, private and public insurance payments, and public funds collected and channeled through a variety of public and private agencies. The mix varies from state to state, resulting in an ad hoc distribution of cost that fails to meet any coherent standard of fairness (Newborn Screening Task Force 2000). This situation is part of a larger problem of pervasive inequity in the distribution of care and of cost in the U.S. health care system as a whole. How can policymakers create a fair financing and delivery structure for newborn screening within an unfair health care system?

Information, Consent, and Privacy

One of the most controversial issues in newborn screening is its mandatory status. Normally, a parent must give informed consent before a child can receive medical treatment, but newborn screening generally takes place without explicit consent. Parents are generally assumed to have the right to be informed about screening, the right to refuse screening, and the right to confidentiality and privacy protections for information contained in newborn screening results (Newborn Screening Task Force 2000); however, conceptual and practical issues arise when translating this assumption into ethically sound policy.

Parents may have a right to information, but what kind and when? Must parents be given detailed information about all the conditions that are included in the screening before it takes place, or is it ethically acceptable to provide detailed information only to those parents who are notified of a positive result? How can screening programs ensure that parents understand the difference between screening and diagnostic tests, the possibility of false positive and false negative results, and the difference between affected and carrier status? What methods of delivering the essential information and counseling are both ethical and cost-effective, especially for the ACMG's list of conditions, which includes conditions whose clinical significance is poorly understood even by specialists?

Given the limited information available about many conditions on the newborn screening list, the importance of ongoing investigation and evaluation is widely acknowledged. In the past, the assumption has been that full informed consent is required when newborns are subjected to screening tests that are investigational or in development and identifiers are not removed from specimens. What procedures should be in place to provide information to parents about their newborn's participation in such research and to obtain valid parental consent?

Newborn screening does not consume a newborn's entire blood sample, and the stored samples are a useful and sought-after resource for research that is unrelated to newborn screening. Appropriate information and consent policies are needed for these situations also. Is it necessary to obtain parental consent for future research uses at the time of screening? If necessary, is initial parental consent sufficient for all possible uses, or should consent be required for some or all uses at the time of use? Is parental consent sufficient for as long as the samples are useful, or should the child's own consent be required after the child reaches a certain age (e.g., 18 or 21)?

What constitutes ethically acceptable protection of privacy and confidentiality in the storage and use of personal data from screening programs? Public concern about the privacy of medical information is growing as medical records become increasingly computerized. In fact, the security of medical information has never been as good as many people suppose, and computerized biomedical data systems could provide greater protection for privacy if properly designed; however, this will not happen in the absence of carefully constructed public policies on privacy and confidentiality.

Currently, state policies related to information, consent, and privacy vary widely. Two states (Maryland and Wyoming) use some form of informed consent model for the basic newborn screening tests. Most of the rest permit parental refusal of routine newborn screening, but the underlying rationale for the right to refuse is unclear and the terms under which it may be exercised vary both across and within states. Often, parents receive little advance information and are barely aware that testing is taking place, let alone that they can refuse it (Newborn Screening Task Force 2000). There is also wide variation in policies on parental consent to research, the storage of bloodspots, and the availability of bloodspots for use in research and quality assurance.

Consultation and Decision Making

To what extent do current consultation and decision-making structures encourage or discourage the introduction of ethically acceptable policies on fairness, information, consent, and privacy? There is consensus in the newborn screening literature that screening policy should not be left to medical and scientific experts alone. Obviously, decisions about the design of newborn screening programs depend as much on basic ethical and social values as on technical considerations and quantitative data. There is less clarity about just what the process of consultation and decision making should be. Members of groups concerned about particular conditions, members of the executive and legislative branches of government, researchers, health care professionals, representatives of communities particularly affected by specific conditions, and the general public—all should be involved, but their respective roles are unclear.

One key issue is the appropriate distribution of government responsibility for newborn screening programs across the local, state, and federal levels. What are the arguments for and against making newborn screening decisions at the state level? What role should the federal government play?

Another issue is the role of groups advocating on behalf of particular genetic conditions. The earliest newborn screening programs for PKU were put in place before there was consensus in the medical and scientific community about their benefits, largely as a result of intense lobbying by citizens working to prevent mental retardation. Citizen activism organized around particular conditions (e.g., cystic fibrosis [American Academy of Pediatrics and Ad Hoc Committee Task Force on Neonatal Screening 1983], MCAD, and other disorders of fatty acid or amino acid metabolism) has been and remains an important influence on newborn screening policy. How can decision making be structured to achieve a fair balancing of resources across the entire spectrum of health needs, without undue bias in favor of conditions with particularly skilled advocates?

Still another issue is the role that the for-profit companies that develop and/or perform tests should play in newborn screening policy decisions. What is the nature and extent of their influence now, and how is it likely to evolve over time? Is this influence appropriate, and, if not, what should be done to balance it?

Race, Ethnicity, and Socioeconomic Status

Finally, the role of race, ethnicity, and socioeconomic status in newborn screening policy is an issue of overarching importance, one that must be woven into the discussion of each of the other areas of analysis. For example, what is the effect of race and ethnicity on the distribution of genetic conditions, and what role should variations in the distribution by race/ethnicity play in test selection? When a condition does have a significantly higher incidence in one racial/ethnic group, should testing be targeted to that particular group or is it better to screen all newborns?

How are individual views about the importance of access to newborn screening services and the meaning and relevance of the genetic information it yields affected by race, ethnicity, and socioeconomic factors? What do the answers to these questions imply about the kind of information that should be provided to parents before testing is done and when a newborn's test is positive for a genetic condition?

In the area of consultation and decision making, what does it mean to engage in community consultation, where communities are defined in relation to race or ethnicity? Are there successful models of ethical consultation with such communities on test selection, access to screening and supportive services, and the meaning and relevance of the genetic information obtained? What are the characteristics of such models?

In this book, we consider all four areas together and focus on the relationships among them. When ethicists focus on a particular issue in isolation, the interrelationships among ethical issues can be neglected; the result may be a sweeping recommendation that seems impractical to policymakers. We believe that when the issues are considered together, with explicit attention to practical implementation and input from people with extensive experience in newborn screening, this outcome is less likely.

For example, the issue areas of fairness, consultation and decision making, and race, ethnicity, and socioeconomic status are closely linked. Assessment of fairness in the distribution of newborn screening costs and benefits is a matter of both substance and process. Where there is consensus on the characteristics that a policy must have to make it fair, the implications of these shared values for program policies can be determined and policies assessed on that basis. Where there are clashing values, or conflicting analyses of the policy implications of shared values (e.g., because of differing assessments of the scientific evidence or of the evidence on economic and social costs), fairness requires fair processes for choosing among them. Moreover, given the history of racial and ethnic discrimination in the United States, explicit attention must be given to race and ethnicity in the identification of shared values and fair processes for resolving or accommodating differences in values and assessments of evidence.

The area of information, consent, and privacy is also linked to the area of fairness in the distribution of resources and the area of race, ethnicity, and socioeconomic status. When every newborn in the United States is screened for genetic conditions, the provision of even minimal information to parents has significant cost implications, especially as the number and complexity of disorders screened for increases. Designing and managing newborn screening databases so that the privacy and confidentiality of newborns and their families are protected also requires substantial resources. The requirement that researchers obtain full informed consent from every family for every research use of newborn screening samples at the time of use might make some socially beneficial research projects prohibitively expensive. There may be differences among groups defined by race, ethnicity, and socioeconomic status in the importance they attach to being informed about screening and what they want to know, the extent to which they wish to protect personal information from disclosure, and how they feel about participating in research. Thus, how the costs and benefits of information, privacy, and consent policies are distributed is of ethical importance in making policy.

The chapters that follow address these questions in all their complexity, and the final chapter presents our conclusions and recommendations for the future.

REFERENCES

American Academy of Pediatrics and Ad Hoc Committee Task Force on Neonatal Screening C. F. F. 1983. Neonatal screening for cystic fibrosis: position paper. *Pediatrics* 72 (6): 741–45.

American College of Medical Genetics. 2006. Newborn screening: toward a uniform screening panel and system. *Genet Med* 8 (Suppl 1): 1–252S.

Howse, J. L., and Katz, M. 2000. The importance of newborn screening. *Pediatrics* 106 (3): 595.

National Institutes of Health. 2000. Phenylketonuria (PKU): screening and management. *NIH Consens Statement* 17 (3): 1–33.

New York State Task Force on Life and the Law. 2001. Newborn screening. In *Genetic Testing and Screening in the Age of Genomic Medicine*, pp. 141–77. New York: New York State Task Force.

Newborn Screening Task Force. 2000. Serving the family from birth to the medical home: a report from the Newborn Screening Task Force convened in Washington DC, May 10–11, 1999. *Pediatrics* 106 (2 Pt 2): 383–427.

Pass, K. A., Lane, P. A., Fernhoff, P. M., Hinton, C. F., and Panny, S. R. 2000. US newborn screening system guidelines II: follow-up of children, diagnosis, management and evaluation. Statement of the Council of Regional Networks for Genetic Services (CORN). *J Pediatr* 137 (4 Suppl): 1–46.

Secretary's Advisory Committee on Genetic Testing. 2000. *Enhancing the Oversight of Genetic Tests: Recommendations of the SACGT.* Bethesda, MD: National Institutes of Health.

Wilson, J. M. G., and Jungner, G. 1968. *Principles and Practice of Screening for Disease.* Geneva: World Health Organization.

CHAPTER 2

Fair Distribution of Newborn Screening Costs and Benefits

MARY ANN BAILY, PH.D.

Some of the most difficult debates on newborn screening policy involve conflicts over the use of resources. Policymakers speak of budgetary priorities, cost-effectiveness, and stewardship, while advocates speak of moral priorities and the infinite value of a child's life. In fact, because resources are scarce and the range of socially useful things that could be done with them is wide, stewardship and priority setting cannot be avoided. The central issue is, How can we allocate the available resources so that everyone is treated fairly? Specifically, what does fairness in the distribution of the costs and benefits of newborn screening mean, and how should newborn screening programs be structured to achieve it?

The centrality of distributional fairness is particularly obvious in discussions of which conditions to include in a newborn screening test panel. This long-standing policy issue has become more challenging as advances in screening technologies and in the understanding of the origin and treatment of genetic conditions increase the number of conditions that are candidates for screening (Newborn Screening Task Force 2000; Therrell 2001). At a general level, the issue is the extent of our collective moral obligation to the health of the next generation, and whether and to what extent it translates into a moral obligation to spend communal resources to identify and treat genetic conditions in individual newborns.

There are also more specific distributional questions. Is it fair to have (as we do in the United States) newborn screening programs that vary from one state to another, so that a child with a particular genetic condition is identified and successfully treated in one state, while a child with the same condition who happens to be born in another state is not identified and dies or suffers catastrophic consequences (Stoddard and Farrell 1997; Mitka 2000)? What role should variations in the incidence of a condition across groups defined by geography, race, ethnicity, or socioeconomic class play in decisions about what to test for? What is a fair balance between the financial and emotional costs to many families of receiving false positive or ambiguous screening results, and the benefits to a single true positive child and to society of early identification and treatment of a debilitating disease?

There are also fairness issues in the financing and delivery of newborn screening tests and supportive services. A screening program is much more than laboratory tests (Pass et al. 2000; Therrell 2001). It also includes diagnosis, short-term follow-up, long-term treatment and management, parent and professional education, and program evaluation. Creating and paying for an integrated system in which all parents receive appropriate information and their newborns receive appropriate care has always been a challenge in the U.S. context, given the array of uncoordinated financing and delivery structures. Achieving a fair distribution of the system's cost is even harder. To fund the system, current programs rely on a varying mix of parental payments, private and public insurance payments, and public funds collected and channeled through a range of public and private organizations. The resulting ad hoc distribution of cost fails to meet any coherent standard of fairness. This situation is part of a larger problem of pervasive inequity in access and in the distribution of cost in the overall U.S. health care system.

This chapter considers the nature of fairness in the newborn screening context and asks what policies tend to support it. To assess policies, we need to consider fairness as a matter of both substance and process. Where there is consensus on aspects of fairness, the implications for program policies can be identified and policies assessed on that basis. Where there are clashing values, or where there are conflicting analyses of the policy implications of common values (e.g., because of different interpretations of scientific evidence or evidence on economic and social costs), fairness requires fair processes for choosing among them.

In newborn screening, ethical and social values are so important that all agree that policy decisions should not be left to medical and scientific experts alone. There is less clarity about just what the process of consultation and decision making should be. How should responsibility for newborn screening programs be allocated across local, state, and federal levels of government? What should be the role of groups of consumers and health professionals advocating on behalf of a particular genetic condition, such as cystic fibrosis or a specific metabolic disease? What should be the role of companies that stand to profit from the use of their tests in newborn screening programs? How can decision making be structured to achieve a fair balancing of resources across the entire spectrum of need, without undue bias in favor of conditions that have exceptionally skilled and motivated advocates? To what extent are the tools of cost-effectiveness and cost-benefit analysis, often used to make decisions about health programs, compatible with the goal of achieving distributional fairness?

Rationales for Public Health Programs: Efficiency and Equity

To develop a basic equity framework for the assessment of newborn screening policies that is useful for thinking about fairness, we begin by considering the standard justifications for public health programs. Classic public health programs include activities such as the provision of safe water supplies, the control of infectious disease through immunization and venereal disease treatment, research into the causes and cures of disease, and the development and dissemination of information about behaviors that promote good health. These activities produce diffuse benefits for many people, so it makes sense to organize and finance them collectively, through government. The argument for government action is that better results are achieved for less money by acting collectively than could be achieved through individual actions; this can be termed an *efficiency* argument.

Fairness (equity) issues inevitably arise in such programs. The money to pay for them must come from some combination of taxation and user fees. The justification for using public funds is that taxpayers will benefit; however, fairness questions may arise about the specific distribution of a program's costs and benefits. For example, should public funds for an immunization program be local, state, or federal? Should fees be charged and, if so, should they be income-scaled? In publicly funded research programs, are researchers focusing too much on the health problems of white males and not enough on those of other population groups? Are there circumstances in which it is appropriate and fair to focus health promotion services on specific groups defined by income, race/ethnicity, or place of residence?

Public health also includes activities that directly influence the distribution of personal health care across individuals. These activities are more likely to have *equity* as their primary rationale. Many publicly funded health programs exist to provide access to health care for people who cannot afford to pay for it. Historically, local governments were expected to take responsibility for ensuring that some basic care was available to the very poor; the locally funded public hospital serving as "provider of last resort" was the most visible evidence of this. Currently, Medicare, Medicaid, and other federal, state, and local programs provide some free or subsidized personal health care services to certain groups of the population.

Policy analysts are often uncomfortable with programs designed to intervene directly in the distribution of specific goods and services on fairness grounds. They prefer to address fairness through the distribution of general purchasing power. From this perspective, the societal equity goal should be to achieve a fair distribution of purchasing power through taxes and transfers (such as social security and welfare payments). Because people have different personal situations and preferences, it is appropriate that they make different tradeoffs when they spend their fair share of purchasing power on goods and services. If poor people cannot afford basic food, shelter, or health care, the basic level of income should be raised until the goods considered basic necessities are affordable, but if some choose not to purchase them, that is their choice.

In the case of health care, however, most people seem to have a special concern about the distribution of health care separate from the distribution of purchasing power, and they seem to expect the government to make health care distribution a matter of specific policy concern.[1] The next section describes a conceptual framework for characterizing this concern and explores its implications for health policy.

Defining Equitable Access to Health Care

The conceptual framework is based on the work of the President's Commission for the Study of Ethical Problems in Medicine and Biomedical and

Behavioral Research (1983) as presented in its report *Securing Access to Health Care*. The commission's charge was to study the ethical implications of differences in the availability of health services across groups defined by place of residence, income, and race/ethnicity. To do this, the commission sought to identify the basic American values concerning equity in access to health care that were implicit in health policy, make these values explicit, and explore their practical implications. The resulting framework was not (and was not intended to be) original. The basic framework has been set forth in many places in both the health policy literature on health system design and the bioethics literature on justice and health care. Philosophical arguments can be advanced as justifications for this approach to equity, but they are not repeated here because our objective is not to defend or attack the framework. Rather, our claim is that it is the dominant approach to equity in the United States and therefore an appropriate basis for considering fairness in newborn screening.

The commission's report begins by asking what it is about health care that makes its distribution a matter of equity or justice when the distribution of most other goods is not. It answers that health care is of special importance because of its role in relieving suffering, preventing premature death, restoring normal functioning, increasing opportunity, providing information about a person's condition, and giving evidence of mutual empathy and compassion. In recognition of this special importance, many countries throughout the world, including the United States, acknowledge a societal moral obligation to achieve fairness, or equity, in access to health care for all.

The translation of this societal obligation into practical policy is a critical social and political task. How should "equitable access to health care" be interpreted? Access to what? At what cost? In this country, the commission's report concludes, the interpretation that best reflects American values as expressed in health policy debates over the years is access to "an *adequate level of care* without *excessive burden*" (President's Commission 1983, p. 4; emphasis added). The key characteristic of the concept of an adequate level is its explicit acknowledgment of limits on the extent of the societal obligation, limits that arise out of the inherent scarcity of the resources a society has available to it.

The concept of an adequate level is most easily appreciated by comparing it with other ways of defining the required level of care. For example, equitable access could be defined as access to whatever care would be of benefit. This definition ignores the reality that the benefits of health care vary in importance, from the preservation of life to the elimination of minor inconvenience, and that some highly beneficial care is extremely costly. To guarantee universal access to all the care that is of any benefit would be prohibitively expensive and would compromise the ability to spend resources on other important social goods. In economic terminology, the *opportunity cost* of devoting such a large share of societal resources to health care would be too great. An alternative, guaranteeing access only to needed care, seems to avoid this problem, but only until one attempts to specifically define "need." In the health care context, "medical need" often refers to any medical condition for which a health care service might be effective. This in turn translates to everything of benefit, and again the opportunity cost is excessive.

A third possibility is to define equitable access as equal access: what matters is not what everyone gets but that everyone gets the same. (Equality is, of course, interpreted relative to health state; that is, if anyone with a certain liver disease can get a liver transplant, everyone with that disease should be able to get one.) This approach seeks to avoid the task of specifying the guaranteed level; however, it cannot succeed because, given the inevitable differences in incomes and personal preferences, people in the same health state are likely to opt for different levels of care. Maintaining equality would require leveling up to the highest amount chosen or down to some lower amount. Leveling up again translates to everything of benefit, or more (because some people may use care that is not medically beneficial). Leveling down requires society to choose the level that will be guaranteed and then to prohibit people's use of their own resources to buy additional care. This would be considered an unacceptable restriction on liberty in the United States and would be difficult to enforce.

By default, therefore, one arrives at the definition of equity as access to an *adequate level* of care: a level of care that is less than all beneficial care and doesn't necessarily satisfy all needs completely, but is enough to achieve sufficient well-being, opportunity, information, and evidence of interpersonal concern to allow a reasonably satisfying life and a peaceful death. Care above this level has no special moral status. People who want more than the adequate level of care can have it, but society has no obligation to help them get it (although there are practical reasons why a society might choose to encourage the consumption of particular health services, just as there are for other consumer goods).

The companion concept of *excessive burden* refers to the cost of meeting the societal obligation to achieve equitable access. Guaranteeing access to adequate care doesn't necessarily mean providing free care. On the other hand, expecting the sacrifice of everything important to obtain health care would be inconsistent with the reasons for accepting the existence of a societal obligation to ensure access. The intermediate position is that people should be able to obtain an adequate level of care without having to bear an excessive burden, whether in money or in other costs, such as waiting and travel time.

Given the unequal distribution of income and of ill health, if no one is to bear an excessive burden to obtain care, some will have to pay less than the full cost of their own care and others will have to pay more. Equity requires that the final distribution of the total cost of guaranteeing access to an adequate level of care should not impose an excessive burden on anyone. As with defining "adequacy," deciding what "excessive" means and distributing the total cost fairly requires difficult value judgments; however, the framework's logic clearly requires that the cost of care should be distributed from the unhealthy to the healthy and from the poor to the rich, and that the total cost be spread nationally. Finally, because there is no moral obligation to guarantee access to care above the adequate level, there is no obligation to redistribute the cost of care above the adequate level, although such sharing may sometimes be desirable.

Responsibility for Achieving Equitable Access

If health care has special importance to individual well-being, we might argue that individuals should bear personal responsibility for securing access to it. Individuals do have some responsibility for their own access but, given the nature of health and health care, they cannot ensure access to adequate care simply by their own individual actions. Collective action, including political action, is required to achieve equitable access.

Health care, especially modern scientific health care, is a social product, not something individuals can produce for themselves. Moreover, unlike other basic needs such as the need for food, clothing and shelter, the need for health care is distributed unevenly and unpredictably across individuals and the cost of securing care can be high relative to income. Individuals cannot control their health status through their own efforts and thereby avoid this cost. Individual behavior affects health, but the effects are complex and poorly understood and behavior is not always the result of informed and voluntary choice. Given the potential size of the cost, most people also cannot ensure their ability to pay for adequate care for all health conditions they may incur unless there is some social mechanism for spreading the cost.

Private social mechanisms for spreading health care costs exist—namely, private health insurance and private charity—but they are inherently insufficient to achieve equity. There are many reasons why a private health insurance market, by itself, cannot achieve equitable access. For example, in a private insurance market, premiums are adjusted not in accord with income but in accord with individual risk (to the extent that risk can be predicted from information such as age and personal and family health history). This results in lack of access to adequate care for some of the poor and the high-risk and excessive burdens to obtain care for others. Private charity can fill in some gaps, but it, too, has never been sufficient to ensure adequate care. Lack of generosity plays a role, but also important is that charitable action requires the coordinated efforts of many people to be effective, especially if the goal is a stable guarantee of adequate care for all those who cannot obtain it for themselves. Lacking assurance that the donations of others will be forthcoming, people may fail to express their generous impulses or may direct them to other causes.

Because private mechanisms cannot achieve equitable access to health care, the ultimate responsibility for ensuring that the societal obligation is met falls on government, which exists to serve as an instrument for collective action. Although local and state governments may play important roles, the federal government is the logical level of government to take overall responsibility, for several reasons. First, the obligation is society-wide, not limited to particular states and localities. Second, only the federal government has the ability to secure reliable resources and to ensure that the total cost of achieving equitable access is spread fairly across the whole society. Finally, there must be oversight and coordination at the national level to ensure that the societal obligation is met.

Determining the Content of the Adequate Level

This analysis identifies a central question for health policy: how should a society determine the content of the adequate level? Countries around the world are struggling with this question. The logic of the argument for basing health policy on this concept of adequate level does not give a definitive answer, but it does indicate some characteristics that an adequate level must have.

Because the benefits of health care must be weighed against the benefits of competing uses for resources, the adequate level varies with the availability of resources in the society; richer societies can be expected to set a higher standard of adequacy than poor societies. In the assessment of the benefits and costs of care for possible inclusion in the adequate level, "benefits and costs" should be understood broadly as the positive and negative effects, or the good and bad consequences, including those that would be difficult, maybe impossible, to measure satisfactorily.

The importance of health care (the extent to which it is special) depends on an individual's health state; therefore, adequacy must be defined in relation to health status. Defining adequate care for a health condition requires specification of both the amount and the quality of health care to be received. For some conditions, adequacy may mean no treatment, and quality may not be the highest possible. Therefore, an adequate level is best understood as an entire standard of care, not an insurance benefit package that only lists the categories of services covered. Such a list is insufficient just as a list of the names of foods would be insufficient to specify an adequate diet, in the absence of information about the quantities and qualities of each food and who is to be fed.

Adequate care does not include all potentially beneficial care, but it can allow for some choice. A range of reasonable-cost treatment options for a condition can be included in the guaranteed standard of care to accommodate different patient preferences. In adjusting the definition of adequacy to available resources, the values and priorities of a society's members are important in guiding the tradeoffs among different kinds of health benefits and between health benefits and other social goods. Therefore, determining the content of the adequate level of care should not be left to health professionals.

Because adequacy depends on technology, resource availability, and individual and societal values and preferences, it is not something that can be permanently defined. Rather, there must be an ongoing process that allows the definition to evolve over time in response to changes in technology, resources, and preferences.

Given that the obligation to guarantee health care is society-wide, the standard for an adequate level should be national and the total cost should be spread nationally. The societal obligation toward someone who is poor and sick does not depend on where that person lives. Neither should a person's fair share of the cost of care for those who can't afford the full cost depend on geographic proximity. Americans travel frequently from one state to another, and, over the course of their lives, many Americans reside in multiple states. Defining a common national level and spreading the cost nationally provides a common safety net for all Americans, whatever their stage in life or place of residence, and avoids practical problems that would undermine equity. For example, if both the standard of care and its financing are determined at the state or local level, the more needy people a community has, the fewer tax resources it has to pay for their care and the leaner the standard of care it may be able to offer. Incentives may be created for the needy to move in search of adequate care, leading to a possible "race to the bottom" in the content of the guaranteed level. If the standard of care is determined nationally but state and local governments are required to pay for it (the "unfunded mandate" approach), the result will be an unfair distribution of the cost, because need and ability to pay are not evenly distributed geographically.

In a nationally coordinated and funded system, state and local governments may still play important roles. State (and local) public health officials know the health status, care priorities, and health care delivery circumstances of the populations they serve and should therefore be part of the national process that determines the content of the adequate level of care. The desirability of adjusting the delivery of care to local conditions is an argument for state (and local) government involvement in administration of the health care programs employed to guarantee adequate care.

A Multitier System?

The framework described above implies that a "multitier" health care system is not unfair in itself as long as the bottom (guaranteed) tier provides an adequate level of care and the cost of the entire system is distributed fairly. There are practical problems with a multitier system, however. The obvious problem is that people may acknowledge the societal obligation in principle but, in practice, financially shortchange the system designed to fulfill it.

Thus, there is an efficiency argument for a universal social insurance system that complements the ethical argument for a guaranteed adequate level of care. Arrow (1963) outlined the basis for this in a classic article on the economics of the private health insurance market. He demonstrated that in a world of uncertainty, private health insurance cannot give people protection against change in their risk status over time, and he concluded that there is a strong case for collective action to provide nonmarket mechanisms for bearing risk, such as social insurance.

In other words, it is in the self-interest of ordinary Americans to support social insurance for a standard of care that they find personally satisfactory (which may be more than the level of care they consider to be ethically required). In this way, they can be sure that the coverage they want for themselves and those they care about remains available and affordable no matter what happens to their incomes or health status. This goal can be achieved by establishing a health care system with universal coverage and a cost-conscious bottom tier that is not only morally adequate but also generous enough that the average person in the population considers the care satisfactory and only occasionally feels the desire to purchase more. Such a system can be a public-private partnership, as long as the necessary coordination is in place.

Equity in Today's Health Care System

In nearly all countries, including the United States, the government plays a significant role in the provision of access to health care. Other industrialized countries have created organized health care systems under government supervision in which close to universal access is provided to a level of care that at least approximates an adequate level. As noted above, all are struggling with the issue of how to determine whether the care provided is in fact adequate; however, the debates take place in a comprehensive system in which a cost-conscious standard of care has already been established. Unfortunately, the United States has not yet achieved this. The U.S. health care system is a patchwork of uncoordinated public and private financing and delivery structures that fail to meet the equity standard outlined here, for any reasonable definition of adequacy and excessive burden.

Some argue that the lack of progress toward equitable access creates serious doubt as to whether Americans believe in a societal obligation to achieve it. Others hold that both the rhetoric and the content of U.S. health policy over the years demonstrate the existence and influence of this belief; the problem is a political stalemate on the appropriate means to achieve equitable access, one that seems to be difficult to resolve (Daniels, Light, and Caplan 1996). Perhaps the major factor in this stalemate is the long-standing American distrust of government involvement in personal health care, especially federal government involvement. There is a fundamental contradiction in U.S. political culture between recognition of a collective obligation to achieve equitable access to health care and lack of confidence in the one institution (the federal

government) placed to provide the coordination and oversight required to fulfill it. It is against this background that this chapter considers the issue of fair
distribution of the costs and benefits of newborn screening.

Applying the Basic Equity Framework to Newborn Screening

Although newborn screening can yield benefits for families and for society
as a whole, the primary rationale for such screening has traditionally been the
immediate, direct benefits to the newborn. Policy has been based on a few generally accepted principles. Mandated public screening should be restricted to
serious conditions for which there is a reliable test, sufficient prevalence, and
effective early treatment. The test should entail a reasonable use of resources
to achieve the identified benefits to the child. Every child tested should receive
adequate follow-up and continuing treatment without regard to the family's
ability to pay, although fees may be imposed on parents who are deemed able
to pay (Newborn Screening Task Force 2000). States have interpreted these
principles differently, however, leading to the current variation in programs
across the country.

In the language of the equity framework, the rationale for guaranteeing
access to screening and follow-up treatment for the chosen conditions is that
such care is part of the adequate level and is therefore morally required. The
societal obligation to screen the newborn can be derived from the overall societal obligation to achieve equitable access discussed above or, more narrowly,
from the special societal obligation to protect the well-being of children that is
a feature of U.S. law and policy (i.e., the obligation to protect children's well-
being implies an obligation to guarantee adequate health care to children
without excessive burden on their families) (Holtzman 1997; Brock 2001;
Nichols 2007). Under either rationale, we can argue that it is appropriate to
use the basic equity framework outlined above to examine fairness issues in
newborn screening.[2]

The contradiction noted earlier remains, however. The U.S. health care
system does not in fact guarantee children's access to adequate care. Public
newborn screening programs single out certain health conditions for special consideration, and the states differ in the conditions chosen. The equity
framework implies that conditions with similar treatment costs and similar
effects on the child, family, and society should have similar status with respect to the adequate level. Yet, because decisions about publicly funded new-

born screening are not made within the context of an entire standard of care guaranteed to children, a child may be guaranteed screening and follow-up care for a rare genetic metabolic disease through a state newborn screening program but be unable to get adequate and affordable care for severe asthma. The special urgency of detection and care and the claimed efficiency advantages of a universal screening program from which parents can only opt out can be cited as justifications for the exceptional treatment of the rare disorder. Nevertheless, a basic fairness question remains because there are many health services that might offer greater benefits to children at lower cost than newborn screening.

The preferred remedy to this inequity would be to guarantee an adequate level of health care to all children and to distribute the cost fairly so that no one bears an excessive burden. Decisions about newborn screening programs would then be made in the context of the broader social process of defining the adequate level. If this remedy is not feasible, the relevant question is, given the social and political constraints that prevent guaranteeing adequate care to all children, what newborn screening policy is the best with respect to fairness? Some might argue that fairness would be served by modifying the principle that restricts the program to conditions requiring early treatment, and screening newborns for more conditions, so that more children with congenital conditions would be guaranteed timely diagnosis, treatment, and long-term management. But it seems fairer to maintain the current rule unless and until we are ready to explore the definition of the entire adequate level of care for children and the place of newborn screening within it.

Fairness within Newborn Screening Programs

Turning from fairness across the whole range of children's health care to fairness within newborn screening programs, we can group the major fairness issues under three headings: selection of tests; financing and delivery of screening, follow-up, diagnosis, and treatment and management services; and research and evaluation.

Selection of Tests

The observed variation in test panels across states is currently considered a major equity problem. To many, it seems unfair that a child with a genetic condition is identified and successfully treated in one state, while in another state a child with the same condition is not identified and goes without treatment. According to the equity framework, the adequate level of care is based on a society's level of resources and is assumed to be the same regardless of place of residence (although geographically isolated people may have to bear extra travel costs). The a priori case for uniformity seems even stronger for children's health care than for adult care. If the adequate level is determined at a local, state, or regional level, it could be argued that adults can choose their location and can participate in the social process to define the guaranteed standard in that location. This argument is not, of course, applicable to a newborn.

On the other hand, the cost of testing should be considered in selecting which conditions to test for. Incidence variations can be associated with differences in the cost per identified case within a particular region (including both screening costs and costs related to false positives) (Gessner, Teutsch, and Shaffer 1996; Panepinto et al. 2000). Whether and to what extent it is fair to allow this cost variation to affect test panels is a controversial issue. We can consider several points here.

Geographic variation does not seem to be a valid justification for current state-level variations in test panels, in principle or in practice. It is not the geographic location per se that affects a newborn's risk of having a particular genetic condition. The incidence variations occur because population subgroups with different distributions of genetic conditions are concentrated geographically. These geographic variations are not correlated with state borders, however. High and low geographic concentrations of particular conditions can occur within states that have a low overall incidence of the condition. Moreover, the Newborn Screening Task Force's report noted that at the time it was meeting, in the nine states that did not have universal testing for sickle cell disease (SCD) because of low incidence, the incidence of SCD was higher than that of galactosemia, a condition those states did test all infants for (Newborn Screening Task Force 2000).

It might be possible to develop a testing plan based on geographic divisions that does match incidence patterns. Even if such a design were considered fair in principle, however, keeping it fair in practice would be difficult because the geographic distribution of genetic conditions changes over time with population shifts related to economic change and immigration.

Because certain genetic conditions are associated with race or ethnicity, it is tempting to define subgroups of the population on the basis of race and ethnicity and tailor the choice of screening tests to these subgroups. This is not inherently unfair; adequate care should be defined in relation to health status, which includes risk for a particular health condition (President's Commission for the Study of Ethical Problems in Medicine and Biomedical and Behavioral Research 1983). The strategy is problematic in practice, however, because race and ethnicity are socially constructed concepts that do not map onto underlying genetic makeup as closely as popular perception suggests (Juengst 1998; Lee, Mountain, and Koenig 2001). The history of newborn screening for SCD has demonstrated the complexity in targeting screening programs to specific racially and ethnically defined groups (Bowman 1994; Joiner 2000; see also chapters 3 and 8).

If newborn screening is not universal, logic suggests that there should be valid science-based reasons for definition of the subgroups to be tested and that the testing design should make economic sense. Careful cost analysis is essential (Sprinkle, Hynes, and Konrad 1994) because new technologies are changing the structure of screening costs. Tandem mass spectrometry (MS/MS) and DNA-based testing have high fixed costs, but the marginal cost to add an additional test to the standard test panel is low (Levy and Albers 2000). Once universal newborn screening for any condition has been established, using these technologies, the actual screening cost to test all newborns for an additional condition may not be very different from the cost of defining high-incidence subgroups and testing them separately. There may be a good case on fairness grounds for basing test selection for publicly funded newborn screening programs on national incidence rates and testing all newborns in the United States for the entire panel.

Follow-up costs for additional false positives must be considered, however. The costs related to false positives include not only the resource costs of the notification and definitive diagnosis but also the costs in time and anxiety that fall directly on the family—costs that are difficult to measure and cannot be easily redistributed to the entire population. Policymakers must find a fair balance between the burdens on families whose newborns have false positive screening results and the benefits of identifying additional true positives and increasing the perceived fairness of the system (Kwon and Farrell 2000).

With funding from the Health Resources and Services Administration (HRSA), the American College of Medical Genetics (ACMG) recently completed a major report recommending that all states screen all newborns for a core list of 29 conditions (American College of Medical Genetics 2006). In addition to reporting these results, the ACMG group recommends that parents also be informed if an infant has one of 25 secondary, "report only" conditions—which do not meet the group's criteria for inclusion in a uniform screening panel but are automatically identified in the screening and follow-up process for the 29 conditions in the core list.

The ACMG report has been severely criticized for its methodology, content, and working process. The critics argue that the methodology was highly idiosyncratic and did not conform to established standards for evidence-based reviews; that the report has insufficient discussion of many important ethical, legal, and social issues that are relevant to such a significant expansion of programs; and that the working group had extensive expertise in metabolic genetics and laboratory medicine but lacked expertise in evidence-based medicine, bioethics, primary care, and health economics. Moreover, advocacy groups such as the March of Dimes were promoting the report's recommendations for the uniform panel months before members of the policy community and the public were allowed to see the report and assess the methods used to develop the recommendations (Botkin et al. 2006; see also chapters 7 and 10 for further discussion of the ACMG group's work).

One surprising aspect of the ACMG report is its departure, with little discussion or justification, from the principle that mandatory screening should be done only when the condition causes serious harm to the newborn that can be avoided if the condition is diagnosed and treated immediately after birth, before symptoms appear. This omission occurred even though this criterion had guided newborn screening from its inception, and the highly respected Newborn Screening Task Force had reaffirmed it only a few years before the ACMG began its work (Newborn Screening Task Force 2000; Bailey et al. 2006; Grosse et al. 2006).

For conditions that do not meet this criterion, the case for making screening mandatory does not hold. More important for the topic of this chapter, it is unclear that screening and treatment for these conditions must be provided to all children on equity grounds. In other words, it isn't clear that the screening belongs in the morally required "adequate level" of care or, even if it does, that it deserves higher priority than other morally required care not currently guaranteed to children in our fragmented health care system (see chapter 5).

Financing and Delivery of Screening and Associated Services

As the Newborn Screening Task Force report and other sources document (Newborn Screening Task Force 2000; U.S. General Accounting Office 2003), there are substantial variations across states in the content of follow-up care and in the way programs are financed. Within states, also, the quantity and quality of follow-up services received by individual children and their families varies. The cost of the programs is distributed in an arbitrary manner that imposes excessive burdens on some families and fails to distribute the burden of the total cost of the system equitably across the entire nation.

Two important factors producing this situation are the variability in states' public health capacity and the structure of children's access to health care. Because the states differ greatly in population size, land area, per capita income, and other characteristics, their public health programs also differ, resulting in major discrepancies in their newborn screening programs. The structure of the financing and delivery system itself also contributes to unfair distribution of services and costs. Newborn screening programs began as testing programs under the direction of state public health laboratories; follow-up, diagnosis, and treatment services evolved over time and were funded in an ad hoc manner. As newborn screening expanded, states shifted some of the responsibility for the funding and delivery of screening-related health services to the larger health care system. To the extent that a child had coverage, services now came from the child's regular sources of care and were paid for by payers such as Medicaid and private insurance. States used various strategies of cost shifting and separate funding to cover services for the uninsured and underinsured.

Data on the structure of health insurance coverage for children (Kaiser Commission on Medicaid and the Uninsured 2007) show that about three-fifths have private insurance and a little over one-quarter are covered under Medicaid or the State Children's Health Insurance Program (SCHIP), a program that subsidizes coverage for low-income children either under Medicaid or under a separate state plan created for low-income children not eligible for Medicaid. About 12 percent of children have no insurance at all. Medicaid has a particularly strategic place in newborn screening because it pays for more than one-third of all births. In this complex system, the probability that a child has coverage, the standard of care that the coverage provides access to, and the distribution of the cost of care that falls directly on the family all vary significantly with income, race/ethnicity, citizenship, and place of residence. Low-income, minority, and noncitizen children are significantly more likely to be uninsured and to receive less than adequate care. The percentage of uninsured children varies by state, from 5.3 percent in Michigan to 20.5 percent in Texas.

The equity framework highlights the importance of defining a minimum level of services required for screened conditions. Evaluation of the performance of state public health programs and state Medicaid and SCHIP programs requires clarity on the minimum level that should be provided to the children who depend on these programs for care. Clarity on what is minimally required is also important for private insurance. Coverage under private insurance varies tremendously, and there are economic reasons why genetic conditions tend to be badly served in a private health insurance system. For example, managed care plans must compete on the basis of the relationship between the standard of care they offer and the premium. The market rewards plans that skimp on care categories that are important to small numbers of patients with high-cost, chronic conditions. A plan that offers excellent care to such patients runs the risk of attracting members with higher than average costs; skimping on such care has the opposite effect. Establishing clear standards as to what is minimally required does not eliminate the problem but at least provides the necessary benchmarks for designing policies to eliminate inequities in access.

Financial incentives created by the structure of financing for services related to newborn screening significantly influence the delivery of services and therefore the distribution of the benefits. Financing also determines the final distribution of program cost. Currently, state newborn screening programs receive some federal funds through block grants. Medicaid's cost is shared by the states and the federal government according to a formula related to per capita state income. SCHIP is also financed by a combination of federal and state funds. Reliance on state funding raises equity issues over and above the general point that the cost of adequate care should be shared nationally. State tax structures are regressive compared with federal tax structures (i.e., the tax burden falls more heavily on lower-income groups). State revenues also vary more with economic conditions, because states cannot run budget deficits. Given that state obligations for public welfare, unemployment compensation, and Medicaid tend to increase when the state economy is depressed, this can be a serious problem for state health programs.

Recent dramatic expansions in the number of conditions included in many state newborn screening programs are putting additional strain on financing and service delivery structures that were already far from satisfactory. Policymakers must give serious attention to the issue of equitable financing of newborn screening. For example, what concrete actions can be taken to make financing more equitable within existing state programs? What concrete actions can be taken to ensure more equitable sharing of the cost of newborn screening nationally? Are there changes that could be made in Medicaid at the national level to provide better funding for newborn screening? Could the federal government simply take over the financial responsibility for newborn screening? Could we move to a system of universal coverage of children through incremental expansion of Medicaid, SCHIP, and private insurance?

Research and Evaluation

To make good decisions about whether newborn screening should be mandated for a particular condition, policymakers need extensive information on the nature and distribution of congenital conditions, their consequences for individuals and society, and the availability and effectiveness of treatment. Historically, this information has been developed in an unsystematic way. Some conditions have received far more attention than others, and even for the conditions that have been extensively studied, there are serious information gaps. These gaps are apparent in the ACMG's newborn screening report (see chapter 10).

Research funding strategies that encourage the development of information on the full range of congenital conditions in the population would help to promote fairness in newborn screening in the long run. This could be done through individual, freestanding, time-limited research projects. Such projects are inherently expensive, however. A more economical approach would be to build ongoing research and evaluation into the routine management of newborn screening programs.

An important issue for society is the extent to which newborns and their families should be expected to cooperate in research and quality improvement activities. It can be argued that members of society have an obligation to accept a fair share of the burden of these activities in health care because they benefit from past research and effective program administration, and, to carry the argument further, that it is fair to include them in minimal-risk research and evaluation without their specific consent. (See chapters 12, 13, and 14 for various perspectives on the ethical issues raised by the use of newborn screening bloodspots and data on screened infants for research purposes.)

Fair Decision Making about Newborn Screening

The equity framework provides guidance on the broad outlines of the adequate level of care and the key characteristics of a process for defining specific content, but it does not say what the actual standard of care should be. Bioethicists have noted with some frustration that many philosophical theories of justice in health care support the concept of a societal obligation to guarantee adequate care, but none provides specific guidance on the content of such care. There must be a fair social decision-making process to resolve the inevitable disagreements (Daniels 1994, 2000, 2001).

The U.S. health care system lacks this decision-making process, and the introduction and evolution of newborn screening is an example of what can happen without it. As noted in chapter 1, newborn screening began in the 1960s with development of the Guthrie blood test for phenylketonuria (PKU). A few states developed voluntary screening programs; over time, more states introduced PKU testing and made it mandatory, partly in response to intensive grassroots lobbying by children's advocates. Mandated PKU screening was controversial because it was established before there was clear evidence of benefits. The federal government (the Maternal and Child Health Bureau) funded research to aid in establishing the PKU test's effectiveness and provided other assistance to states for the development of genetics-related child health services (see chapter 9), but newborn screening remained a state public health program. Over time, as states added new tests to their screening panels, newborn screening policy continued to conform to the so-called extemporaneous model in which independent market, professional practice, legal, and consumer forces drive decision making in an ad hoc manner (Wilfond and Nolan 1993).

In recent years, the limitations of the extemporaneous model have become increasingly apparent. As new knowledge and new technologies continue to affect the newborn screening environment, states face increasing pressure to expand their programs from health professionals, consumer advocates, and for-profit suppliers of screening services and technologies. To respond appropriately to the pressure, states need a more systematic, evidence-based decision-making process that incorporates attention to underlying normative issues.

Against this background, we examine here the roles of government, other stakeholders, and technical tools for economic evaluation in promoting fairness in the newborn screening policy process.

The Roles of Different Levels of Government

Currently, newborn screening decisions are made at the state level and considerable variation among state programs persists. The Newborn Screening Task Force called for coordination of newborn screening policy at the national level (Newborn Screening Task Force 2000; Cunningham 2002). This is consistent with the equity framework, which implies that the state is the wrong level for financing and for determining the basic panel of tests and the content of adequate follow-up care (although it may be the right level for making administrative decisions about program implementation).

Many agree that national coordination of policy is important for achieving distributional fairness in newborn screening. The major obstacle to coordination is financing. One possibility would be for the overall decision making and financing of newborn screening to become a federal government responsibility. The federal government could also take over program administration, or (more likely) the states could retain responsibility for managing the program and integrating it into existing state public health activities. This would represent a radical change in the status quo, however, and is probably not feasible. A transfer of full financial responsibility is unlikely to be politically acceptable, and if the federal government attempted to impose a national newborn screening policy on the states without financing, it would have to overcome the intense state opposition to unfunded mandates.

Alternatively, states could voluntarily seek to coordinate newborn screening activities. Since the beginning of newborn screening, there have been limited state coalitions to take advantage of economies of scale and increased case detection. Some states have managed to achieve successful coalitions for MS/MS testing as well. For example, the Massachusetts-based New England Newborn Screening Program also provides services to Maine, New Hampshire, Vermont, and Rhode Island. Each state in the New England program makes its own decision about which tests to include in its test panel, however. As noted, states are currently facing strong pressure from parent advocacy groups, instrument manufacturers, private laboratories, and others to expand their newborn screening programs, and forming a united front might make it easier for states to deal with the pressure. But without a way to share the financing of newborn screening equitably on a national basis, states are likely to find that achieving full cooperation continues to be difficult (Stoddard and Farrell 1997).

An intermediate position is a voluntary federal-state partnership. This could take the form of an agreement on a required minimum set of tests and the content of the required follow-up care, reached through a process that involves state and federal decision makers as well as other stakeholders and includes a plan for shared federal-state financing to support it. Any financing scheme must be careful to include the entire newborn screening system in an equitable way.

An important step in this direction was taken in 2004, when the federal government[3] funded the establishment of seven Genetics and Newborn Screening Regional Collaborative Groups (RCs) and a National Coordinating Center (NCC). NCC is funded under a cooperative agreement between HRSA and the ACMG, and has a central office and an advisory committee consisting of the seven RCs and representatives of national organizations such as the American Academy of Pediatrics, the Association of Public Health Laboratories, the National Society of Genetics Counselors, the March of Dimes, and the Genetic Alliance. The RCs and NCC are intended to provide a structure for states to cooperate with one another and with appropriate public and private organizations to improve quality and access in services related to newborn screening.[4]

The Roles of Other Stakeholders

According to the equity framework, ongoing input on the values and priorities of the members of society is important in determining the content of the adequate level of care related to newborn screening and adjusting it over time. This could be done through a national newborn screening advisory body, which could determine the minimum panel of tests and the minimum standards for education, follow-up, diagnosis, and treatment for screened conditions. Ideally, the advisory body would be a standing committee (newborn screening advisory committee, NBSAC) that could develop expertise over time and respond to changing conditions.

The Children's Health Act of 2000 provided for an advisory committee on heritable disorders in newborns and children (106th Congress 2007); the committee was eventually chartered as the Advisory Committee on Heritable Disorders and Genetic Diseases in Newborns and Children and was directed "to advise and guide the Secretary regarding the most appropriate application of universal newborn screening tests, technologies, policies, guidelines and programs for effectively reducing morbidity and mortality in newborns and children having or at risk for heritable disorders" (U.S. Department of Health and Human Services 2005, p. 1). The committee's first meeting was in June 2004. The committee endorsed the ACMG report to the secretary of Health and Human Services; it promotes the expansion of states' newborn screening programs to conform to the report's recommendations and is developing a systematic process for evaluating proposals to add more conditions to the uniform panel. The committee also plays a role in continuing assessment, technical assistance, and policy development related to the full range of newborn screening support services.

The Newborn Screening Task Force also recommended that states establish ongoing NBSACs that include parents, health care professionals, third-party payers, appropriate government agencies, and "other concerned citizens" (Newborn Screening Task Force 2000). In the mid-1990s, a survey showed that about two-thirds of the states already had NBSACs and about half of the states had advisory committees with consumer representation (Hiller, Landenburger, and Natowicz 1997). State committees can be a source of the information about the values and concerns of the state's population required for state participation in the national newborn screening advisory process. They can also advise on local implementation issues and be a vehicle for consultation and advocacy with communities especially affected by newborn screening.

An advisory committee, whether at the state or federal level, can be constituted in a variety of ways, with a variety of conceptualizations of the roles of its members. For example, committee members may see their roles in terms of a "representative" model or a "perspectives" model. In the first, the members of the committee consider themselves representatives of a group of stakeholders and therefore feel a responsibility to reflect the views of their "constituency," although in fact the committee member is usually selected through an informal process and uses only an informal process to consult with a stakeholder group. In the second, the members of the committee consider themselves reflectors of a particular perspective. They may also feel a responsibility to explain the perspective accurately but are likely to feel somewhat freer to participate in discussion and decision making based on their own opinions. There is no clear differentiation between these two models, and some committee members may find themselves moving back and forth between them in their behavior on the committee. Ideally, members of advisory committees need guidelines to help them understand their role, both in general terms and in the context of the particular committee on which they serve.

There is an inherent potential bias in that the people motivated to serve on a time-consuming committee may have a particularly strong self-interest in the decisions, at times biasing the decision-making process. It is therefore important that committees make a systematic effort to gather information on values in general, and distributional values in particular, from the general public and from important subgroups, such as groups defined by race and ethnicity. A wide variety of methods are available for use by advisory committees or public health departments in gathering information about societal values and preferences as input into health care policies. The methods differ as to whether they provide respondents with information as part of the consultation, and whether the respondents are able to engage in deliberation or discussion to arrive at their views. The following are some examples (Jordan et al. 1998):

Citizens' juries. Groups of jurors selected to represent public or local opinion. They sit for a given period of time during which experts give evidence on a topic and jurors ask questions and debate issues.

User consultation panels. Groups of representatives selected from a locality or population, with members rotated to ensure a diversity of views. Panel members receive information on topics decided on in advance and participate in a discussion that is often led by a moderator.

Focus groups. Usually semistructured discussion groups of six to eight participants led by a moderator, with focus on specific topics. Debate and discussion are encouraged.

Questionnaire surveys. Forms distributed by mail or at a site such as a physician's waiting room. Surveys allow collection of information from a large sample of respondents and examination of the relation between variables; they are most appropriate when the issues are already known in some detail.

Opinion surveys of standing panels. Periodic questionnaire surveys of large, sociologically representative samples (typically 1000 or more) of a population.

For newborn screening policy, methods that provide respondents with information and give them the opportunity to deliberate seem most appropriate, because the issues in genetics and priority setting are not well understood by the public (Gutmann and Thompson 1997). In the United States, the public meetings organized by Oregon Health Decisions (Fleck 1994) to debate health care priorities in the context of Medicaid reform and the focus groups set up by American Health Decisions to identify American values in end-of-life care (Tyler and American Health Decisions 1997) are examples of efforts to engage the public in informed, deliberative consultation. (For additional discussion of state NBSACs and their role in the formation of policy in the United States, see chapter 7.)

A striking feature of the newborn screening policy landscape is the importance of forceful advocacy by parents of affected children, health care professionals who treat affected children, and child health advocacy organizations such as the March of Dimes. These advocates have lobbied federal and state advisory committees and used internet sites and more traditional media in attempts to persuade state legislatures and the general public to support expanded newborn screening. In some states, individual parents have been the critical factor in major changes in newborn screening programs. (See chapter 4 for additional discussion of the role of advocates and chapter 6 for a narrative of the experience of one state, Tennessee.)

In newborn screening policy discussions, frequent reference is made to "what parents want." In practice, however, this usually means "what some of the parents of children already identified as having a particular genetic condition are advocating for." We have little evidence of what parents in general want. Many aren't even aware of the existence of the disorders screened for until they are told about them during pregnancy or, even later, when they receive a positive result. We don't know how important they think screening is, and if we were to ask parents, or taxpayers in general, about this, the question would have to be properly framed. It should not be phrased, "Do you want to refuse screening for your newborn?" or "Do you think screening newborns for genetic disorders is a good idea?" The wording should make it clear that screening has benefits but also an opportunity cost, and it should provide examples of the benefits that might be obtained if newborn screening resources were devoted to alternative uses.

Private, for-profit companies have also played a significant and at times troubling role in shaping newborn screening policy. Frequently, the influence is exerted through consumers and health professionals. Direct marketing of tests to these groups by the laboratories that provide them is an important factor in motivating advocacy for the addition of new tests to public newborn screening test panels.

In some states, private laboratories seek permission to market their services to mothers in the hospital and "piggyback" on the state screening process. Should this be allowed? Does it raise fairness problems? On the one hand, the equity framework suggests that it is not automatically unfair for people to choose to buy additional testing for their infants with their own money. On the other hand, allowing the private testing to be combined with public program education, testing, and follow-up may send the message that the private tests are more valuable than they really are, creating a public perception of inequity and distorting decisions about the public screening program.

Private companies have sometimes been aggressive in their attempts to influence state policy directly. For example, in the mid-1990s, the Massachusetts Department of Public Health came under intense pressure to introduce MS/MS into its newborn screening program from NeoGen, a for-profit company that pioneered the use of the new technology in screening newborns for a wide range of metabolic disorders. An article by Atkinson et al. (2001) describes the public consultation and decision-making process that led to the state's 1997 decision to adopt the new technology and shaped the details of its new program. When the state's advisory committee chose its existing test provider, the university-based New England Newborn Screening Program, to implement the new testing and required hospitals to submit samples to this program, rather than contracting directly with NeoGen or allowing individual hospitals to choose NeoGen, the company sued the state on the grounds that it was violating antitrust law. (The suit was unsuccessful.)

The relationship between public and private testing is a key feature of newborn screening policy and requires careful management. There is nothing inherently wrong with contracting with private for-profit or not-for-profit entities to supply services under public health programs, but states must take great care in writing the contracts. In contracting for newborn screening services, a state must structure the contract to be part of a comprehensive strategy designed to ensure that the whole spectrum of services, not just the testing itself, will be provided and paid for in an equitable way, that access to services and financing will be stable over time, and that data generated by the program will be available to the state for ongoing quality improvement and socially beneficial research. The states and the federal government must also take care to avoid bias in newborn screening policy resulting from the influence of companies on public decision making, whether directly through lobbying or indirectly through educational outreach and financial support to parent advocacy groups and health care professionals.

The Role of Economic Evaluation Techniques

The principal tools for economic evaluation of public programs are cost-benefit analysis and cost-effectiveness analysis. Cost-benefit analysis (CBA) is "an analytic tool for estimating the net social benefit of a program or intervention as the incremental benefit of the program less the incremental cost with all benefits and costs measured in dollars," where the incremental cost is "the cost of the program less the cost of the alternative it is being compared with" (Gold et al. 1996, pp. 395, 399). A CBA systematically identifies all of the positive and negative effects of a program, assigns them dollar values, and computes the net value. If the dollar values capture the true social value of each effect, programs can be selected according to their net value. All programs that produce positive net value and are not mutually exclusive are worth doing, and, among those that are mutually exclusive, the one with the highest net value is the best. The methodology is general; because all program effects are valued in dollars, programs in education, health, or transportation are all put on a common footing for comparison.

Unfortunately, assigning dollar values to effects is difficult. Some program inputs have market prices that reflect the opportunity cost of using them in the program, but calculating the opportunity cost of other inputs (e.g., the time costs of people who do not work for money) is more difficult. Valuing benefits is especially challenging. Economic theory suggests that the benefits should be valued according to the preferences of the people who will receive them, but public programs are usually public because their benefits cannot be efficiently produced and allocated by private markets. Therefore, there is no easy way to determine what people would be willing to pay for the benefits. Analysts must rely on answers to hypothetical questions on surveys (notoriously unreliable) or indirect evidence from market behavior toward products producing similar benefits. Also—and this, for many people, is more important—willingness to pay will depend on income; thus, when benefits are measured according to willingness to pay, CBA tends to favor programs that benefit the rich.

Valuing health benefits in dollars is particularly troublesome. People cannot easily answer hypothetical questions about what they would pay for changes in the risk of death or disability, and a measure of benefit that is biased in favor of the rich seems especially unfair in the health context. To many people, the very idea of valuing life or valuing health in dollars seems repugnant. Therefore, CBA is rarely used in assessing health programs.

The alternative, cost-effectiveness analysis, differs from CBA primarily in not even attempting to value effects on health in dollar terms. CEA is "an analytic tool in which costs and effects of a program and at least one alternative are calculated and presented in a ratio of incremental cost to incremental effect. Effects are health outcomes, such as cases of a disease prevented, years of life gained, or quality-adjusted life years, rather than monetary measures as in cost-benefit analysis" (Gold et al. 1996, p. 395). By giving program cost in dollars per unit of health outcome, CEA avoids attaching an *explicit dollar value* to a health outcome, but, in doing so, it gives up the ability to directly compare health programs with nonhealth programs. Also, unless a program is cost-saving (produces the same or greater benefits at lower cost than the alternative), a decision about whether to implement it defines an *implicit dollar value*. If the program costs more but produces more of the positive health outcome, the yes or no decision implies that the greater benefits are or are not worth at least as much as the additional cost.

Comparisons of health programs that produce multiple effects on health in different combinations (more of one, less of another) are difficult to make using CEA. Unfortunately, in comparing health programs, this is the typical case. Analysts need a measure that combines the effects (e.g., effects on both the quality and the length of life) into a single quantitative measure of program effectiveness. The measure most commonly used is the quality-adjusted life-year (QALY), defined as "a measure of health outcome which assigns to each period of time a weight, ranging from 0 to 1, corresponding to the health-related quality of life during that period, where a weight of 1 corresponds to optimal health, and a weight of 0 corresponds to a health state judged equivalent to death; these are then aggregated across time periods" (Gold et al. 1996, p. 405). The weights come from a complex methodology in which individuals are asked about their tradeoffs among health states in order to elicit preferences over a set of standard health states and place the health states on a continuum from 0 to 1. The weights of individuals' responses are then aggregated into social weights and used to translate program health effects into QALYs. The incremental cost-effectiveness of a project is the ratio of the additional QALYs it produces per dollar of additional cost compared with the alternative.

Although CEA does not value health effects in dollars, it engages in a less obvious type of valuation by using the utilities people attach to different health states to construct the social weights used to transform time in health states into QALYs. When a CEA measures effectiveness in QALYs, the analysis is sometimes referred to as a cost-utility analysis (CUA) to highlight the fact that the methodology is somewhere between a CBA and a CEA, using purely physical units of health output.

In assessing the value of CEA to people who must make practical decisions, commentators have distinguished between its use as an organizing framework for the collection and interpretation of information and its use as a mechanical decision rule. The first use is strongly supported, while the second is not. When one is making decisions, simple common sense recommends careful attention to the costs and benefits of each alternative. In a policy context, a decision maker must do the following: define the policy problem and objectives; make sure that the most appropriate alternatives are being considered; describe input-output relationships in each alternative; identify, measure, and value costs; identify and measure effectiveness; account for the timing of costs and benefits; allow for uncertainty; and present and interpret the findings. CEA offers a detailed methodology for carrying out these necessary steps—a methodology that has been significantly improved and standardized by a U.S. Public Health Service–appointed expert panel, the Panel on Cost Effectiveness in Health and Medicine (Gold et al. 1996). A well-performed CEA can provide valuable information and structure to the decision-making process.

Nevertheless, there is a firm consensus that CEAs are "an aid to decision-making, not a complete procedure for making decisions" (Gold et al. 1996, p. 22). Performing a CEA is a challenging task. A number of authors have noted the relatively low quality of the existing CEA literature (Gerard 1992; Kernick 1998; Pollitt 2001; Jefferson and Demicheli 2002). If CEAs are to be useful, the quality should be higher; however, these analyses require resources and how precise to make them is a judgment call that requires weighing benefits and costs in itself. On these practical grounds alone, it would be inappropriate to make the "bottom line" of a CEA the authority for making decisions.

More important, a CEA does not—and in its current form cannot—incorporate all the societal values that are relevant to a decision. The most important value it fails to capture is the subject of this chapter: fairness in the distribution of program costs and benefits. In its basic form, CEA does not take distribution into account. If fair distribution matters, the analyst must gather additional information about who will benefit and who will pay, and judge whether the result is equitable.

There is an extensive recent literature in ethics and economics on the distributional issue in economic evaluation. Much of the literature focuses on the use of CEAs that measure output in QALYs to make priority-setting decisions in real health care systems. Much of it originates in the United Kingdom, Canada, and Europe, because priority setting is both more urgent and more straightforward in organized national health systems.

In these systems, the people who managed resources were acutely aware of opportunity cost and were sure that some services yielded better value for money than others, but found it difficult to agree about which services should have priority. They could not help wishing for a decision tool that could produce decisions automatically without constant agonizing over priorities. They did not believe there could be a value-free, technical way to make allocation decisions, but they hoped to find a technique that could take a few societal value judgments with wide support and translate them into specific allocation decisions.

With this hope, they made what seemed to be an uncontroversial assumption: the goal of public expenditures on health care is to improve health. They combined this with a second uncontroversial assumption—that resources are scarce—and had a decision rule: in making health care spending decisions, the goal should be to maximize population health, while taking due account of resource scarcity. But how does one measure the amount of health a program produces? The QALY was invented to answer this question, so the rule became: make decisions about expenditures on health programs to maximize the number of QALYs produced given the available resources. If shifting resources from one program to another would increase the number of QALYs gained, it should be done.

There has been a lively and often acrimonious debate about the ethical implications of the use of QALYs in public decision making, the final rule stated above, and possible alternative goals and rules (e.g., Harris 1988, 1991, 1995, 1996; Cubbon 1991; Wagstaff 1991; Williams 1992, 1995; Menzel 1995; Singer et al. 1995; Hope 1996; McKie et al. 1996; Farrar et al. 1997; Seedhouse 1997; Powers and Faden 2000, 2006; Donaldson, Birch, and Gafni 2002; Brock 2004; Amundson 2005; Bickenbach 2005; Nord 2005). In retrospect, it is odd—for several reasons—that so many people thought (and some still think) that maximizing QALYs is the appropriate normative social goal in health policy.

First, people want more from health care than health improvement; for example, they also want information and caring. Someone with a symptom that could be either a condition that will go away without treatment or a fatal condition that has no treatment is likely to want a physician to tell him which it is and, if the news is bad, to care for him during the dying process. Second, even if health improvement is all that matters and QALYs measure it well, maximizing the total number of QALYs without regard to distribution would not be the right social goal. Maximizing total national income would not maximize social well-being if it all went to one person—why should QALYs be different? If anything, the case for considering distribution at the time of deciding whether to begin a project is stronger for health programs than for other kinds of public investments. Public health expenditures produce QALYs and distribute them to particular people; they cannot be redistributed after the fact. As with the distribution of monetary benefits, people are likely to have complex and conflicting views on what constitutes fairness in the distribution of QALYs, but the distribution surely matters.

Why, then, was there such an intense debate? The economists provoked criticism by engaging in a pattern of behavior typical to economics. Because they did not have a good solution to the distributional fairness problem, they minimized it or ignored it completely. Contrary to popular perception, economists are concerned about the value judgments implicit in economic models, even when the people who construct them try to be as value-neutral as possible (Hausman and MacPherson 1996); however, they often acknowledge questionable value judgments and inherent flaws and then use the models anyway. The implicit assumption seems to be that important decisions must be made and a flawed system for making them is better than no system.

The ethics side of the debate also had problems. The basic point made by many ethicists—that distribution matters and maximizing QALYs is not consistent with important distributional values—is correct. However, some went further and rejected the fundamental legitimacy of the cost-containment effort (La Puma and Lawlor 1990). They tended to focus on patient autonomy and see priority-setting techniques as ethically unacceptable interference in physician-patient decision making—depriving the patient of the ability to ask for and the doctor to provide whatever they think would be of benefit. These ethicists seemed unwilling to acknowledge that in the situations in which economic evaluation techniques are used for priority setting, the patient is usually paying less than the full cost, often much less, and the impact of physician-patient decisions on the people who have to contribute the resources is of moral significance.

The fundamental insight in priority setting in health care is that individuals do not behave as if their own lives and health are infinitely valuable. They make tradeoffs between their health and other important things in their lives when they are allocating their personal resources. The resources for public programs that save lives and improve health do not materialize from outer space. They come from individual members of society through compulsory taxation. If individuals make tradeoffs between health and other goals, surely society should, too, because it is individual members of society who are ultimately paying the bill. This is the insight that is fundamental to the basic equity framework summarized above.

How should the tradeoffs be made? Standard normative models in economics begin by assuming that the well-being of society as a whole is based on the well-being of its individual members as they themselves define it. Social welfare is assumed to be a function of individual evaluations of states of society, and the distributional debate takes place over how to aggregate the individual utilities: for example, whether to give greater weight to programs that benefit those who are less well-off to begin with. These models are of limited use in the context of equity in health care as framed in this chapter. Once one accepts that there are concerns about the distribution of health care and health that are not based on making people better off according to their own preferences and, further, that these concerns are not simply other types of preferences (the preferences of the people putting up the money about what they want other people to have) but have ethical content, one is firmly outside the realm of standard welfare economics.

Moral philosophy provides insight into the nature of the problem, but, as noted, philosophical theories aren't specific enough about what is morally required to help health care managers decide exactly what to do. Moral philosophy does say that individual preferences are morally relevant to priority setting—both the preferences of the people receiving care about what they want and the preferences of the people paying for care about what costs they are willing to share. Preferences are also practically relevant because there must be a collective decision-making process and, in a democracy, the preferences of the voters matter. Nevertheless, popular values cannot have automatic ultimate authority, because they can be morally wrong. What is needed is a complex political compromise on a matter of moral importance. In other words, no simple priority-setting decision tool is available at the moment and there isn't likely to be one in the near future.

There is intense interest in the distributional issue in the economic evaluation of health care. The ethical criticism has forced health economists to be more than usually conscious of the value implications of their techniques. The extensive literature includes conceptual discussion of the different distributional values that make ethical sense (e.g., Menzel et al. 1999; Moatti 1999; Nord 1999; Matchar 2000; Tsuchiya 2000; Dolan and Olsen 2001; Williams 2001; Walker and Siegel 2002; Brock 2004; Amundson 2005; Bickenbach 2005; Nord 2005; Powers and Faden, 2006), empirical exploration of the extent to which these distributional values are held by real people (Nord, Richardson, et al. 1995; Nord, Street, et al. 1996; Richardson and Nord 1997; Bala et al. 1998; Tsuchiya 1999; Ubel 1999; Olsen 2000; Ubel, Baron, et al. 2000; Ubel, Nord, et al., 2000; Cuadras-Morato, Pinto-Prades, and Abellan-Perpinan 2001; Ubel, Baron, and Asch 2001), and analytical work on ways to introduce distributional values into the methodology of CEA (Dolan 1998; Anand 1999; Brouwer and Koopmanschap 2000; Johannesson 2001; Rodriguez-Miguez and Pinto-Prades 2002). At the moment, there is agreement that distributional issues are important and that maximizing QALYs without regard to distribution is not an appropriate normative rule, but there is no agreement yet on a simple, practical alternative approach.

In the meantime, the question under discussion here is the use of CEA in decisions about newborn screening policy. If CEA is interpreted as primarily a method of organizing information about the consequences of a particular policy choice, then it is not just useful in making newborn screening policy, it is essential. In particular, the decision about whether to mandate addition of a test to a newborn screening panel in a public health program is one that requires systematic analysis of the costs and benefits of the decision at the societal level. At times, the analysis may seem to be disregarded and the final decision made on other grounds. Nevertheless, the process of doing a CEA from the societal perspective is useful because it encourages clinicians to get better data on outcomes and provides an alternative to the CEAs of private stakeholders, such as companies that market equipment, laboratories that market tests, and groups advocating on behalf of particular genetic conditions.

At the same time, CEA must not be used as a mechanical decision rule, for all the reasons discussed above. Policy experts caution against overstating the value of the numbers and emphasize the importance of presenting results in terms of ranges, not precise estimates. They also emphasize the need for sensitivity analysis to explore the limits of the CEA conclusions and to identify the kinds of additional data that are particularly important to collect to make good policy decisions. They stress the importance of taking the resource cost of the analysis into account when structuring the CEA and making decisions about the level of detail and precision to seek. Moreover, before using CEAs of newborn screening tests to make policy decisions, it would be prudent to have them vetted by a panel of CEA experts to ensure that the analyses are methodologically sound (for a comprehensive review of the use of CEA analysis in the newborn screening context, see chapter 3). Finally, policymakers should not forget that in its current form, CEA does not take distributional fairness into account. Therefore, distributional values must be factored in separately after information about the size and distribution of the benefits and costs of newborn screening has been developed.

Conclusion

As policymakers respond to the pressure to expand and reshape newborn screening programs, one of their most challenging tasks is to work toward greater fairness in the distribution of the costs and benefits of screening. In this chapter, we have presented a framework for thinking about fairness and applied it in the newborn screening context. We have explored the framework's implications for test selection, financing, and delivery of services, research and evaluation, the locus of decision making, and the use of CEA and CUA. In the process, we have identified areas that require further work so that this policy challenge can be successfully met.

ACKNOWLEDGMENT AND DISCLAIMER

This chapter is based on a paper produced with funding from the Maternal and Child Health Bureau in the Health Resources and Services Administration (HRSA Order No. 01-0538(P); Requisition Reference No. 01-MCHB-70A). Revision and expansion of the paper was funded under grant 5R HG002579 from the National Human Genome Research Institute in the National Institutes of Health. The statements and opinions are those of the author and do not represent the policies of the Department of Health and Human Services or its agencies or offices.

NOTES

1. Other industrialized countries have government-regulated health care systems that provide universal access to a comprehensive standard of health care. The United States does not have such a system, but there is popular support for an array of public programs and policies (such as public hospitals, Medicaid, and the Emergency Medical Treatment and Active Labor Act) whose aim is to ensure access to important health care for people who cannot afford to purchase it themselves.

2. Note that some people who are not sure whether there is a societal moral obligation to guarantee adequate care to adults may be more easily convinced that there is such an obligation toward children.

3. The funding agency was the Genetic Services Branch of the Maternal and Child Health Bureau of HRSA.

4. For more information, see www.nccrcg.org/.

REFERENCES

106th Congress. 2007. Title XXVI of the Children's Health Act of 2000, Screening for Heritable Disorders. Washington, DC: U.S. Congress.

American College of Medical Genetics. 2006. Newborn screening: toward a uniform screening panel and system. *Genet Med* 8 (Suppl 1): 1–252S.

Amundson, R. 2005. Disability, ideology, and quality of life: a bias in biomedical ethics. In *Quality of Life and Human Difference*, ed. D. Wasserman, J. Bickenbach, and R. Wachbroit, pp. 101–24. New York: Cambridge University Press.

Anand, P. 1999. QALYs and the integration of claims in health-care rationing. *Health Care Anal* 7 (3): 239–53.

Arrow, K. J. 1963. Uncertainty and the welfare economics of medical-care. *Am Econ Rev* 53 (5): 941–73.

Atkinson, K., Zuckerman, B., Sharfstein, J. M., Levin, D., Blatt, R. J., and Koh, H. K. 2001. A public health response to emerging technology: expansion of the Massachusetts newborn screening program. *Public Health Rep* 116 (2): 122–31.

Bailey, D. B. Jr., Beskow, L. M., Davis, A. M., and Skinner, D. 2006. Changing perspectives on the benefits of newborn screening. *Ment Retard Dev Disabil Res Rev* 12 (4): 270–79.

Bala, M. V., Wood, L. L., Zarkin, G. A., Norton, E. C., Gafni, A., and O'Brien, B. 1998. Valuing outcomes in health care: a comparison of willingness to pay and quality-adjusted life-years. *J Clin Epidemiol* 51 (8): 667–76.

Bickenbach, J. 2005. Disability and health systems assessment. In *Quality of Life and Human Difference*, ed. D. Wasserman, J. Bickenbach, and R. Wachbroit, pp. 237–66. New York: Cambridge University Press.

Botkin, J. R., Clayton, E. W., Fost, N. C., Burke, W., Murray, T. H., Baily, M. A., Wilfond, B., Berg, A., and Ross, L. F. 2006. Newborn screening technology: proceed with caution. *Pediatrics* 117 (5): 1793–99.

Bowman, J. E. 1994. Genetic screening: toward a new eugenics? In *"It Just Ain't Fair": The Ethics of Health Care for African Americans*, ed. A. Dula and S. Goering, pp. 165–78. Westport, CT: Praeger.

Brock, D. W. 2001. Children's rights to health care. *J Med Philos* 26 (2): 163–77.

———. 2004. Ethical issues in use of cost effectiveness analysis for prioritization of health care resources. In *Handbook of Bioethics: Taking Stock of the Field from a Philosophical Overview*, ed. G. Khushf, pp. 353–80. Dordrecht, The Netherlands: Kluwer.

Brouwer, W. B., and Koopmanschap, M. A. 2000. On the economic foundations of CEA: ladies and gentlemen, take your positions! *J Health Econ* 19 (4): 439–59.

Cuadras-Morato, X., Pinto-Prades, J. L., and Abellan-Perpinan, J. M. 2001. Equity considerations in health care: the relevance of claims. *Health Econ* 10 (3): 187–205.

Cubbon, J. 1991. The principle of QALY maximisation as the basis for allocating health care resources. *J Med Ethics* 17 (4): 181–84.

Cunningham, G. 2002. The science and politics of screening newborns. *N Engl J Med* 346 (14): 1084–85.

Daniels, N. 1994. Four unsolved rationing problems: a challenge. *Hastings Cent Rep* 24 (4): 27–29.

———. 2000. Accountability for reasonableness. *BMJ* 321 (7272): 1300–1301.

———. 2001. Justice, health, and healthcare. *Am J Bioeth* 1 (2): 2–16.

Daniels, N., Light, D., and Caplan, R. L. 1996. *Benchmarks of Fairness for Health Care Reform*. New York: Oxford University Press.

Dolan, P. 1998. The measurement of individual utility and social welfare. *J Health Econ* 17 (1): 39–52.

Dolan, P. A., and Olsen, J. A. 2001. Equity in health: the importance of different health streams. *J Health Econ* 20 (5): 823–34.

Donaldson, C., Birch, S., and Gafni, A. 2002. The distribution problem in economic evaluation: income and the valuation of costs and consequences of health care programmes. *Health Econ* 11 (1): 55–70.

Farrar, S., Donaldson, C., Macphee, S., Walker, A., and Mapp, T. 1997. Creativity and sacrifice: two sides of the coin. A reply to David Seedhouse. *Health Care Anal* 5 (4): 306–9.

Fleck, L. M. 1994. Just caring: Oregon, health care rationing, and informed democratic deliberation. *J Med Philos* 19 (4): 367–88.

Gerard, K. 1992. Cost-utility in practice: a policy maker's guide to the state of the art. *Health Policy* 21 (3): 249–79.

Gessner, B. D., Teutsch, S. M., and Shaffer, P. A. 1996. A cost effectiveness evaluation of newborn hemoglobinopathy screening from the perspective of state health care systems. *Early Hum Dev* 45 (3): 257–75.

Gold, M. R., Siegel, J. E., Russell, L. B., and Weinstein, M. C. 1996. *Cost-Effectiveness in Health and Medicine*. New York: Oxford University Press.

Grosse, S. D., Boyle, C. A., Kenneson, A., Khoury, M. J., and Wilfond, B. S. 2006. From public health emergency to public health service: the implications of evolving criteria for newborn screening panels. *Pediatrics* 117 (3): 923–29.

Gutmann, A., and Thompson, D. 1997. Deliberating about bioethics. *Hastings Cent Rep* 27 (3): 38–41.

Harris, J. 1988. Life: quality, value and justice. *Health Policy* 10 (3): 259–66.

———. 1991. Unprincipled QALYs: a response to Cubbon. *J Med Ethics* 17 (4): 185–88.

———. 1995. Double jeopardy and the veil of ignorance—a reply. *J Med Ethics* 21 (3): 151–57.

———. 1996. Would Aristotle have played Russian roulette? *J Med Ethics* 22 (4): 209–15.

Hausman, D. M., and MacPherson, M. S. 1996. *Economic Analysis and Moral Philosophy*. New York: Cambridge University Press.

Hiller, E. H., Landenburger, G., and Natowicz, M. R. 1997. Public participation in medical policy-making and the status of consumer autonomy: the example of newborn screening programs in the United States. *Am J Public Health* 87 (8): 1280–88.

Holtzman, N. A. 1997. Genetic screening and public health. *Am J Public Health* 87 (8): 1275–77.

Hope, T. 1996. QALYs, lotteries and veils: the story so far. *J Med Ethics* 22 (4): 195–96.

Jefferson, T., and Demicheli, V. 2002. Quality of economic evaluations in health care. *BMJ* 324 (7333): 313–14.

Johannesson, M. 2001. Should we aggregate relative or absolute changes in QALYs? *Health Econ* 10 (7): 573–77.

Joiner, C. H. 2000. Universal newborn screening for hemoglobinopathies [letter; comment]. *J Pediatr* 136 (2): 145–46.

Jordan, J., Dowswell, T., Harrison, S., Lilford, R. J., and Mort, M. 1998. Health needs assessment: whose priorities? Listening to users and the public. *BMJ* 316 (7145): 1668–70.

Juengst, E. T. 1998. Group identity and human diversity: keeping biology straight from culture. *Am J Hum Genet* 63 (3): 673–77.

Kaiser Commission on Medicaid and the Uninsured. 2007. *Health Insurance Coverage in America: 2006 Data Update*. Menlo Park, CA: Henry J. Kaiser Family Foundation.

Kernick, D. P. 1998. Economic evaluation in health: a thumb nail sketch. *BMJ* 316 (7145): 1663–65.

Kwon, C., and Farrell, P. M. 2000. The magnitude and challenge of false-positive newborn screening test results. *Arch Pediatr Adolesc Med* 154 (7): 714–18.

La Puma, J., and Lawlor, E. F. 1990. Quality-adjusted life-years: ethical implications for physicians and policymakers. *JAMA* 263 (21): 2917–21.

Lee, S. S., Mountain, J., and Koenig, B. A. 2001. The meanings of "race" in the new genomics: implications for health disparities research. *Yale J Health Policy Law Ethics* 1 (Spring 2001): 33–69.

Levy, H. L., and Albers, S. 2000. Genetic screening of newborns. *Annu Rev Genomics Hum Genet* 1:139–77.

Matchar, D. B. 2000. Treating QALYs with a heavy dose of social values: is the cure worth the cost? *Med Care* 38 (9): 889–91.

McKie, J., Kuhse, H., Richardson, J., and Singer, P. 1996. Double jeopardy, the equal value of lives and the veil of ignorance: a rejoinder to Harris. *J Med Ethics* 22 (4): 204–8.

Menzel, P. T. 1995. QALYs: maximisation, distribution and consent. A response to Alan Williams. *Health Care Anal* 3 (3): 226–29.

Menzel, P., Gold, M. R., Nord, E., Pinto-Prades, J. L., Richardson, J., and Ubel, P. 1999. Toward a broader view of values in cost-effectiveness analysis of health. *Hastings Cent Rep* 29 (3): 7–15.

Mitka, M. 2000. Neonatal screening varies by state of birth. *JAMA* 284 (16): 2044–46.

Moatti, J. 1999. Ethical issues in the economic assessment of health care technologies. *Health Care Anal* 7 (2): 153–65.

Newborn Screening Task Force. 2000. Serving the family from birth to the medical home: a report from the Newborn Screening Task Force convened in Washington DC, May 10–11, 1999. *Pediatrics* 106 (2 Pt 2): 383–427.

Nichols, L. M. 2007. The moral case for covering children (and everyone else). *Health Aff (Millwood)* 26 (2): 405–7.

Nord, E. 1999. *Cost-Value Analysis in Health Care: Making Sense out of QALYS.* New York: Cambridge University Press.

———. 2005. Values for health states in QALYs and DALYs. In *Quality of Life and Human Difference*, ed. D. Wasserman, J. Bickenbach, and R. Wachbroit, pp. 125–41. New York: Cambridge University Press.

Nord, E., Richardson, J., Street, A., Kuhse, H., and Singer, P. 1995. Maximizing health benefits vs egalitarianism: an Australian survey of health issues. *Soc Sci Med* 41 (10): 1429–37.

Nord, E., Street, A., Richardson, J., Kuhse, H., and Singer, P. 1996. The significance of age and duration of effect in social evaluation of health care. *Health Care Anal* 4 (2): 103–11.

Olsen, J. A. 2000. A note on eliciting distributive preferences for health. *J Health Econ* 19 (4): 541–50.

Panepinto, J. A., Magid, D., Rewers, M. J., and Lane, P. A. 2000. Universal versus targeted screening of infants for sickle cell disease: a cost-effectiveness analysis. *J Pediatr* 136 (2): 201–8.

Pass, K. A., Lane, P. A., Fernhoff, P. M., Hinton, C. F., and Panny, S. R. 2000. US newborn screening system guidelines II: follow-up of children, diagnosis, management and evaluation. Statement of the Council of Regional Networks for Genetic Services (CORN). *J Pediatr* 137 (4 Suppl): 1–46.

Pollitt, R. J. 2001. Newborn mass screening versus selective investigation: benefits and costs. *J Inherit Metab Dis* 24 (2): 299–302.

Powers, M., and Faden, R. 2000. Inequities in health, inequalities in health care: four generations of discussion about justice and cost-effectiveness analysis. *Kennedy Inst Ethics J* 10 (2): 109–27.

———. 2006. *Social Justice: The Moral Foundations of Public Health and Health Policy.* New York: Oxford University Press.

President's Commission for the Study of Ethical Problems in Medicine and Biomedical and Behavioral Research. 1983. *Securing Access to Health Care: A Report on the Ethical Implications of Differences in the Availability of Health Services.* Washington, DC: Government Printing Office.

Richardson, J., and Nord, E. 1997. The importance of perspective in the measurement of quality-adjusted life years. *Med Decis Making* 17 (1): 33–41.

Rodriguez-Miguez, E., and Pinto-Prades, J. L. 2002. Measuring the social importance of concentration or dispersion of individual health benefits. *Health Econ* 11 (1): 43–53.

Seedhouse, D. 1997. The inescapable prejudice of health economics: a reply to Farrar, Donaldson, Macphee, Walker and Mapp. *Health Care Anal* 5 (4): 310–14.

Singer, P., McKie, J., Kuhse, H., and Richardson, J. 1995. Double jeopardy and the use of QALYs in health care allocation. *J Med Ethics* 21 (3): 144–50.

Sprinkle, R. H., Hynes, D. M., and Konrad, T. R. 1994. Is universal neonatal hemoglobinopathy screening cost-effective? *Arch Pediatr Adolesc Med* 148 (5): 461–69.

Stoddard, J. J., and Farrell, P. M. 1997. State-to-state variations in newborn screening policies. *Arch Pediatr Adolesc Med* 151 (6): 561–64.

Therrell, B. L. 2001. U.S. newborn screening policy dilemmas for the twenty-first century. *Mol Genet Metab* 74 (1–2): 64–74.

Tsuchiya, A. 1999. Age-related preferences and age weighting health benefits. *Soc Sci Med* 48 (2): 267–76.

———. 2000. QALYs and ageism: philosophical theories and age weighting. *Health Econ* 9 (1): 57–68.

Tyler, B. A., and American Health Decisions. 1997. *The Quest to Die with Dignity: An Analysis of Americans' Values, Opinions and Attitudes Concerning End-of-Life Care*. Appleton, WI: American Health Decisions.

Ubel, P. A. 1999. The challenge of measuring community values in ways appropriate for setting health care priorities. *Kennedy Inst Ethics J* 9 (3): 263–84.

Ubel, P. A., Baron, J., and Asch, D. A. 2001. Preference for equity as a framing effect. *Med Decis Making* 21 (3): 180–89.

Ubel, P. A., Baron, J., Nash, B., and Asch, D. A. 2000. Are preferences for equity over efficiency in health care allocation "all or nothing"? *Med Care* 38 (4): 366–73.

Ubel, P. A., Nord, E., Gold, M., Menzel, P., Prades, J. L., and Richardson, J. 2000. Improving value measurement in cost-effectiveness analysis. *Med Care* 38 (9): 892–901.

U.S. Department of Health and Human Services. 2005. Advisory Committee on Heritable Disorders and Genetic Diseases in Newborns and Children Charter. ftp://ftp.hrsa.gov/mchb/genetics/charter.pdf.

U.S. General Accounting Office. 2003. Newborn Screening Characteristics of State Programs. www.gao.gov/new.items/d03449.pdf.

Wagstaff, A. 1991. QALYs and the equity-efficiency trade-off. *J Health Econ* 10 (1): 21–41.

Walker, R. L., and Siegel, A. W. 2002. Morality and the limits of societal values in health care allocation. *Health Econ* 11 (3): 265–73.

Wilfond, B. S., and Nolan, K. 1993. National policy development for the clinical application of genetic diagnostic technologies: lessons from cystic fibrosis. *JAMA* 270 (24): 2948–54.

Williams, A. 1992. Cost-effectiveness analysis: is it ethical? *J Med Ethics* 18 (1): 7–11.

———. 1995. Economics, QALYs and medical ethics—a health economist's perspective. *Health Care Anal* 3 (3): 221–26.

———. 2001. The "fair innings argument" deserves a fairer hearing! Comments by Alan Williams on Nord and Johannesson. *Health Econ* 10 (7): 583–85.

CHAPTER 3

Cost-Effectiveness as a Criterion for Newborn Screening Policy Decisions

SCOTT D. GROSSE, PH.D.

Decisions about which disorders to include in newborn screening panels can be based on a variety of considerations. This chapter discusses the strengths and limitations of economic evaluation methods, relative to other decision-making criteria, for selecting the disorders to include in public health programs of newborn bloodspot screening. It does not address the application of economic evaluation methods to other types of newborn screening decisions, including hearing screening, specimens other than dried bloodspots, supplementary newborn screening tests offered outside the public health context, or the choice of laboratory methods and diagnostic cut-offs.

A justification for economic evaluation is the principle of *opportunity cost*, defined as the value of what could be done if resources were otherwise employed. Decision makers should ask whether funding an intervention is the best use of resources. For example, suppose an intervention costs $2 million per year and is expected to prevent two deaths each year. Could other interventions not currently funded save more lives at a similar or lower cost? Other outcomes besides preventing mortality are important, but this example gives a sense of the concept of opportunity cost. A health intervention is cost-effective (provides good value for money) if it compares favorably with other policies in terms of the ratio of desired outcomes to resources expended. Absolute cost or affordability is a separate issue.

The first section is an overview of cost-effectiveness analysis methods. The core of the chapter then provides a critical review of the use of economic criteria in decision making about newborn screening and reviews the recent literature on economic evaluations of newborn screening, including screens for phenylketonuria, congenital hypothyroidism, galactosemia, biotinidase deficiency, congenital adrenal hyperplasia, sickle cell disease, medium-chain acyl-CoA dehydrogenase deficiency, and cystic fibrosis. The major findings are:

- Cost-effectiveness is a criterion for newborn screening decisions in the United Kingdom but not in the United States, except in three states (Washington, California, and Arizona) that require an internal cost-benefit analysis of proposed newborn screening regulations.
- It is difficult to document that results of cost-effectiveness analysis have had an impact on decisions on newborn screening panels in either country in recent decades.

The chapter concludes with a discussion of why economic studies do not seem to have been influential in newborn screening policy decisions. This chapter can serve as a case study of the limited use of cost-effectiveness analysis to inform health policy decisions (Neumann 2005).

Cost-Effectiveness Analysis

The two main types of economic evaluation are *cost-effectiveness analysis* (CEA) and *cost-benefit analysis* (CBA). A CEA divides the difference in net costs by the difference in health outcomes to yield a cost-effectiveness ratio as the summary measure. For example, a CEA might report that an intervention costs $10,000 per life-year saved. A CBA converts health outcomes into monetary benefits. This chapter focuses on CEA because it is the dominant contemporary economic evaluation approach in public health, except in regulatory analysis, where CBA has long been favored (Robinson 2004; Grosse, Teutsch, and Haddix 2007).

Cost-effectiveness analysis compares interventions in terms of the relative cost to achieve a desired outcome. *Cost* refers to the resources required to provide an intervention or to care for someone with a particular condition. For example, the cost of screening includes the costs of laboratory testing, follow-up, diagnosis, and treatment relative to the costs of diagnosis and treatment in the absence of routine screening. The *direct costs* of treatment include medical, special education, and care-giving costs. The costs to be included depend on the analytical perspective. In the health system perspective, only medical costs are included, whereas in the societal perspective all direct costs should be included. The lost economic production of an individual who dies prematurely or experiences morbidity or disability is commonly referred to as *indirect costs*, although this term is potentially confusing because it is also used in accounting studies to refer to overhead costs.

If, for a given pair of interventions, one is both more effective and less costly, it is said to "dominate" the other. After excluding dominated interventions, analysts calculate the *incremental cost-effectiveness ratio* (ICER) for each pair of alternatives in which one intervention is both more effective and more costly. An ICER divides the difference in average net cost of one intervention compared with another by the incremental units of outcome (e.g., additional numbers of life-years saved).[1] Costs and outcomes in future years are discounted to present values using a *discount rate*.[2] An intervention that dominates the status quo is said to be *cost-saving* and no ICER is calculated. Only a minority of health care interventions both reduce total costs and improve health outcomes (Graham et al. 1998; Maciosek et al. 2006).

Cost-effectiveness analysis can facilitate the systematic comparison of policies or programs in terms of relative cost per unit of achieved health outcome, on average. For example, suppose that screening for disorder A prevents 2000 premature deaths each year at an average cost of $50,000 per life-year saved (total cost $100 million per year) and that screening for disorder B prevents 50 premature deaths each year at an average cost of $10,000 per life-year saved (total cost $500,000 per year). Because the interventions deal with distinct populations, it is not possible to calculate an ICER comparing the two. Although screening for disorder B seems more cost-effective, screening for disorder A might also be considered good value relative to other potential uses of resources. It is also useful to present disaggregated information on the distribution of costs and outcomes to determine who benefits and who loses from a policy (Coast 2004).

When CEA results do not guide health policy decision making, it is not that costs do not matter, but that costs are not systematically considered relative to expected outcomes. In the U.S. health policy context, lack of use of CEAs to guide the allocation of resources seems to reflect a discomfort with acknowledging the inevitability of rationing of resources and a lack of strong incentives to adopt the use of CEA in decision making (Garber 2004; Luce 2005; Neumann 2005). It also might reflect a tendency for decision makers to rely more on what has been termed "colloquial" types of evidence, such as personal vignettes from affected individuals and expert testimony, than on quantitative evidence (Lomas et al. 2005).

Outcome Measures

Cost-effectiveness analysis can be used to calculate either health outcomes directly or intermediate outcomes such as the cost per case of disease detected or averted. Intermediate outcomes can be useful for comparing screening strategies for the same disorder but not for interventions that target different disorders. Knowing that detecting a case of disorder X costs less than detecting a case of disorder Y tells us nothing about the relative value of case detection for the two disorders. Because health is multidimensional, analysts must choose which health outcome to analyze. Analysis of mortality, described in terms of life-years saved or gained, places no value on the prevention of morbidity or disability.

The quality-adjusted life-year (QALY) is a preference-based measure of health that integrates mortality and morbidity based on the perceived desirability or utility of health states relative to death and perfect health. A utility weight (or utility score) of 1.0 represents "perfect" health, and 0 represents death (Gold, Stevenson, and Fryback 2002; Hammitt 2002). A CEA that uses QALYs as the outcome measure is commonly referred to as a *cost-utility analysis* (CUA), which presumes that QALYs measure utility.

Concerns about the validity of QALY estimates hinder their acceptance by decision makers. No single approach is used to calculate utility weights for health states, and different methods can yield different estimates (Hammitt 2002). In particular, the consistency and validity of QALY estimates for children have been questioned (Griebsch, Coast, and Brown 2005). Generic instruments used to calculate QALY weights have not been validated for children younger than five years of age, and parent proxy respondents are typically used (Tilford 2002). Ethical challenges to the validity of QALYs for disabling conditions need to be considered (Siegel and Clancy 2003).

Interpretation

The results of CEAs must be interpreted to determine whether an intervention yields good value for money. An intervention can be considered relative to another intervention or to a threshold or benchmark value. Commonly, U.S. analysts use a benchmark of $50,000 per discounted life-year or QALY gained, or use multiple benchmarks such as $50,000 and $100,000 per QALY gained (Weinstein 1995; Owens 2002; Evans, Tavakoli, and Crawford 2004). The U.K. National Institute for Health and Clinical Excellence (NICE) is reported to use a benchmark equivalent to $50,000 per QALY (Devlin and Parkin 2004; Evans, Tavakoli, and Crawford 2004).

League tables that report ICERs for diverse interventions show that ICERs vary from negative (cost-saving) to millions of dollars spent per life-year saved (Graham et al. 1998; Neumann 2005). Certain clinical services are funded despite high ICERs because decision makers choose to prevent devastating harm for a relatively small number of individuals and because the total amount of money involved is limited (Berger and Teutsch 2005). For example, enzyme replacement therapy for individuals with symptomatic Gaucher disease, a rare, often lethal lysosomal storage disorder, typically costs between $100,000 and $200,000 per patient per year (Clarke, Amato, and Deber 2001).

Differences in methods make it challenging to compare results from CEA studies. To advance comparability, guidelines for CEAs have been published (Siegel and Clancy 2003). In the United States in 1996, the Panel on Cost-Effectiveness in Health and Medicine made recommendations for reference-case CEAs (Gold et al. 1996). These include adopting a societal perspective, in which all costs, including those incurred by individuals and families, are taken into account; discounting future costs and outcomes, using a 3 percent discount rate; and using the QALY as a common metric. Adherence to CEA guidelines is inconsistent, although improving over time (Neumann 2005).

Newborn Screening Criteria and Cost-Effectiveness

Decision makers routinely cite the Wilson and Jungner criteria for population screening, published by the World Health Organization (Wilson and Jungner 1968). The criteria relate to incidence, adequate understanding of natural history, opportunity for detection before serious symptoms, existence of a suitable and acceptable test, an accepted and effective treatment, and the availability of infrastructure for diagnosis and treatment. None of the criteria were clearly defined. Accordingly, different observers can reach divergent conclusions as to whether a specific condition meets each criterion (Grosse and Gwinn 2001). For example, in 1997, two reports on screening for inborn errors of metabolism disagreed on whether there was an adequate understanding of the natural history of medium-chain acyl-CoA dehydrogenase deficiency (MCAD) (Pollitt et al. 1997; Seymour et al. 1997).

The Wilson and Jungner screening criteria are ambiguous on the subject of cost-effectiveness. One of the 10 criteria states: "The costs of case-finding (including diagnosis and treatment of patients diagnosed) should be economically balanced in relation to possible expenditure on medical care as a whole" (Wilson and Jungner 1968, p. 67). This criterion does not provide guidance on what "economically balanced" might entail. A narrow interpretation is that it refers to net savings from screening and early treatment (Pollitt et al. 1997). Although analyses of screening for phenylketonuria (PKU) and congenital hypothyroidism (CH) have found screening to be cost-saving (Lord et al. 1999), whether other screening tests are generally cost-saving in terms of reduced direct costs is a subject of disagreement (Grosse 2005; Carroll and Downs 2006; Grosse, Teutsch, and Haddix 2007). Other interpretations of this criterion have been much broader (Wildner 2003).

In contrast to the conventional approach to evaluating screening tests, which addresses criteria one at a time (Wilson and Jungner 1968), CEA simultaneously evaluates multiple criteria. The relative cost-effectiveness of screening all newborns for a given disorder depends on several factors:

- Incidence of the disorder
- Frequency with which the disorder is detected early in the absence of screening
- Frequency of adverse outcomes in the absence of screening
- Potential harms resulting from early detection or false positives
- Reduction in adverse outcomes with early detection and treatment
- Sensitivity and specificity of the screening tests
- Costs of screening, follow-up, and confirmatory testing
- Costs avoided by providing early treatment

Under the traditional criterion-based approach, disorders with low incidence have typically been rejected for population-based screening, because of the large number that must be screened to identify one case. With CEA, even for a very rare disorder, if the cost to screen is moderate and the improvement in outcomes is dramatic, screening could still provide acceptable "value for money." For example, screening for a disorder with an incidence of 1 in 100,000 births, a fatality rate of 50 percent without screening, an 80 percent reduction in mortality with early treatment, a screening cost of $5 per test, and a cost to treat of $200,000 per case could result in a cost per life-year saved of less than $50,000 (Lindegren et al. 2004). Similarly, a new analysis of potential newborn screening for severe combined immunodeficiency disorder (SCID), with more refined estimates (e.g., incidence of 1 in 50,000 births, treatment cost of $450,000), concludes that a screening test that costs $5 and has a false positive rate of 0.4 percent could result in a cost of less than $50,000 per QALY saved (McGhee, Stiehm, and McCabe 2005).

In the United Kingdom, the National Screening Committee (2004), which is responsible for making screening policy recommendations to the National Health Service in England and Wales, has elaborated on the Wilson and Jungner criteria with a set of 22 criteria. Criterion number 16 states: "The opportunity cost of the screening programme (including testing, diagnosis and treatment, administration, training and quality assurance) should be economically balanced in relation to expenditure on medical care as a whole (i.e. value for money)." This expansion clarifies that the criterion refers to cost-effectiveness. The National Screening Committee did not set a decision rule for determining "value for money" nor require a formal CEA, although NICE does.

In the United States, each state sets its own criteria for selecting disorders for officially designated newborn screening panels. Most states rely on recommendations from state advisory committees, although in some cases screening policies have been determined by legislation or executive decision (Stoddard and Farrell 1997). At least two states, Massachusetts and Wisconsin, include a cost criterion for the selection of newborn screening panels. In both states this criterion specifies that the cost of screening for an additional test being considered must be "reasonable" or "comparable" to other screening tests already in place, typically $2 to $5 per test (Stoddard and Farrell 1997; Atkinson et al. 2001). Neither state requires an assessment of the balance of costs and benefits to society or the health care system as a whole, only the costs to the screening laboratory.

Washington State has an explicit requirement for evidence of a positive balance of costs and benefits for the addition of a new screening test to the state's newborn screening panel. This criterion is not restricted to newborn screening but refers to all regulations issued by the state government. The Washington Administrative Procedure Act states: "Before adopting a rule . . . an agency shall: determine that the probable benefits of the rule are greater than its probable costs, taking into account both the qualitative and quantitative benefits and costs and the specific directives of the statute being implemented" (Revised Code of Washington 34.05.328 §[1][b]).

The Washington State Newborn Screening Advisory Committee in 2001 established five screening criteria. The algorithm set by the advisory committee was that if a test were considered to meet the first four criteria—prevention potential and medical rationale; treatment available; public health rationale; and available technology—then both CBA and CEA would be conducted. The rationale was that economic evaluations are costly in terms of staff time and should be done only if there are adequate epidemiological data. Although the legislation cited above implies the use of CBA, some members of the advisory committee wanted CEA results to be calculated using cost per life-year saved as the outcome measure, as well as CBA results calculated without monetized life-years. They thought that such outcomes might be easier for decision makers to interpret.

Arizona also has a statute that requires submission of an economic impact statement before a rule-making, which includes rulings on newborn screening panels. The statute does not specify a method of economic evaluation. Further, the statute does not require positive net benefit, only that decision makers should be provided with relevant economic data (Ruthann Smejkal, personal communication, July 15, 2005). Certain other state programs that do not have requirements for economic evaluations, notably the program in California, do have a policy to prepare internal CBAs to inform legislators before requests to raise the per-infant fee charged to hospitals to cover the cost of screening (Cunningham 2004).

The federal Maternal and Child Health Bureau of the Health Resources and Services Administration commissioned the American College of Medical Genetics (ACMG) to develop criteria and a scoring scheme for a core newborn screening panel to be recommended to states. An expert panel convened by the ACMG constructed a list of 19 screening criteria (American College of Medical Genetics 2005). As others have noted (Botkin et al. 2006; Grosse, Boyle, et al. 2006), cost-effectiveness was not among the criteria, although a CEA of newborn screening for selected disorders was commissioned (Carroll and Downs 2006). Two of the ACMG criteria relate to costs: (1) a test with overall analytical cost of less than $1 per test per condition, and (2) a cost of treatment for the disorder of less than $50,000 per patient per year. However, these criteria are not equivalent to cost-effectiveness. A screening test that costs $50 per infant would receive the same score as a test that costs $2 per infant, which seems of dubious value. A screening test for a disorder with an expensive treatment, such as SCID, might well provide good value for money (Lindegren et al. 2004; McGhee, Stiehm, and McCabe 2005). Also, a societal assessment of cost-effectiveness should include downstream costs, including costs to the follow-up system, health care providers, education system, and families (Wildner 2003).

The exclusion of cost-effectiveness as a criterion for newborn screening tests is not tantamount to ignoring costs, but it can lead to costs being considered in an unsystematic fashion. On the other hand, setting cost-effectiveness as a criterion could lead to the production of estimates based on inadequate data so as to meet arbitrary cost-effectiveness thresholds. Using cost-effectiveness as a criterion for unbiased and informed decision making requires sufficient financing for rigorous analyses to be funded and conducted by organizations that do not have an interest in the promotion of specific interventions.

Economic Evaluations of Newborn Screening
Data Needs

The frequency of adverse outcomes in the absence of screening is a necessary input for CEAs of screening. Although a randomized controlled trial (RCT) is considered the gold standard for evidence of effectiveness (Dezateux 2003), RCTs in newborn screening have been done only for cystic fibrosis. Observational studies are subject to biases. For example, if cases detected through screening manifest a wider spectrum than clinically detected cases, the frequency of adverse outcomes in a screened cohort might seem lower. Conversely, mortality might be understated in case series if cases that result in death before diagnosis go unrecognized. One unbiased method is the retrospective analysis of stored residual bloodspots (Liebl et al. 2003). Two studies analyzed large (~100,000) individually identified samples of stored bloodspot specimens for CH (Alm et al. 1984) and MCAD (Pourfarzam et al. 2001). To determine the frequency of deaths in cases of undiagnosed disease, one can analyze specimens associated with unexplained death (Dott et al. 2006; Strnadova et al. 2007).

Calculation of QALYs requires data on utility weights for health states. For example, a CEA of screening for CF used estimates of preference weights for health states associated with levels of lung function (Simpson et al. 2005). It is common to use published utility weights for sequelae such as neurological impairments due to causes other than metabolic disorders, but there is a lack of agreement on appropriate weights (Grosse, Teutsch, and Haddix 2007). Studies have used widely varying QALY weights for children with mental retardation or intellectual disability: 0.06 (Insinga, Laessig, and Hoffman 2002), 0.15 to 0.30 (Schoen et al. 2002), 0.39 to 0.56 (Carroll and Downs 2006), 0.38 to 0.67 (Feuchtbaum and Cunningham 2006; Tran, Banerjee, and Li 2006), and 0.65 (Venditti et al. 2003). The first two estimates, which imply quality of life closer to death than to perfect health, were taken from studies of adults with neurological deficits, a population of questionable relevance to children with developmental disabilities. Two studies also specified QALY weights of 0.74 to 0.79 for children with "mild" impairment (Carroll and Downs 2006; Tran, Banerjee, and Li 2006).

One of the biggest data gaps is in information on the costs of diagnosis and treatment in the absence of screening. For example, four children treated for propionic acidemia at a pediatric center in New Hampshire during 1994 to 1998 incurred average charges for inpatient critical care of $136,000 (Filiano, Bellimer, and Kunz 2002).

Another gap is in the data on costs of delayed diagnoses, because diagnostic codes are not recorded until a test is ordered. Anecdotal accounts of "diagnostic odysseys" involve repeated visits to specialists, laboratory tests, and hospital admissions before the establishment of a diagnosis (Kharrazi and Kharrazi 2005). Most CEAs have excluded such costs, although certain studies have included informed guesses (Washington State 2003). Estimates of averted hospitalizations before diagnosis can make screening seem more cost-effective, as shown in two recent CEAs of screening for CF (Simpson et al. 2005; van den Akker-van Marle et al. 2006).

Phenylketonuria and Congenital Hypothyroidism

Before the development of dietary treatment for PKU in the 1950s and newborn screening for PKU in the 1960s, 95 percent of individuals with PKU were reported to have an IQ of less than 50 (American Academy of Pediatrics 1996). In the early years of screening, CBAs concluded that the saved costs resulting from avoided institutionalization for mental retardation substantially exceeded the costs of screening and treatment (Cunningham 1969; Steiner and Smith 1973; Webb 1973; Van Pelt and Levy 1974). Subsequent analyses have adopted the same assumptions and yielded equivalent conclusions (Barden, Kessel, and Schuett 1984; Dagenais, Courville, and Dagenais 1985; U.S. Congress Office of Technology Assessment 1988; Hisashige 1994; Pollitt et al. 1997; Lord et al. 1999; Geelhoed et al. 2005; Carroll and Downs 2006).

Screening for PKU is less likely to be cost-saving than previous analyses concluded, for several reasons (Grosse 2005). First, individuals with mental retardation are less likely to be institutionalized than in the past, resulting in much lower direct costs of care, even considering the costs of special education services and lost productivity (Honeycutt, Grosse, and Dunlap 2003; Centers for Disease Control and Prevention 2004). Second, it is now recommended that the expensive dietary therapy be pursued for life. Third, children born to mothers with inadequately treated PKU (maternal PKU) are at risk for birth defects and mental retardation (Kirkman and Frazier 1996). Most critically, the assumption that, in the absence of screening, children with PKU will develop irreversible mental retardation does not seem to be correct (Koch et al. 1999; Levy 2000).

When screening for CH was introduced in the 1970s, economic evaluations concluded that this would generate even greater economic benefits than screening for PKU. CH is more common than PKU and much less expensive to treat. One often-cited CBA reported an estimate of an average of $7.80 in direct costs saved per dollar spent on screening (Layde, Von Allmen, and Oakley 1979). A subsequent analysis made similar assumptions about effectiveness but used actual data on screening costs in Wisconsin; that study reported a more realistic ratio of $2.55 in direct costs averted per dollar spent on screening (Barden and Kessel 1984). An economic evaluation by the U.S. Congress Office of Technology Assessment (1988) reported similar estimates.

These economic evaluations of CH screening overstated the percentage of children who would require care for severe mental retardation in the absence of screening. Layde, Von Allmen, and Oakley (1979) cited two small studies (Raiti and Newns 1971; Klein, Meltzer, and Kenny 1972) reporting that 15 percent of all children with CH had an IQ below 35. In fact, only 2 of 87 children (2.3%) in the two studies had an IQ below 35. Subsequent analyses have repeated this error (Barden and Kessel 1984; U.S. Congress Office of Technology Assessment 1988; Geelhoed et al. 2005).

Another common but incorrect assumption in economic studies of screening for CH was that children diagnosed with CH as a result of screening have the same risk of mental retardation as children with clinically diagnosed CH. However, in cases of CH that come to clinical attention the children are likely to be more severely affected. For example, in Sweden, a retrospective study of 100,239 stored bloodspots collected before the initiation of screening for CH found that of 31 children who screened positive for CH and could be tracked, 5 of 15 children (33%) with a clinical diagnosis of CH had cognitive assessments below the normal range, whereas none of the 16 children who had not had a clinical diagnosis of CH had test scores below the normal range (Alm et al. 1984). The latter group displayed milder cognitive impairments and behavioral abnormalities (Alm et al. 1984; Pollitt et al. 1997); screening and treatment are likely to be of benefit even for children with CH that would not have resulted in a clinical diagnosis.

Not all CEAs have overstated the risk of mental retardation in CH in the absence of screening. An earlier economic evaluation of newborn screening for CH took into account evidence that few children with CH required institutional care in the absence of screening. Smith and Morris (1979) calculated a 1.4 to 1 ratio of averted direct costs to screening costs. More recently, Carroll and Downs (2006) assumed that 4 percent of children with CH would develop moderate or severe "developmental delay," equivalent to an IQ below 70, and an additional 27 percent would have a lesser delay. Nevertheless, screening for CH was still estimated to be cost-saving (Carroll and Downs 2006). However, the cost parameter for "severe developmental delay" in that study included both the direct and indirect costs for individuals with mental retardation (Centers for Disease Control and Prevention 2004). It is contrary to recommended practice to include the costs of lost productivity in a CEA that uses QALYs as the outcome measure, because of potential double-counting of disability in QALYs and lost earnings (Gold et al. 1996).

Galactosemia and Biotinidase Deficiency

Screening tests for disorders other than PKU and CH introduced in the 1960s and 1970s were not found to be cost-saving. The U.S. Congress Office of Technology Assessment (1988) report concluded that adding screening for galactosemia and maple syrup urine disease (MSUD) would entail additional costs, but no attempt was made to assess the value of detecting those disorders. A U.K. study of inborn errors of metabolism concluded that screening for galactosemia, biotinidase deficiency, and MSUD would *not* be cost effective in the U.K. context (Pollitt et al. 1997). The later timing of the collection of dried bloodspot specimens in the United Kingdom, generally occurring six or more days after birth, lessens the opportunities for presymptomatic detection of galactosemia (Pollitt et al. 1997).

Classic galactosemia is a relatively rare condition, with a prevalence at birth of 1 in 40,000 to 1 in 60,000. The primary benefit of screening for galactosemia is a reduction in the risk of early mortality, but the probability of sudden death in the absence of early detection is uncertain. The probability of death in classic galactosemia is not well established, but is said to be 20 to 30 percent (Pollitt et al. 1997). A study from Germany reported the death rate for children up to three years of age in an unscreened cohort as approximately 40 percent (Schweitzer-Krantz 2003). On the other hand, a Norwegian study reported one infant death in a cohort of 16 children (6%), although one or more cases of neonatal septicemia in which the deceased child was not diagnosed with galactosemia were probably missed (Hansen et al. 1996). Although a spectrum of disabilities is associated with galactosemia, mental retardation is not necessarily preventable by early identification and treatment (Levy and Albers 2000; Schweitzer-Krantz 2003). Consequently, the degree of cost-effectiveness of screening for galactosemia is uncertain. Carroll and Downs (2006) calculated a cost-effectiveness ratio of $94,000 per life-year saved. They assumed a 14 percent death rate in galactosemia in the absence of screening, although the source cited (Badawi et al. 1996) referred to mortality in a screened cohort.

Biotinidase deficiency is even less common than galactosemia, about 1 in 90,000 births according to Carroll and Downs (2006), who projected screening for this disorder to be cost-saving. They assumed relatively high frequencies of impairments: 76 percent with hearing loss, 70 percent with seizure disorder, 50 percent with vision loss, and 50 percent with "severe developmental delay" (i.e., mental retardation), the effects of which were assumed to be additive. That is, they took estimates of total costs for children with each disorder, many of whom had multiple impairments, and multiplied them by each frequency. This resulted in a substantial overestimate of costs in the absence of screening, because the cost estimates were related to average costs of individuals with a given impairment, not the incremental cost of each impairment excluding comorbidities. Furthermore, Carroll and Downs assumed no mortality in biotinidase deficiency, which could further overstate projected cost-savings because children who die in infancy incur no long-term costs of care.

The Washington State Department of Health in 2002 conducted CBA/CEA assessments of screening for galactosemia and biotinidase deficiency (Grosse et al. 2003; Washington State 2003). Both disorders were estimated to cost between $25,000 and $30,000 per life-year saved (Grosse et al. 2003) and the screenings were found to generate net economic benefit (Washington State 2003). The rate of mortality in cases of galactosemia without screening was projected to be 33 percent, based on clinical experience at the University of Washington (Washington State 2003). The Washington analysis projected 50 percent mortality in cases of biotinidase deficiency, in contrast to the analysis of Carroll and Downs (2006), which assumed no mortality.

Congenital Adrenal Hyperplasia

Another disorder for which cost-effectiveness is uncertain is congenital adrenal hyperplasia (CAH). The primary rationale for screening, and the only one that has been included in economic evaluations, is prevention of deaths through the detection of salt-wasting CAH. Salt-wasting CAH carries a risk of death from acute salt-wasting crisis in the absence of early recognition and management. The number of deaths associated with salt-wasting CAH is not well established, but the risk is reported to most likely be 5 percent or less in populations with high levels of health care (Grosse and Van Vliet 2007a, 2007b; Strnadova et al. 2007), and only about 1 in 20,000 infants have salt-wasting CAH. Consequently, the cost-effectiveness of CAH screening might rest on other benefits of early detection, including correct sex assignment in cases of ambiguous genitalia, but reliable estimates of long-term outcomes are lacking.

Two cost-effectiveness analyses of screening for CAH reached differing conclusions. In the United States, a recent CEA that assumed the rate of mortality in untreated salt-wasting CAH to be 13 percent calculated an ICER of approximately $20,000 per QALY (Carroll and Downs 2006). Actually, the results were in terms of life-years, because no reduction in health-related quality of life was assumed to occur for CAH. Another U.S. CEA calculated that if the mortality rate without screening were 4 percent or less, the ICER of screening for CAH would be greater than $100,000 per life-year saved (Yoo and Grosse

2005). Finally, a Finnish CEA of screening assumed 16 to 25 percent mortality among children with salt-wasting CAH (Autti-Ramo et al 2005) but did not report the ICER of screening for CAH.

Sickle Cell Disease

Screening for sickle cell disease (SCD) and other hemoglobin variants has been the subject of several CEAs, which have focused on comparing strategies of universal screening versus selective screening of infants from ethnic groups with an elevated prevalence of SCD (Grosse, Olney, and Baily 2005). In 1991, one study contended that screening infants in a low-prevalence population would cost an extraordinary $450 billion per life saved (Tsevat et al. 1991). Subsequent analyses that factored in costs and errors in ethnic identification concluded that universal screening for SCD could be cost-effective in states with relatively large African American populations (Gessner, Teutsch, and Shaffer 1996; Panepinto et al. 2000). With $50,000 per life-year saved as a threshold, universal screening would be cost-effective in states with more than 9 percent of births among African Americans, as well as in the United States as a whole (Panepinto et al. 2000). Decision makers focused on the last finding and supported universal screening in all states, even those with few infants affected by SCD (Grosse, Olney, and Baily 2005). Two U.K. health technology assessment reports also addressed universal and targeted newborn screening. One report concluded that universal screening would meet conventional cost-effectiveness thresholds in just 5 to 7 percent of the 150 health districts with the highest prevalence of SCD (Zeuner et al. 1999). The other report had similar findings, but chose not to use a decision rule (Davies et al. 2000). The latter study, which argued in favor of universal screening on nonquantitative grounds, proved more influential (Grosse, Olney, and Baily 2005).

Comparisons of universal with selective or targeted screening have been hindered by a lack of program data on the yield and cost of ethnically targeted screening. The sensitivity of selective screening was assumed to be 80 percent in three studies (Gessner, Teutsch, and Shaffer 1996; Davies et al. 2000; Panepinto et al. 2000) and 94.5 percent in another study (Zeuner et al. 1999). A higher sensitivity of selective screening means fewer additional cases detected by universal screening.

The CEAs for sickle cell disease all projected a reduction in mortality on the basis of RCT results showing an 84 percent decrease in episodes of pneumococcal sepsis with oral antibiotic prophylaxis (Gaston et al. 1986), but did not incorporate any estimate of the prevention of deaths through closer medical monitoring, parent education about the importance of seeking immediate medical care, and immediate antibiotic treatment for febrile illnesses (Gill et al. 1995). They also did not incorporate reductions in disability. Therefore, important potential, albeit unproven, benefits of screening were omitted.

On the other hand, immunizations have lowered the cost-effectiveness of early detection of SCD by preventing many infections that would otherwise have been prevented by antibiotic prophylaxis. In 2000, the U.S. Food and Drug Administration approved a seven-valent pneumoccocal conjugate vaccine (PCV7) for use in children under two years of age. The PCV7 reduced the burden of invasive pneumoccocal diseases among young black children in Tennessee by more than 80 percent (Talbot et al. 2004). Although antibiotic prophylaxis is still needed to protect against pneumoccocal infection that cannot be prevented by PCV7 (Adamkiewicz et al. 2003), the cost-effectiveness of newborn screening in terms of prevention of lethal sepsis is less favorable in the United States than it was before 2000.

Tandem Mass Spectrometry Screening and MCAD

The use of MS/MS technology to screen for metabolic diseases has been the focus of numerous cost-effectiveness analyses. CEAs published through 2006 include five from the United States (Insinga, Laessig, and Hoffman 2002; Schoen et al. 2002; Venditti et al. 2003; Carroll and Downs 2006; Feuchtbaum and Cunningham 2006) and one each from the United Kingdom (Pandor et al. 2004, 2006), Canada (Tran, Banerjee, and Li 2006), and Finland (Autti-Ramo et al. 2005). All assumed that the infrastructure for bloodspot screening was already in place and did not include the fixed costs of this infrastructure. The primary focus was MCAD, which is the most common of the disorders newly detectable through use of MS/MS and the one with the best data on outcomes. Most experts believe that 12 to 25 percent of children with MCAD die by the age of three years in the absence of screening, that 16 to 33 percent of survivors with severe symptoms experience developmental delays, and that deaths and intellectual disability due to MCAD are largely preventable by screening and early treatment (Pandor et al. 2004). However, the number of cases of disability associated with MCAD is uncertain. A systematic review concluded that intellectual disability occurs in 5 to 10 percent of children with MCAD not detected at birth (Grosse, Khoury, et al. 2006).

Furthermore, a recent study from Australia found no cognitive impairment in children with MCAD who were born in states without screening, which presumably reflected improved clinical awareness (Wilcken et al. 2007). Also, in that study, the differential in mortality up to age four years that was attributable to screening was about 10 to 13 percent (Grosse and Dezateux 2007), consistent with the 12 percent fatality rate reported in a retrospective study of stored bloodspots in the United Kingdom (Pourfazam et al. 2001).

One CEA analyzed data from the Wisconsin newborn screening program that used MS/MS to screen for MCAD (Insinga, Laessig, and Hoffman 2002). Data indicated an average incremental laboratory screening cost of $4 per birth, including the prorated cost of equipment, reagents, and staff time. A conservative "base-case" scenario, in which it was assumed that 50 percent of children with diagnosed MCAD had a mortality risk of 16 percent, that 3 percent of children with MCAD detected through screening would die, and that 5 percent of children would experience severe impairment without screening, yielded an ICER of screening of $41,862 per QALY. Using alternative QALY weights for severe impairment from other studies as discussed above, the base-case ICER would have been greater than $50,000 per QALY. A best-case scenario with assumptions more favorable to screening (100% of children experiencing a 16% mortality risk, 100% of deaths preventable) was associated with an ICER of $6,008 per QALY. This study was the only CEA published through 2006 that assumed routine treatment of MCAD patients with L-carnitine dietary supplements, a therapy that lacks high-quality evidence of improved outcomes but is recommended for all MCAD patients in Wisconsin, though not in most other states (Rhead 2006).

A second analysis assumed that programs were already using MS/MS to screen for just PKU, which was true for two states as of 2003, and were considering using this technology to screen for MCAD as well (Venditti et al. 2003). The study concluded that adding MCAD would reduce overall costs. The investigators assumed that 75 percent of children with MCAD would become symptomatic and that 64 percent of those (i.e., 64% of 75%) would experience comas unless their MCAD was detected by screening. Although net costs were estimated to be negative, the study also estimated QALY gains.

A third investigation analyzed a hypothetical MS/MS screening for amino acid and fatty acid oxidation disorders (Schoen et al. 2002). Based on an assumed screening cost of $15 per specimen and an average diagnostic cost of $6 for MSUD, homocystinuria, MCAD and other fatty acid oxidation disorders, glutaric acidemia type I, methylmalonic acidemia, and propionic acidemia, it was concluded that MS/MS screening would be cost-effective. That analysis had serious limitations, including a 10-fold overstatement of the incidence of MSUD. Schoen et al. assumed only a 2 percent mortality rate and no developmental disability resulting from MCAD in the absence of screening. MCAD was projected to reduce undiscounted life-years per case by 1.0 and discounted life-years by only 0.1; the latter is a calculation error because if a death is avoided in infancy, the number of discounted life-years is essentially the same as undiscounted life-years.

The Washington State Department of Health in 2002 conducted CBA/CEA assessments of screening with tandem mass spectrometry for MCAD, homocystinuria, and MSUD (Grosse et al. 2003; Washington State 2003). The CBA concluded that screening for all three disorders would yield a net economic benefit based on the value of lives saved. The analysis concluded that MSUD met a cost-effectiveness threshold of $50,000 per life-year saved, but that MCAD and homocystinuria had ICERs in excess of that threshold (Grosse et al. 2003). The state advisory committee had already concluded that these three disorders met the epidemiological criteria for inclusion in the state screening panel, and it relied on the CBA results to satisfy the economic criterion (Washington State 2003). A CBA prepared in Arizona with assistance from Washington State also concluded that adding MCAD screening would yield net economic benefits (Green et al. 2002).

A U.K. health technology assessment study included a CEA of the use of MS/MS in screening for metabolic disorders (Pandor et al. 2004, 2006). The study concluded that using MS/MS to screen for both PKU and MCAD would be cost-saving. The point estimates assumed that 70 percent of children with MCAD would become symptomatic without screening, that 12 percent of those children (i.e., 12% of 70%) would experience neurological disability, that without screening 20 percent of all affected children would die, and that no deaths or impairments would occur with screening. The finding of cost-savings resulted from two key assumptions. First, the cost of laboratory screening was calculated to be lower than in the United States, less than $2.50 per test. Second, it was projected that most of the additional laboratory costs would be offset by fewer false positive screening results for PKU.

A recent health technology assessment study from Canada that adopted epidemiological assumptions similar to those used by Insinga, Laessig, and Hoffman (2002) in Wisconsin, including 16 percent mortality and 10 percent probability of mental retardation in the absence of screening, concluded that MS/MS screening for MCAD would be highly cost-effective, at approximately C$2500 per QALY in the base-case analysis (Tran, Banerjee, and Li 2006; Tran et al. 2007). The range of cost-effectiveness ratios was C$1000 for the most favorable set of assumptions and C$12,000 for the least favorable set of assumptions. However, the study assumed a surprisingly low incremental cost of MS/MS screening for PKU and MCAD of C$2.40 per test, which was attributed to the Nova Scotia screening laboratory. Because that laboratory screens only 10,000 births per year, the equipment cost alone would seem to be higher than that estimate.

A Finnish study modeled screening for MCAD, long-chain hydroxyacyl-CoA dehydrogenase deficiency (LCHAD), glutaric aciduria type 1 (GA1), PKU, and CAH (Autti-Ramo et al. 2005). The ICER for the panel as a whole was projected to be between 5,500 and 25,500 euros per QALY. The assumptions made for MCAD outcomes in the absence of screening—40 percent mortality and 60 percent disability among survivors—far exceed estimates in the scientific literature. A distinctive feature of this study was an attempt to calculate QALY weights for each disorder based on a range of attributes, not just cognitive impairments. Specifically, the QALY weights for "severe handicap" were calculated to be 0.49 for LCHAD, 0.50 for GA1, and 0.76 for MCAD.

Two CEAs published in 2006 modeled the use of MS/MS screening in the United States. First, Feuchtbaum and Cunningham (2006) projected that the ICER for MS/MS screening for a variety of disorders would be less than $2500 per QALY. The unit cost of MS/MS screening was calculated to be $10, based on program data. Assuming that in the absence of screening 12 percent of all children with metabolic disorders detectable by MS/MS would experience severe impairment at a cost of $1 million per child, screening was projected to be cost-saving. The estimated numbers of deaths and neurological impairments were aggregated for all disorders. Second, Carroll and Downs (2006) calculated that screening for MCAD would be cost-saving, despite a cost estimate of $16 per laboratory test. This result is attributable in large part to a rather high estimate of the cost of caring for a patient with late-treated MCAD, in excess of $300,000. However, the source cited (Washington State 2003) actually estimated a cost of $12,000 for hospitalization due to metabolic crisis. A recent study from Australia found no difference in hospitalization rates for children with MCAD in states with or without screening (Wilcken et al. 2007). In addition, Carroll and Downs (2006) assumed 20 percent mortality and 20 percent occurrence of developmental delay or cerebral palsy among survivors in the absence of screening, both of which are much higher than more recent estimates of 10 percent and zero, respectively, in Australia (Grosse and Dezateux 2007; Wilcken et al. 2007).

Cystic Fibrosis

A CEA of newborn screening for cystic fibrosis (CF) in the United Kingdom projected an ICER of approximately $12,000 per QALY (Simpson et al. 2005). The study assumed that earlier detection of CF is associated with delayed progression of lung disease, better lung function, and better health-related quality of life. However, a systematic review concluded that there is no evidence that newborn screening for CF results in either better lung function or better health-related quality of life (Grosse et al. 2004).

A recent CEA of newborn screening for CF in the Netherlands projected that screening on the basis of immunoreactive trypsinogen alone would result in a cost-effectiveness ratio of a little over $30,000 per life-year saved (van den Akker-van Marle et al. 2006). The Dutch study assumed an absolute reduction in childhood mortality consistent with the finding in the United States that newborn screening is associated with a difference in risk of death up to 10 years of age of 2 percentage points (Grosse, Rosenfeld, et al. 2006). Newborn screening for CF was shown to be potentially cost-saving if it were assumed that screening would result in reduced numbers of births affected by CF and fewer sweat tests ordered for children without CF (van den Akker-van Marle et al. 2006). The latter is consistent with the findings from Wisconsin that following the introduction of newborn screening for CF, an observed decrease in the requisitioning of sweat tests ordered by clinicians for respiratory workups offset much of the cost of screening (Rosenberg and Farrell 2005).

An unpublished CBA prepared by the Washington State Department of Health (2005) projected economic benefits from three sources: (1) savings due to avoided deaths, valued at $4 million each, based on preliminary estimates from Grosse, Rosenfeld, et al. (2006) as discussed above; (2) savings due to one hospitalization avoided per child with CF, on average, valued at $26,720 per child, based on a French study (Siret et al. 2003); and (3) savings of $22,352 per child, based on the questionable assumption that all second and follow-up visits for children with CF are the result of a "diagnostic odyssey."

Discussion

The literature on cost-effectiveness in newborn screening is plagued by a lack of reliable data on the numbers of adverse outcomes prevented by screening. Published CEAs have used widely varying assumptions about the percentages of affected children with long-term disability in the absence of screening, ranging from 4 to 100 percent for CH and from zero to 60 percent for MCAD. The rate of mortality in the absence of screening has been assumed in different studies to be as low as zero and as high as 50 percent for biotinidase deficiency, with equivalent ranges of 2 to 40 percent for MCAD, 2 to 25 percent for CAH, and 14 to 33 percent for galactosemia. The lack of agreement among CEAs indicates the uncertainty in this area. Without good evidence of the magnitude of effectiveness, estimates of cost-effectiveness are inherently speculative. CEAs in this field could be improved if they were based on systematic reviews of the relevant scientific literature, as has been done in a few cases (Pandor et al. 2004, 2006; Tran, Banerjee, and Li 2006; Tran et al. 2007) and is true in general of evidence-based public health (Brownson et al. 2003).

What conclusions can we draw about the cost-savings or cost-effectiveness of screening for particular disorders? The newborn screening cost-effectiveness literature provides more information for certain conditions than others. Screening for PKU can be cost-saving, although this conclusion is not based on data on long-term outcomes in unscreened cohorts receiving dietary treatment. Screening for CH is also universally regarded as cost-saving (Grosse 2005), and this conclusion seems fairly solid because it is supported even by studies that have avoided overstating the frequency of disability in the absence of screening (Smith and Morris 1979).

In particular, screening for MCAD seems either cost-saving or cost-effective, although this depends in part on how the screening is implemented and the level of clinical awareness. The unit cost of adding screening for MCAD to an existing panel that did not use MS/MS is reported to range from $2 to $20 per specimen. Screening for MCAD is potentially cost-saving if the screening cost is very low, avoided costs of care are large, and costs of carnitine supplementation are not included. Screening does not necessarily reduce costs of hospitalization or disability associated with MCAD, as indicated by recently reported Australian data (Wilcken et al. 2007).

Even more challenging is to reliably estimate the economic impact of using MS/MS to screen for disorders for which evidence on long-term outcomes is less clear. Furthermore, no analyses have considered the expansion of newborn screening in comparison with competing demands for scarce child health resources. Issues such as who bears the costs, who receives the benefits, and access to long-term care and counseling have not been addressed.

Policymakers have made limited use of economic criteria and results to decide which tests to include in newborn screening panels in the United States, other than in Washington State, California, and Arizona. Even in those states, economic evaluations have been performed internally by health department staff to support decisions reached on the basis of other criteria, so as to satisfy legal or political requirements to show economic appropriateness. In Washington, the final decision to add CF to the state screening panel was reached after health department staff produced estimates of net economic benefit (Washington State 2005). Subsequently, the California health department adapted the same economic analysis to justify adding CF to its screening panel. In addition, the California decision to use MS/MS to screen for a large number of disorders and not just MCAD was supported by a CBA conducted within the health department (Cunningham 2004). That analysis did not calculate the incremental costs and benefits for individual disorders and did not document the evidence underlying the assumptions of effectiveness.

Although CEAs of newborn screening have been conducted at the national level in the United Kingdom for each disorder considered for inclusion, their influence seems to have been limited. The finding in a report (Pandor et al. 2004) that screening with MS/MS was cost-effective for a subset of disorders did not lead to routine implementation. The National Screening Committee has another criterion, that RCT evidence is required to document benefits in terms of mortality or morbidity, and this criterion has trumped the economic criterion. The 2001 decision to introduce newborn screening for CF in England overruled a previous finding of insufficient evidence to justify newborn screening for CF, even though no evidence of cost-effectiveness of screening newborns for CF was submitted. Finally, the National Health Service adopted universal hemoglobinopathy screening in part out of a concern that members of ethnic minorities were less likely to be screened with a selective screening program (Sassi, Le Grand, and Archard 2001).

The explanation for the overall lack of influence of CEAs in decisions on newborn screening panels suggested by advocates of expanded screening is that policymakers do not believe cost to be a legitimate factor in rationing access to potentially life-saving interventions aimed at children (Howse and Katz 2000). In response, it has been noted that policymakers do consider cost: many life-saving interventions targeted to children, such as bicycle helmets and child-restraint devices, receive limited funding. Further, newborn screening and follow-up care compete for resources with other life-saving interventions (Hinman 2001). In reality, policymakers who are uncomfortable dealing with costs and rationing do, implicitly, address costs. Which services get funded is often a matter of advocacy, colloquial evidence, and politics rather than priority setting on the basis of scientific evidence and resource constraints. Many policymakers have limited appreciation for quantitative evidence (Lomas et al. 2005).

The lack of reliance on economic evaluations in newborn screening decisions presumably also reflects other factors. Policymakers might not believe that CEAs identify all important costs and benefits or measure them accurately. One of the inherent limitations of economic evaluation methods is that any benefits or risks of harm that cannot be readily quantified are excluded from the analysis (Ackerman and Heinzerling 2004). As Albert Einstein famously said, not all that counts can be counted. Also, policymakers might not understand or appreciate the value of CEA findings, although they might cite CEA findings that justify decisions reached on other grounds. This situation is not unique to CEA; decision makers often overlook the results of evidence-based reviews in favor of other types of information (Helfand 2005). A more rational and transparent decision-making process should address standards of evidence and involve a broad range of stakeholders in a deliberative process (Berger and Teutsch 2005; Lomas et al. 2005; see also chapters 2 and 10).

Economic evaluations often are conducted before adoption of a policy. Prospective or *ex ante* analyses necessarily involve simulation modeling of expected outcomes and costs. Such analyses cannot yield definitive findings on cost-effectiveness. Often, the findings of prospective CEAs or CBAs turn out to be either excessively optimistic or overly conservative. One of the most useful functions of a CEA is to make explicit assumptions of effectiveness and to identify areas of uncertainty for which additional data are needed to inform policy decisions.

Policymakers should regard economic evaluation as an ongoing process and should commission *ex post* evaluations based on program cost data and surveillance of outcomes. Without effectiveness, there can be no cost-effectiveness. It is essential for newborn screening to be accompanied by systems to collect information on long-term outcomes. Newborn screening panels should be periodically reassessed based on a continuous process of data collection and analysis.

Conclusion

It is possible to steer a middle course between insisting that cost-effectiveness should be the only criterion for newborn screening tests and excluding it from decision making. If properly done, with critical scrutiny of data and assumptions, economic evaluation can inform policymakers of the implications of their options, including who is expected to bear the costs and reap the benefits. Although CEA methods pose ethical challenges, excluding cost-effectiveness as a consideration is also ethically problematic. Ultimately, cost is an issue of fairness as well as efficiency, because to say that cost does not matter involves favoring certain interventions over other interventions that might be of greater benefit but would not be funded because of limited resources. Optimizing the public's health through newborn screening requires careful and open consideration of evidence of effectiveness, risks, and resource constraints.

ACKNOWLEDGMENTS AND DISCLAIMER

I gratefully acknowledge the following individuals who provided comments on drafts of this chapter, in addition to participants in the "Ethical Decision-Making for Newborn Genetic Screening" project: John Adams, Ingeborg Blancquaert, Cathy Carruthers, Lauren Cipriano, Phaedra Corso, Michael Glass, James Gudgeon, Harry Hannon, Nora Henrikson, Cynthia Hinton, Mercy Mvundura, Peter Neumann, Lijing Ouyang, Scott Ramsey, Lisa Robinson, Danielle Ross, Ruthann Smejkal, Steven Teutsch, and John Thompson. I take responsibility for all statements, including any errors and lack of clarity that remain. The findings and conclusions in this chapter are mine and do not necessarily represent the views of the Centers for Disease Control and Prevention.

NOTES

1. ICER = $(C_1 - C_0)/(E_1 - E_0)$, where the numerator is the difference in net costs and the denominator is the difference in health outcomes.

2. The formula for present value (PV) is $PV = FV/(1 + r)^t$, where FV is future value, r is the discount rate, and t is the number of years in the future.

REFERENCES

Ackerman, F., and Heinzerling, L. 2004. *Priceless: On Knowing the Price of Everything and the Value of Nothing.* New York: New Press.

Adamkiewicz, T. V., Sarnaik, S., Buchanan, G. R., Iyer, R. V., Miller, S. T., Pegelow, C. H., Rogers, Z. R., Vichinsky, E., Elliott, J., Facklam, R. R., O'Brien, K. L., Schwartz, B., Van Beneden, C. A., Cannon, M. J., Eckman, J. R., Keyserling, H., Sullivan, K., Wong, W. Y., and Wang, W. C. 2003. Invasive pneumococcal infections in children with sickle cell disease in the era of penicillin prophylaxis, antibiotic resistance, and 23-valent pneumococcal polysaccharide vaccination. *J Pediatr* 143 (4): 438–44.

Alm, J., Hagenfeldt, L., Larsson, A., and Lundberg, K. 1984. Incidence of congenital hypothyroidism: retrospective study of neonatal laboratory screening versus clinical symptoms as indicators leading to diagnosis. *BMJ* 289 (6453): 1171–75.

American Academy of Pediatrics, Committee on Genetics. 1996. Newborn screening fact sheets. *Pediatrics* 98 (3): 473–501.

American College of Medical Genetics. 2005. *Newborn Screening: Toward a Uniform Screening Panel and System.* Rockville, MD: Maternal and Child Health Bureau.

Atkinson, K., Zuckerman, B., Sharfstein, J. M., Levin, D., Blatt, R. J., and Koh, H. K. 2001. A public health response to emerging technology: expansion of the Massachusetts newborn screening program. *Public Health Rep* 116 (2): 122–31.

Autti-Ramo, I., Makela, M., Sintonen, H., Koskinen, H., Laajalahti, L., Halila, R., Kaariainen, H., Lapatto, R., Nanto-Salonen, K., Pulkki, K., Renlund, M., Salo, M., and Tyni, T. 2005. Expanding screening for rare metabolic disease in the newborn: an analysis of costs, effect and ethical consequences for decision-making in Finland. *Acta Paediatr* 94 (8): 1126–36.

Badawi, N., Cahalane, S. F., McDonald, M., Mulhair, P., Begi, B., O'Donohue, A., and Naughten, E. 1996. Galactosaemia—a controversial disorder. Screening & outcome: Ireland 1972–1992. *Ir Med J* 89 (1):16–17.

Barden, H. S., and Kessel, R. 1984. The costs and benefits of screening for congenital hypothyroidism in Wisconsin. *Soc Biol* 31 (3–4): 185–200.

Barden, H. S., Kessel, R., and Schuett, V. E. 1984. The costs and benefits of screening for PKU in Wisconsin. *Soc Biol* 31 (1–2): 1–17.

Berger, M. L., and Teutsch, S. 2005. Cost-effectiveness analysis: from science to application. *Med Care* 43 (7 Suppl): 49–53.

Botkin, J. R., Clayton, E. W., Fost, N. C., Burke, W., Murray, T. H., Baily, M. A., Wilfond, B., Berg, A., and Ross, L. F. 2006. Newborn screening technology: proceed with caution. *Pediatrics* 117 (5): 1793–99.

Brownson, R. C., Baker, E. A., Leet, T. L., and Gillespie, K. N. 2003. *Evidence-Based Public Health.* Oxford: Oxford University Press.

Carroll, A. E., and Downs, S. M. 2006. Comprehensive cost-utility analysis of newborn screening strategies. *Pediatrics* 117 (5 Pt 2): S287–95.

Centers for Disease Control and Prevention. 2004. Economic costs associated with mental retardation, cerebral palsy, hearing loss, and vision impairment—United States, 2003. *MMWR Morb Mortal Wkly Rep* 53 (3): 57–59.

Clarke, J. T., Amato, D., and Deber, R. B. 2001. Managing public payment for high-cost, high-benefit treatment: enzyme replacement therapy for Gaucher's disease in Ontario. *CMAJ* 165 (5): 595–96.

Coast, J. 2004. Is economic evaluation in touch with society's health values? *BMJ* 329 (7476): 1233–36.

Cunningham, G. C. 1969. Two years of PKU testing in California: the role of the laboratory. *Calif Med* 110 (1): 11–16.

———. 2004. Cost-benefit analysis of MS-MS in newborn screening in California. Report presented to the Advisory Committee on Heritable Disorders and Genetic Diseases in Newborns and Children, Washington, DC, September 22, 2004. http://mchb.hrsa.gov/programs/genetics/committee/2ndmeeting.htm.

Dagenais, D. L., Courville, L., and Dagenais, M. G. 1985. A cost-benefit analysis of the Quebec Network of Genetic Medicine. *Soc Sci Med* 20 (6): 601–7.

Davies, S. C., Cronin, E., Gill, M., Greengross, P., Hickman, M., and Normand, C. 2000. Screening for sickle cell disease and thalassaemia: a systematic review with supplementary research. *Health Technol Assess* 4 (3): 1–99.

Devlin, N., and Parkin, D. 2004. Does NICE have a cost-effectiveness threshold and what other factors influence its decisions? A binary choice analysis. *Health Econ* 13 (5): 437–52.

Dezateux, C. 2003. Newborn screening for medium chain acyl-CoA dehydrogenase deficiency: evaluating the effects on outcome. *Eur J Pediatr* 162 (Suppl 1): S25–28.

Dott, M., Chace, D., Fierro, M., Kalas, T. A., Hannon, W. H., Williams, J., and Rasmussen, S. A. 2006. Metabolic disorders detectable by tandem mass spectrometry and unexpected early childhood mortality: a population-based study. *Am J Med Genet A* 140 (8): 837–42.

Evans, C., Tavakoli, M., and Crawford, B. 2004. Use of quality adjusted life years and life years gained as benchmarks in economic evaluations: a critical appraisal. *Health Care Manage Sci* 7 (1): 43–49.

Feuchtbaum, L., and Cunningham, G. 2006. Economic evaluation of tandem mass spectrometry screening in California. *Pediatrics* 117 (5 Pt 2): S280–86.

Filiano, J. J., Bellimer, S. G., and Kunz, P. L. 2002. Tandem mass spectrometry and newborn screening: pilot data and review. *Pediatr Neurol* 26 (3): 201–4.

Garber, A. M. 2004. Cost-effectiveness and evidence evaluation as criteria for coverage policy. *Health Aff (Millwood)* Suppl Web Exclusives: W4–96.

Gaston, M. H., Verter, J. I., Woods, G., Pegelow, C., Kelleher, J., Presbury, G., Zarkowsky, H., Vichinsky, E., Iyer, R., and Lobel, J. S. 1986. Prophylaxis with oral penicillin in children with sickle cell anemia: a randomized trial. *N Engl J Med* 314 (25): 1593–99.

Geelhoed, E. A., Lewis, B., Hounsome, D., and O'Leary, P. 2005. Economic evaluation of neonatal screening for phenylketonuria and congenital hypothyroidism. *J Paediatr Child Heath* 41 (11): 575–79.

Gessner, B. D., Teutsch, S. M., and Shaffer, P. A. 1996. A cost effectiveness evaluation of newborn hemoglobinopathy screening from the perspective of state health care systems. *Early Hum Dev* 45 (3): 257–75.

Gill, F. M., Sleeper, L. A., Weiner, S. J., Brown, A. K., Bellevue, R., Grover, R., Pegelow, C. H., and Vichinsky, E. 1995. Clinical events in the first decade in a cohort of infants with sickle cell disease. Cooperative Study of Sickle Cell Disease. *Blood* 86 (2): 776–83.

Gold, M. R., Siegel, J. E., Russell, L. B., and Weinstein, M. C. 1996. *Cost-Effectiveness in Health and Medicine*. New York: Oxford University Press.

Gold, M. R., Stevenson, D., and Fryback, D. G. 2002. HALYS and QALYS and DALYS, oh my: similarities and differences in summary measures of population health. *Annu Rev Public Health* 23:115–34.

Graham, J. D., Corso, P. S., Morris, J. M., Segui-Gomez, M., and Weinstein, M. C. 1998. Evaluating the cost-effectiveness of clinical and public health measures. *Annu Rev Public Health* 19:125–52.

Green, D., Smejkal, R., Carruthers, C., and Thompson, J. D. 2002. An initiative to expand newborn screening in the State of Arizona: cost-benefit analysis. Paper presented to the Newborn Screening and Genetic Testing Symposium, Phoenix, AZ, November 4–7.

Griebsch, I., Coast, J., and Brown, J. 2005. Quality-adjusted life-years lack quality in pediatric care: a critical review of published cost-utility studies in child health. *Pediatrics* 115 (5): e600–614.

Grosse, S. D. 2005. Does newborn screening save money? The difference between cost-effective and cost-saving interventions. *J Pediatr* 146 (2): 168–70.

Grosse, S. D., Boyle, C. A., Botkin, J. R., Comeau, A. M., Kharrazi, M., Rosenfeld, M., and Wilfond, B. S. 2004. Newborn screening for cystic fibrosis: evaluation of benefits and risks and recommendations for state newborn screening programs. *MMWR Recomm Rep* 53 (RR-13): 1–36.

Grosse, S. D., Boyle, C. A., Kenneson, A., Khoury, M. J., and Wilfond, B. S. 2006. From public health emergency to public health service: the implications of evolving criteria for newborn screening panels. *Pediatrics* 117 (3): 923–29.

Grosse, S. D., Carruthers, C.A., Thompson, J.D., and Glass, M. 2003. The use of economic appraisal in framing newborn screening policy recommendations in Washington State. Paper presented at Improving Outcomes through Health Technology Assessment, ISTAHC 2003, Canmore, Canada, June 24.

Grosse, S. D., and Dezateux, C. 2007. Newborn screening for inherited metabolic disease. *Lancet* 369 (9555): 5–6.

Grosse, S., and Gwinn, M. 2001. Assisting states in assessing newborn screening options. *Public Health Rep* 116 (2): 169–72.

Grosse, S. D., Khoury, M. J., Greene, C. L., Crider, K. S., and Pollitt, R. J. 2006. The epidemiology of medium chain acyl-CoA dehydrogenase deficiency: an update. *Genet Med* 8 (4): 205–12.

Grosse, S. D., Olney, R. S., and Baily, M. A. 2005. The cost effectiveness of universal versus selective newborn screening for sickle cell disease in the US and the UK: a critique. *Appl Health Econ Health Policy* 4 (4): 239–47.

Grosse, S. D., Rosenfeld, M., Devine, O. J., Lai, H. J., and Farrell, P. M. 2006. Potential impact of newborn screening for cystic fibrosis on child survival: a systematic review and analysis. *J Pediatr* 149 (3): 362–66.

Grosse, S. D., Teutsch, S. M., and Haddix, A. C. 2007. Lessons from cost-effectiveness research for United States public health policy. *Annu Rev Public Health* 28:365–91.

Grosse, S. D., and Van Vliet, G. 2007a. How many deaths can be prevented by newborn screening for congenital adrenal hyperplasia? *Horm Res* 67 (6): 284–91.

———. 2007b. Outcomes in CAH: need for evidence-based estimates. *Horm Res* 68 (4): 203.

Hammitt, J. K. 2002. QALYs versus WTP. *Risk Anal* 22 (5): 985–1001.

Hansen, T. W., Henrichsen, B., Rasmussen, R. K., Carling, A., Andressen, A. B., and Skjeldal, O. 1996. Neuropsychological and linguistic follow-up studies of children with galactosaemia from an unscreened population. *Acta Paediatr* 85 (10): 1197–1201.

Helfand, M. 2005. Incorporating information about cost-effectiveness into evidence-based decision-making: the evidence-based practice center (EPC) model. *Med Care* 43 (7 Suppl): 33–43.

Hinman, A. R. 2001. The importance of newborn screening. *Pediatrics* 108 (3): 821.

Hisashige, A. 1994. Health economic analysis of the neonatal screening program in Japan. *Int J Technol Assess Health Care* 10 (3): 382–91.

Honeycutt, A. A., Grosse, S. D., and Dunlap, J. L. 2003. Economic costs of mental retardation, cerebral palsy, hearing loss, and vision impairment. In *Using Survey Data to Study Disability*, ed. B. M. Altman, S. N. Barnartt, and G. Hendershot, pp. 207–28. London: Elsevier.

Howse, J. L., and Katz, M. 2000. The importance of newborn screening. *Pediatrics* 106 (3): 595.

Insinga, R. P., Laessig, R. H., and Hoffman, G. L. 2002. Newborn screening with tandem mass spectrometry: examining its cost-effectiveness in the Wisconsin newborn screening panel. *J Pediatr* 141 (4): 524–31.

Kharrazi, M., and Kharrazi, L. D. 2005. Delayed diagnosis of cystic fibrosis and the family perspective. *J Pediatr* 147 (3 Suppl): S21–25.

Kirkman, H. N., and Frazier, D. M. 1996. Maternal PKU: thirteen years after epidemiological projections. *Int Pediatr* 11:279–83.

Klein, A. H., Meltzer, S., and Kenny, F. M. 1972. Improved prognosis in congenital hypothyroidism treated before age three months. *J Pediatr* 81 (5): 912–15.

Koch, R., Moseley, K., Ning, J., Romstad, A., Guldberg, P., and Guttler, F. 1999. Long-term beneficial effects of the phenylalanine-restricted diet in late-diagnosed individuals with phenylketonuria. *Mol Genet Metab* 67 (2): 148–55.

Layde, P. M., Von Allmen, S. D., and Oakley, G. P. Jr. 1979. Congenital hypothyroidism control programs: a cost-benefit analysis. *JAMA* 241 (21): 2290–92.

Levy, H. L. 2000. Comments on final intelligence in late treated patients with phenylketonuria. *Eur J Pediatr* 159 (Suppl 2): S149.

Levy, H. L., and Albers, S. 2000. Genetic screening of newborns. *Annu Rev Genomics Hum Genet* 1:139–77.

Liebl, B., Nennstiel-Ratzel, U., Roscher, A., and von Kries, R. 2003. Data required for the evaluation of newborn screening programmes. *Eur J Pediatr* 162 (Suppl 1): S57–61.

Lindegren, M. L., Kobrynski, L., Rasmussen, S. A., Moore, C. A., Grosse, S. D., Vanderford, M. L., Spira, T. J., McDougal, J. S., Vogt, R. F. Jr., Hannon, W. H., Kalman, L. V., Chen, B., Mattson, M., Baker, T. G., and Khoury, M. 2004. Applying public health strategies to primary immunodeficiency diseases: a potential approach to genetic disorders. *MMWR Recomm Rep* 53 (RR-1): 1–29.

Lomas, J., Culyer, T., McCutcheon, C., McAuley, L., and Law, S. 2005. *Conceptualizing and Combining Evidence for Health System Guidance: Final Report, May 2005*. Ottawa: Canadian Health Services Research Foundation (available at www.chsrf.ca/other_documents/pdf/evidence_e.pdf).

Lord, J., Thomason, M. J., Littlejohns, P., Chalmers, R. A., Bain, M. D., Addison, G. M., Wilcox, A. H., and Seymour, C. A. 1999. Secondary analysis of economic data: a review of cost-benefit studies of neonatal screening for phenylketonuria. *J Epidemiol Community Health* 53 (3): 179–86.

Luce, B. R. 2005. What will it take to make cost-effectiveness analysis acceptable in the United States? *Med Care* 43 (7 Suppl): 44–48.

Maciosek, M. V., Coffield, A. B., Edwards, N. M., Flottemesch, T. J., Goodman, M. J., and Solberg, L. I. 2006. Priorities among effective clinical preventive services: results of a systematic review and analysis. *Am J Prev Med* 31 (1): 52–61.

McGhee, S. A., Stiehm, E. R., and McCabe, E. R. 2005. Potential costs and benefits of newborn screening for severe combined immunodeficiency. *J Pediatr* 147 (5): 603–8.

National Screening Committee. 2004. Criteria for appraising the viability, effectiveness and appropriateness of a screening programme. www.nsc.nhs.uk/uk_nsc/uk_nsc_ind.htm.

Neumann, P. J. 2005. *Using Cost-Effectiveness Analysis to Improve Health Care Opportunities and Barriers.* Oxford: Oxford University Press.

Owens, D. K. 2002. Analytic tools for public health decision making. *Med Decis Making* 22 (5 Suppl): S3–10.

Pandor, A., Eastham, J., Beverley, C., Chilcott, J., and Paisley, S. 2004. Clinical effectiveness and cost-effectiveness of neonatal screening for inborn errors of metabolism using tandem mass spectrometry: a systematic review. *Health Technol Assess* 8 (12): iii, 1–121.

Pandor, A., Eastham, J., Chilcott, J., Paisley, S., and Beverley, C. 2006. Economics of tandem mass spectrometry screening of neonatal inherited disorders. *Int J Technol Assess Health Care* 22 (3): 321–26.

Panepinto, J. A., Magid, D., Rewers, M. J., and Lane, P. A. 2000. Universal versus targeted screening of infants for sickle cell disease: a cost-effectiveness analysis. *J Pediatr* 136 (2): 201–8.

Pollitt, R. J., Green, A., McCabe, C. J., Booth, A., Cooper, N. J., Leonard, J. V., Nicholl, J., Nicholson, P., Tunaley, J. R., and Virdi, N. K. 1997. Neonatal screening for inborn errors of metabolism: cost, yield and outcome. *Health Technol Assess* 1 (7): i–iv, 1–202.

Pourfarzam, M., Morris, A., Appleton, M., Craft A., and Bartlett, K. 2001. Neonatal screening for medium-chain acyl-CoA dehydrogenase deficiency. *Lancet* 358 (9287): 1063–64.

Raiti, S., and Newns, G. H. 1971. Cretinism: early diagnosis and its relation to mental prognosis. *Arch Dis Child* 46 (249): 692–94.

Rhead, W. J. 2006. Newborn screening for medium-chain acyl-CoA dehydrogenase deficiency: a global perspective. *J Inherit Metab Dis* 29 (2–3): 370–77.

Robinson, L. A. 2004. Current federal agency practices for valuing the impact of regulations on human health and safety. Report prepared for the Institute of Medicine Committee to Evaluate Measures of Health Benefits for Environment, Health, and Safety Regulation. www.iom .edu/file.asp?id=24313.

Rosenberg, M. A., and Farrell, P. M. 2005. Assessing the cost of cystic fibrosis diagnosis and treatment. *J Pediatr* 147 (3 Suppl): S101–5.

Sassi, F., Le Grand, J., and Archard, L. 2001. Equity versus efficiency: a dilemma for the National Health Service—if the National Health Service is serious about equity it must offer guidance when principles conflict. *BMJ* 323 (7316): 762–63.

Schoen, E. J., Baker, J. C., Colby, C. J., and To, T. T. 2002. Cost-benefit analysis of universal tandem mass spectrometry for newborn screening. *Pediatrics* 110 (4): 781–86.

Schweitzer-Krantz, S. 2003. Early diagnosis of inherited metabolic disorders towards improving outcome: the controversial issue of galactosaemia. *Eur J Pediatr* 162 (Suppl 1): S50–53.

Seymour, C. A., Thomason, M. J., Chalmers, R. A., Addison, G. M., Bain, M. D., and Cockburn, F. 1997. Newborn screening for inborn errors of metabolism: a systematic review. *Health Technol Assess* 1 (11): i–iv, 1–95.

Siegel, J. E., and Clancy, C. M. 2003. Using economic evaluations in decision making. In *Prevention Effectiveness: A Guide to Decision Analysis and Economic Evaluation*, ed. A. C. Haddix, S. M. Teutsch, and P. S. Corso, pp. 178–98. London: Oxford University Press.

Simpson, N., Anderson, R., Sassi, F., Pitman, A., Lewis, P., Tu, K., and Lannin, H. 2005. The cost-effectiveness of neonatal screening for cystic fibrosis: an analysis of alternative scenarios using a decision model. *Cost Eff Resour Alloc* 3:8.

Siret, D., Bretaudeau, G., Branger, B., Dabadie, A., Dagorne, M., David, V., de Braekeleer, M., Moisan-Petit, V., Picherot, G., Rault, G., Storni, V., and Roussey, M. 2003. Comparing the clinical evolution of cystic fibrosis screened neonatally to that of cystic fibrosis diagnosed from clinical symptoms: a 10-year retrospective study in a French region (Brittany). *Pediatr Pulmonol* 35 (5): 342–49.

Smith, P., and Morris, A. 1979. Assessment of a programme to screen the newborn for congenital hypothyroidism. *Community Med* 1 (1): 14–22.

Steiner, K. C., and Smith, H. A. 1973. Application of cost-benefit analysis to a PKU screening program. *Inquiry* 10 (4): 34–40.

Stoddard, J. J., and Farrell, P. M. 1997. State-to-state variations in newborn screening policies. *Arch Pediatr Adolesc Med* 151 (6): 561–64.

Strnadova, K. A., Votava, F., Lebl, J., Muhl, A., Item, C., Bodamer, O. A., Torresani, T., Bouska, I., Waldhauser, F., and Sperl, W. 2007. Prevalence of congenital adrenal hyperplasia among sudden infant death in the Czech Republic and Austria. *Eur J Pediatr* 166 (1): 1–4.

Talbot, T. R., Poehling, K. A., Hartert, T. V., Arbogast, P. G., Halasa, N. B., Mitchel, E., Schaffner, W., Craig, A. S., Edwards, K. M., and Griffin, M. R. 2004. Elimination of racial differences in invasive pneumococcal disease in young children after introduction of the conjugate pneumococcal vaccine. *Pediatr Infect Dis J* 23 (8): 726–31.

Tilford, J. M. 2002. Cost-effectiveness analysis and emergency medical services for children: issues and applications. *Ambul Pediatr* 2 (4 Suppl): 330–36.

Tran, K., Banerjee, S., and Li, H. 2006. *Newborn Screening for Medium Chain Acyl-CoA Dehydrogenase Deficiency Using Tandem Mass Spectrometry: Clinical and Cost Effectiveness.* Ottawa: Canadian Coordinating Office for Health Technology Assessment.

Tran, K., Banerjee, S., Li, H., Noorani, H. Z., Mensinkai, S., and Dooley, K. 2007. Clinical efficacy and cost-effectiveness of newborn screening for medium chain acyl-CoA dehydrogenase deficiency using tandem mass spectrometry. *Clin Biochem* 40 (3–4): 235–41.

Tsevat, J., Wong, J. B., Pauker, S. G., and Steinberg, M. H. 1991. Neonatal screening for sickle cell disease: a cost-effectiveness analysis. *J Pediatr* 118 (4 Pt 1): 546–54.

U.S. Congress Office of Technology Assessment. 1988. *Healthy Children: Investing in the Future.* Washington, DC: Government Printing Office.

van den Akker-van Marle, M. E., Dankert, H. M., Verkerk, P. H., and Dankert-Roelse, J. E. 2006. Cost-effectiveness of 4 neonatal screening strategies for cystic fibrosis. *Pediatrics* 118 (3): 896–905.

Van Pelt, A., and Levy, H. L. 1974. Cost-benefit analysis of newborn screening for metabolic disorders. *N Engl J Med* 291 (26): 1414–16.

Venditti, L. N., Venditti, C. P., Berry, G. T., Kaplan, P. B., Kaye, E. M., Glick, H., and Stanley, C. A. 2003. Newborn screening by tandem mass spectrometry for medium-chain acyl-CoA dehydrogenase deficiency: a cost-effectiveness analysis. *Pediatrics* 112 (5): 1005–15.

Washington State, Department of Health. 2003. Least burden and cost benefit analysis, newborn screening for metabolic disorders, WAC 246-650. www.sboh.wa.gov/Meetings/Meetings_2003/2003-10_15/documents/Tab09-NBS_analysis.pdf.

———. 2005. Newborn screening for cystic fibrosis economic analysis. Unpublished report. www.sboh.wa.gov/Meetings/2005/12-14/documents/Tab11d-CF_Economic%20Analysis.pdf.

Webb, J. F. 1973. PKU screening—is it worth it? *CMAJ* 108 (3): 328–29.

Weinstein, M. 1995. From cost-effectiveness ratios to resource allocation: where to draw the line? In *Valuing Health Care: Costs, Benefits, and Effectiveness of Pharmaceuticals and Other Medical Technologies*, ed. F Sloan, pp. 77–97. New York: Cambridge University Press.

Wilcken, B., Haas, M., Joy, P., Wiley, V., Chaplin, M., Black, C., Fletcher, J., McGill, J., and Boneh, A. 2007. Outcome of neonatal screening for medium-chain acyl-CoA dehydrogenase deficiency in Australia: a cohort study. *Lancet* 369 (9555): 37–42.

Wildner, M. 2003. Health economic issues of screening programmes. *Eur J Pediatr* 162 (Suppl 1): S5–7.

Wilson, J. M. G., and Jungner, G. 1968. *Principles and Practice of Screening for Disease*. Geneva: World Health Organization.

Yoo, B. K., and Grosse, S. D. 2005. Cost-effectiveness of newborn screening for congenital adrenal hyperplasia: a preliminary analysis. In *Proceedings, National Newborn Screening and Genetic Testing Symposium, Portland, OR*. Washington, DC: Association of Public Health Laboratories.

Zeuner, D., Ades, A. E., Karnon, J., Brown, J., Dezateux, C., and Anionwu, E. N. 1999. Antenatal and neonatal haemoglobinopathy screening in the UK: review and economic analysis. *Health Technol Assess* 3 (11): i–v, 1–186.

CHAPTER 4

An Advocate's Perspective on Newborn Screening Policy

JANNINE DE MARS CODY, PH.D.

I doubt there has ever been a child who, when asked what he or she wanted to be when grown up, said, I want to have a child with a disability so that I can grow up to be an advocate! People do not plan for the role of being such a parent, they do not train for it, they just suddenly realize that their world and their priorities have been turned inside out and they are "not in Kansas any more." In this new role as an advocate, they bring all their previous life experiences with them, whether in business, politics, medicine, or the garden club. While each of these provides some of the essential skills, none provides a complete education in advocacy for children with genetic conditions. Advocates watch and listen, and over time this new Land of Oz begins to make sense. They then find themselves creating websites, organizing conferences, talking to the press, testifying before legislators, and sitting on an array of committees, even on committees making newborn screening policy.

One of the guiding principles of the Genetic Alliance is "meaningful progress in policy, healthcare and research requires proactive consumer participation." (The Genetic Alliance [www.geneticalliance.org] is a coalition of more than 600 advocacy organizations serving 25 million people affected by 1000 genetic conditions.) To have effective consumer participation it is important to build strong relationships between consumer advocates and the many professionals with whom they interact. These relationships are built on an understanding and appreciation of the skills, knowledge, and perspective that each brings to the discussion. This chapter does not discuss whether newborn screening panels should be expanded or how such an expanded panel should be implemented, but discusses the decision-making process and the role that advocates might play in that process.

The goals of this chapter are:

- To discuss how advocates measure success and the unique perspective they bring to the decision-making process.
- To discuss the questions advocates must ask of themselves and others about changes in newborn screening policy.
- To discuss the implications that strong advocacy and professional relationships can have for newborn screening policymaking.

How Advocates Measure Success

Advocates often find themselves on committees or advisory panels with a plethora of professionals. Although these committees are convened to discuss issues of common interest to all parties, the perspectives the advocates bring and the urgencies and pressures they feel are different from those of the professionals. These differences can create tensions unless all parties understand how the others see the world. Let me illustrate this point by recasting a well-known story (Eiseley 1979, p. 169).

> A thoughtful and insightful health care provider was strolling down the beach contemplating the ethical issues that affect newborn screening. She looked down the beach and saw a human figure moving like a dancer. She smiled to herself at the thought of someone dancing to the day and she walked faster to catch up.
>
> As she got closer, she noticed that the figure was that of a young man and that what he was doing was not dancing at all. The young man was reaching down to the shore, picking up small objects, and throwing them into the ocean.
>
> She came closer still and called out, "Good morning! May I ask what you are doing?"

The young man paused, looked up, and replied, "Throwing starfish into the ocean."

"I must ask, then, why are you throwing starfish into the ocean?" asked the somewhat startled health care provider.

To this, the young man replied, "The sun is up and the tide is going out. If I don't throw them in, they'll die."

On hearing this, the health care provider commented, "But, young man, do you not realize that there are miles and miles of beach and there are starfish all along every mile? You can't possibly make a difference!"

At this, the young man bent down, picked up yet another starfish, and threw it into the ocean. As it met the water, he said, "It made a difference to that one."

This young man is an advocate. He is motivated to make a difference, one starfish at a time. Some advocates focus on their personal issues or those of their children—throwing back one starfish at a time. Others work toward helping their organization, composed of others affected by the same condition—organizing a crew to help throw back the starfish along an entire stretch of beach. Still others become advocates serving on committees with professionals—trying to determine how to implement seashore change so that starfish will not be stranded on the beach at low tide. But success for the advocate is still defined by the knowledge that he or she made a difference to someone.

This is not to suggest that making a difference to someone is not part of the motivation of professionals; it most assuredly is. For advocates, though, all the other factors that must be juggled (time, money, personnel) exist, but have different weights. In addition, the advocate's measure of success, to "make a difference to that *one*," is almost opposite to that of public health, which measures success by making changes that can be implemented for populations of people. It is not the measure of success for a company that needs to make a profit. When there are different measures of success, it isn't necessarily the case that one is right and the others wrong; the measures simply reflect fundamentally different perspectives. Given the different perspectives, it is hardly surprising that tensions can arise. But there is common ground. The key to finding that common ground and creating effective partnerships is acknowledging that a wide variety of players with different expertise and perspectives *should* be at the table and that the variety of perspective that each brings is equally valid. This is simply mutual respect.

What Advocates and Organizations Must Learn and What Questions They Must Address

Advocacy usually begins at a personal level. For parents, personal advocacy is working for the betterment of their child's life. An example would be parents trying to find the best possible doctor for their child.

Some people choose to take what they have learned from their personal experience and combine that with what others in their situation have learned and move their advocacy to the next level to help others with the same condition. That level is group advocacy. In this discussion, group advocacy is defined as involving others who have a child with the same or a similar condition. An example of group advocacy might be a disease-based organization creating a set of criteria that will aid their member families in finding the best doctors for their children.

Others may choose to take their advocacy to the next level, which is public advocacy. Public advocacy is more global in perspective and seeks to affect regional or societal systems. One example would be advocates' having their child's condition added to a public health newborn screening panel.

These levels of advocacy are defined not by which person or organization is doing the advocacy, but rather by the level of the question being addressed. An advocacy organization can carry out activities at all three levels. An organization may help an individual family solve a problem, develop practice guidelines for the condition affecting their child, and advocate to Congress for increased funding for government agencies providing assistance to families affected by the condition.

The important point is that as one moves from personal advocacy to group advocacy to public advocacy, the circle of influence as well as the circle of responsibility enlarges. Therefore, how one sets an agenda for making change is dependent on which level of advocacy is being considered. To make a decision in the personal advocacy realm, you need only to consult with yourself, possibly your immediate family, or an advisor of your choice. Group advocacy decision making involves consulting with leaders, who then represent the members of the organization. Public advocacy involves consulting with as many individuals and communities of people as perceive that they have a stake in the matter under discussion. Public advocacy brings a responsibility to determine all the individuals and communities that might be affected and to involve them in the process.

How does one go about addressing the issues around newborn screening? There is not much of a question about the decision-making process in personal advocacy; it's personal. In group advocacy, the first step is to determine the collective personal advocacy experience of the group's members. For the purposes of this discussion, the central question is, would a presymptomatic diagnosis help those affected? The key word is "help" because there is a multitude of ways to define that word. What might be helpful to one person may not be helpful or may even be detrimental to another. Also, those affected include both the child and the family. To gain consensus around this central question, one must ask many other questions.

- Would the treatment plan have been different or expedited if there had been a presymptomatic diagnosis?
- Would reproductive choices regarding subsequent pregnancies have been influenced had an early diagnosis been made for the first child?
- Would the child's health be improved by having a presymptomatic diagnosis? This question relates to secondary conditions as well as the primary condition.
- Would the outcome be significantly changed or would the course of the condition be altered? In cases in which there is no cure or prevention, a slowing of a degenerative disease may be a significantly positive outcome.

Several methods can be used singly or in combination to arrive at a consensus about these questions. The simplest is to survey the membership. This may best be done using a standard mail-out survey or by listserve. When there are issues on which people have diverse or contradictory opinions, follow-up may be needed. An annual conference is an ideal setting; conference calls have become a convenient and affordable mechanism for real-time discussion as well. It is also important to survey the members of the organization's medical or professional advisory board. The board's perspective will be different and may provide insight into additional questions that need to be addressed by the affected individuals or families. The medical advisory board may also be able to alert the organization to the arguments that may be made in opposition to a proposed strategy. This information will be critical for the organization to build a strong case in support of whatever plan they decide to try to implement.

Because medical conditions differ in severity, age of onset, and treatment options, the answers to the above questions will differ from organization to organization. However, there will be other organizations that are simultaneously navigating through the same complex issues. Discussion with these other organizations can provide a perspective on the ways in which each condition is both unique and similar to others. This expansion to understand other advocacy groups' views is an important part of learning about the landscape in which an advocate's organization operates.

If an organization determines that a presymptomatic diagnosis *can* be made (more discussion on this below), the next question is, *should* the condition be screened for? This question moves the discussion from a matter concerning those who are affected and may benefit from screening to public advocacy. It addresses the fact that a screening test, by definition, is applied to a population in which most of the individuals do not have the condition. It also addresses the more practical aspects of testing a large number of people to find the few who are affected. The practical questions that need to be determined by an advocacy organization are:

- Does the severity of the condition, in comparison with the improvements in outcome from presymptomatic testing, justify the costs? Costs are measured in terms of fiscal, medical and psychological outcomes.
- How often will an affected child be identified?
- What is the financial cost of the test?

An organization should be prepared to address these questions in a public forum. The cost-versus-benefit arguments need to be fully explored so that an accurate case can be put forward. Outside expert advice is critical. Members of the organization's medical advisory board are perfect for this role. Additionally, there is no need for a young organization to go through this strategic planning process alone. Other organizations have been through similar processes or are currently going through them. Advocacy organizations can also seek advice from umbrella organizations like the Genetic Alliance for information on building capacity, strategies, and alliances.

Although this discussion is about the screening of newborns, advocacy organizations need to ask themselves how and when population screening might be most effectively performed.

- Should screening be limited to a population that is at higher risk than the general population? This increases the cost-effectiveness of the testing, because the ratio of positive to negative test results would be increased if such a population could be identified. However, there are no conditions that affect exclusively one population of people, so some affected individuals would be missed. The ability to identify groups at higher risk based on racial or ethnic origin is becoming increasingly difficult. This is due to both interracial marriages and the social pressure (either positive or negative) related to being associated with a certain population of individuals.

- Should screening be limited to those with a higher personal risk status? This could include those having an affected family member or a mother with a risk factor such as an environmental or chemical exposure or advanced maternal age.

- Is the screening most appropriately performed on a newborn? If the condition has a later onset, should screening be delayed until school age or until individuals reach adulthood and can make their own decisions about testing?

- Should the test be mandated, or should there be an informed consent process, or something in between? This is one of the more complex questions because of the many factors that must be weighed to arrive at an answer. At one end of the spectrum are conditions that warrant mandated testing because they are severe and essentially curable. At the other end of the spectrum are those conditions that are not treatable, but genetic counseling with the affected child's family could provide important information on the recurrence risk and the cause of death or disability. Most conditions fall somewhere in between.

Each of the above points could elicit a lengthy discussion of the pros, cons, risks, and benefits. However, the last point in particular deserves attention because of the fundamental nature of the question: mandated versus choice in screening. There is already a heated debate on this topic for conditions that are currently included in screening panels, so the possibility of additional tests intensifies this issue. Some advocates take the stand that individuals should be able to make informed choices about their own health care, and that newborn screening should involve an informed consent process. At first, one might expect that every advocate would hold this opinion. However, some parents have a terrible fear in their gut that if they had been offered an option, they might have declined the test and their child might not have been diagnosed. They can imagine themselves being faced with a choice between making their precious newborn baby cry by jabbing him or her for blood versus an extremely remote chance that the infant has a rare condition with a cryptic, unpronounceable name. Because they fear that they might not have made the right choice, they want to protect other parents and ensure they make the "right choice" to have the testing performed. In addition, an argument can be made that if the testing requires a consent process, those who are less educated and more disenfranchised (distrustful of "the system") will be more likely to turn down testing, making informed consent a matter of subtle discrimination. (For additional discussion of the consent issue, see chapters 10, 12, 13, and 14.)

Most of the questions posed above are about whether testing *should* be done. But advocacy groups also need to understand the technical questions about whether testing *can* be done. These questions are not new, the standards have not changed, but organizations need to determine the answers for their condition of interest.

- Is there an existing test that can be applied on a population screening basis? If not, how likely is it that one could be developed? Should an advocacy group fund or advocate for funding the development of such a test?

- If there is such a test, how sensitive is it? How often is an individual who has the condition missed (a false negative)?

- How specific is the test? How often does the test identify a person as having the condition when in fact he or she does not have the condition (a false positive)? This becomes particularly important if a treatment regimen is initiated so that the adverse consequences of the condition are avoided. It becomes difficult to know whether or how severely that person would be affected had he or she not been treated.

When an organization has completed this process, has the answers to the questions, and is ready to make a case that the condition should be added to a newborn screening panel, the battle has barely begun. Because decisions about what tests are included in newborn screening panels are made by individual states, the battle has to be fought in every state.

Some of the most important work a lay advocacy group can do is to influence what comes after a test is adopted as a newborn screening test. Advocacy groups should appreciate better than anyone that a diagnosis is just step one.

A lifetime of living with the condition is ahead of the affected individuals and their families. Some of the most important issues an organization must deal with are:

- Is there appropriate follow-up care for individuals identified by the testing? Is this care timely and provided by a qualified health professional?
- How many cases are missed?
- Are there children who are identified and treated, yet might never have become ill from their condition?
- What is the difference in outcome between missed cases and identified cases?
- What are the gaps in the system of care?
- Are the turn-around times appropriate, from the blood draw to the onset of treatment?

Sometimes advocates are asked to serve on committees or councils. As a committee member it is critical for the advocate to know the role he or she is being asked to play. Advocates may be asked to participate as a representative of the membership of their group, to convey the consensus of the specific membership, and to advocate for the point of view of their membership. Alternatively, they may be asked to play a deliberative role as a member of an advisory group. In this role they are asked to participate because of their unique perspective. This particular role requires advocates to see the bigger picture and think of advocacy not in terms of their personal issue, but in terms of changing the landscape within which their specific advocacy group operates. The transition from a representative role to a deliberative role can be difficult for many advocates.

Often, which role one is asked to serve in can be determined just by sizing up the situation. If asked to participate in a meeting to discuss the possibility of adding three new tests to the newborn screening panel and members of all three advocacy groups are present, the advocate can be certain that the job is to represent the views of his or her specific group's members. If the advocate is the sole advocacy group representative at such a meeting, he or she needs to find out whether the job is to represent the other groups as well or to deliberate on the issues as someone with a consumer perspective. Being effective depends on a clear understanding of the role one is asked to play. (See chapter 7 for further discussion.)

Implications for Newborn Screening Policy

Newborn screening exists thanks to advocacy. The early proponents of newborn screening did not have extensive data from longitudinal double-blind treatment trials to determine efficacy. They had preliminary data that showed dramatic improvements in children with phenylketonuria (PKU) who were on a particular diet. Had conclusive data been required, the program would have been delayed a decade and hundreds of people would now be leading institutionalized instead of independent lives. Advocacy provides the passion and energy to strive to make life better—to take that leap of faith when there is a gap in the data.

In 1968, Wilson and Jungner published a list of criteria for the adoption of a condition for newborn screening (pp. 26–27):

1   The condition sought should be an important health problem.
2   There should be an accepted treatment for patients with recognized disease.
3   Facilities for diagnosis and treatment should be available.
4   There should be a recognizable latent or early asymptomatic stage.
5   There should be a suitable test or examination.
6   The test should be acceptable to the population.
7   The natural history of the condition, including development from latent to declared disease, should be adequately understood.
8   There should be an agreed policy on whom to treat as patients.
9   The cost of the case-finding (including diagnosis and treatment of patients diagnosed) should be economically balanced in relation to possible expenditure on medical care as a whole.
10   Case-finding should be a continuing process and not a "once and for all" project.

I would like to review these criteria, but before doing so I want to make sure the discussion is properly framed. Those who have been immersed in the issue of newborn screening for many years naturally tend to view newborn screening through the window defined by the current application. For example, there is a misconception that because newborn screening is currently a mandated public health program, any new tests must meet the criteria of a mandated public health test. I would like to completely remove these preconceptions from the following discussion. The criteria for testing need to be discussed with regard to the science and medicine. Only then can the process of applying the criteria, whether through a public health program or the private sector, be discussed. This is one area in which advocates can be helpful to the discussion. Because advocates are not a part of the application of newborn screening, they can help to refocus the discussion on the criteria when these are what is actually being discussed. Once the criteria are defined, then the application process that will produce the optimal result can be determined.

Since these criteria were published, medical technology, health care financing, medical therapy, and health care delivery have all changed dramatically. In addition, patient advocacy has increased hand in hand with the expectation that patients or their families will take increasing responsibility for their own medical decisions. Because of these fundamental changes in the medical landscape, the criteria on which newborn screening are based and the practical applications of how screening systems are performed need to be revisited. Additionally, the Wilson and Jungner criteria are full of words with subjective definitions, such as "adequate," "acceptable," "suitable," and "balanced." The changed landscape and the change in who is allowed to be part of the discussion create three main shifts in perspective that modify how the criteria would be addressed differently today. These changed perspectives are:

- The definition of treatment
- The decision-making balance of power
- Increasing consumer orientation

There is an increasing appreciation that treatment does not just mean a complete cure or complete prevention of any disease manifestations. Reducing someone's symptoms is equally important in the absence of any cure. The medical community often seems to believe that if medicine cannot offer a "cure," it is not worthwhile to test for the condition. This is where parents see things differently. While parents would like nothing more than a cure for their child's condition, in the absence of a cure there is still the day-in and day-out of life that must be managed as well as possible. The family has to deal with issues such as risks in future pregnancies, financial planning, educational choices, finding a support group, securing insurance, choice of job, and finding specialists. This affects every aspect of the family's life, and having a diagnosis adds clarity to this struggle. When you know what your child has, then you know what your child doesn't have. Without a diagnosis, you have no idea what is going wrong, what might go wrong, or how to effectively manage problems. While a diagnosis might be for a bad condition, knowing the diagnosis is a good thing. More than 30 conditions can be identified by tandem mass spectrometry (MS/MS). These conditions range from those that are a part of the traditional newborn screening panels to those that can merely be identified as the cause of death of a newborn. The following is a list of some of the possible types of outcomes from a condition identified by MS/MS:

- Effective and established treatment that averts severe disability
- Treatment with questionable efficacy in moderating the effects of a disease
- Identification of the cause of death of a newborn
- Risk awareness for future pregnancies
- Identification of a nonaverage metabolite level with unknown significance

Any of the above scenarios, as well as numerous variations of them, could describe the outcomes of conditions identified by MS/MS. Many parent advocates want a diagnosis for their child's condition regardless of how proven or unproven the treatment regimens. The rationale is that if we do not ever *try* to save these babies we will never learn *how* to save them. These questions will not be answered unless babies with these conditions are identified and there are potential research participants with whom research treatment protocols may be devised and implemented. So to identify a sufficient number of potential participants to generate meaningful results on rare conditions, a huge number of babies need to be screened. We will never get to treatment if we don't start with diagnosis.

The decision-making balance of power in health care has dramatically changed in the last 30 years. Patients are asking for and are being given more and more of the decision-making responsibility for their health care. The availability of health information for the lay public is increasing rapidly. There is now public access to research results via the internet, which has allowed patients and advocacy organizations to become increasingly well informed about the science and medicine that affect them. This information can be gathered without leaving home. Patients are arriving at their doctor's office with medical information from the internet in hand. The balance of power has shifted from physicians' decision to do as they see fit to a shared decision between the patient and the physician.

This change in the power balance goes hand in hand with the advocacy movement. Patients feel empowered to ask questions about additional testing or to get second opinions. Therefore, if the state says it is screening for 5 conditions, patient advocates feel free to ask why it cannot test for 6 conditions or 40 conditions. Some are happy to pay for the extras, but others ask why the extras are not available to everyone. At this point, the balance of power affects public health decisions. Decisions about public health are not based primarily on a feasibility study or a cost-benefit analysis, but are increasingly influenced by the voices of advocates.

The whole consumer and advocacy movement has shifted both the health care and the public health debates. Consumerism has been effective in creating change in science and medicine. But consumerism-based change happens on a purely opportunistic basis, often with a celebrity or wealthy person creating the opportunity. On the one hand it has effectively created change, but on the other hand it requires effective consumers for change to happen. For people with conditions that do not have a master organizer or a celebrity spokesperson, their condition may not receive equal deliberation and consequently equal funding. Media visibility and private money have created an uneven playing field that has spurred more progress on some conditions relative to others.

Layered on top of all of this is the widening gap between the medical "haves" and "have-nots." This is where we get into the application of newborn screening. The increase in health care disparities caused by our inability to solve the health care financing issue pressures public health into attempting to raise the safety net of minimal care in an effort to close that gap. This moves from the purely medical efficacy realm into the social justice realm. How important is it for newborn screening to be a part of public health, or for the testing to be conducted in public health laboratories? In the attempt to find answers to these questions, newborn screening becomes one component, one example, in the complex tug-of-war between socialism and capitalism in health care.

Given these changes in the health care landscape, each of the Wilson and Jungner criteria now has new points to be considered.

1 The condition sought should be an important health problem.
   - How is this defined, and by whom?
   - What weight does the economic burden to society carry?
   - Some conditions are high-impact but low-incidence, and others are low-impact but high-incidence. How should such differences be evaluated?
   - As a society, has our general thinking evolved from an exclusively civic-oriented evaluation of the question to one that is a little fur-

ther along the continuum toward a consumer-oriented evaluation of the question?

2 There should be an accepted treatment for patients with recognized disease.

- You cannot learn *how* to treat if you never *try* to treat. Some conditions may be high-impact and low-incidence, so the only way to identify a large enough cohort is to screen a large number of newborns.
- What is a treatment? Can this mean only an essential cure, so that no signs of disease are apparent if treatment is administered? What about a treatment that provides a better quality of life or a longer even though still shortened lifespan? What about the value of genetic counseling, which can occur only once there is a diagnosis? What if 50 percent of treated children have a significant benefit and the others do not?
- Where and how do we draw the line between matters of private health and matters of public health?

3 Facilities for diagnosis and treatment should be available.

- How are appropriate treatment facilities defined?
- Does a single medical facility have to provide all aspects of care if a multidisciplinary team is required (i.e., centers of excellence), or is it sufficient to have all the necessary providers available in the community?
- Facilities are rarely available before there is a demand for a service, so how reasonable is this requirement? Is it, rather, capability for expansion that is necessary (i.e., a master plan)?

4 There should be a recognizable latent or early asymptomatic stage.

- Do the early stages have to be asymptomatic? Many conditions first become apparent as an initial subtle failure to develop on the typical time frame, which is followed by a "diagnostic odyssey" as the child fails to keep up with developmental milestones. Earlier diagnosis may provide a more optimal intervention, or at the least may prevent an expensive search for a diagnosis.

5 There should be a suitable test or examination.

- Have standards changed?
- Is there a requirement for even higher efficiency and throughput?

6 The test should be acceptable to the population.

- Does this mean a test having "minimal risk" as defined by a human subjects review panel? If so, then this criterion has changed significantly since 1968.

7 The natural history of the condition, including development from latent to declared disease, should be adequately understood.
- In the perfect health care system, early detection means detection before the onset of symptoms. But in today's health care arena with so many uninsured people, early (presymptomatic) detection may mean preventing a long period between the onset of symptoms and a diagnosis, or no diagnosis.
- What if presymptomatic testing and treatment just slow the course of the disease or lessen the severity?

8 There should be an agreed policy on whom to treat as patients.
- In a case where genetic counseling is the only option, are parents considered patients?

9 The cost of the case-finding (including diagnosis and treatment of patients diagnosed) should be economically balanced in relation to possible expenditure on medical care as a whole.
- Does this balance include all the costs, including the cost of social and educational support?

10 Case-finding should be a continuing process, not a "once and for all" project.
- Shouldn't this also include case management?

The Immediate Challenges

In the near future there will be a huge increase in the number of screening tests that can be provided to newborns. The methodologies may be MS/MS or microarray or another, yet unimagined technique. Because these are "bundled" tests, with multiple conditions assessed in one experiment, the issue regarding which tests should be included is actually reversed. We are no longer making arguments about when to *include* a new test for a condition; we must argue about when to *exclude* a test from the panel.

Although many of these health care issues are within the jurisdiction of the states, there needs to be some consistency among states. If federal-level policy does not change, the following is likely to happen:

- There will continue to be large disparities between states in the screening tests performed and the quality of the follow-up care. This could put some states at risk for not providing services equal to those of other states.
- Families with health insurance will learn about expanded newborn screening and have the testing performed privately. Families without health insurance will not learn about or will not be able to afford the expanded private testing. This will result in a disproportionate number of uninsured children with delayed diagnoses and adverse outcomes. The cost of caring for these children will be much more likely to become the responsibility of the state.
- The increased number of affected children identified by expanded screening will create a huge financial burden on an already under-reimbursed clinical service, because even for patients with insurance, the reimbursement is insufficient to cover the cost of counseling and follow-up care.

To maximize the benefits to the health of children, several things need to happen:

- State screening programs need to find a way to coexist with private laboratories that provide similar or expanded service. They need to have comparable quality in testing and follow-up care, which will happen only through federal guidelines and funding.
- There need to be *national* guidelines on newborn screening that include a minimum testing panel and guidelines for follow-up care and reimbursement for that care. National guidelines will not only provide uniformity across the country but also prevent having to address the same questions 50 times.
- Federal support is required to implement expanded screening programs. Expanded programs have a large initial capital investment. The biggest cost will be the cost of sample collection, because more hospital staff with more training will be required, especially if they are obtaining consent. The laboratories will also need additional staff to coordinate the linkages between affected families and their physicians. Additionally, the follow-up care, genetic counseling, and special diets and therapies are expensive.
- Long-term follow-up programs for the affected individuals should be set up, and long-term evaluations of those programs.

Most advocates realize that what they want is unachievable, but they are ready to compromise and make the world better, one starfish at a time. Advocates are at the table to remind everyone why they are all there—because every person at the table wants to make a difference, too. Advocates are also there to provide punctuation. Advocacy ensures that there are only commas in the effort to make things better; there are no periods, because the work is never done. Your reach should always exceed your grasp.

REFERENCES

Eiseley, L. C. 1979. *The Star Thrower*. New York: Times Books.
Wilson, J. M. G., and Jungner, G. 1968. *Principles and Practice of Screening for Disease*. Geneva: World Health Organization.

RESOURCES

The Genetic Alliance (www.geneticalliance.org) is a source of other advocacy organizations.

The National Conference of State Legislatures (www.ncsl.org) is a resource for policy-related issues.

The National Newborn Screening and Genetics Resource Center (www.genes-r-us.uthscsa .edu) is a central resource for information and contacts on newborn screening. It has links to state health departments and information about newborn screening activities in each state.

CHAPTER 5

Newborn Screening for Conditions That Do Not Meet the Wilson and Jungner Criteria

The Case of Duchenne Muscular Dystrophy

LAINIE FRIEDMAN ROSS, M.D., PH.D.

The classic example of population screening in pediatrics is newborn screening for phenylketonuria (PKU), which began in the 1960s. In hindsight, it is easy to be critical of its rapid introduction as a mandatory universal screen and the concomitant iatrogenic problems that were caused by the poor understanding of the natural history of PKU and hyperphenylalaninemic variants and by inadequate data on who needed treatment and for how long (Committee for the Study of Inborn Errors of Metabolism 1975; Reilly 1977). Wilson and Jungner (1968) proposed 10 criteria that new screening programs should fill before they are introduced as a public health measure. Many newborn screening task forces (Committee for the Study of Inborn Errors of Metabolism, 1975; Institute of Medicine 1994; Newborn Screening Task Force 2000) have reaffirmed these criteria, albeit with some minor modifications (National Screening Committee 1998).

Four of the Wilson and Jungner criteria are: (1) the need for an accepted treatment for patients with recognized disease; (2) adequate understanding of the natural history of the condition; (3) an agreed policy on whom to treat as patients; and (4) a test or examination that is acceptable to the population. However, there are advocates who argue for expanding newborn screening even if the programs do not meet some of the traditional screening criteria, particularly when the condition can be identified using multiplex testing methodology such as tandem mass spectrometry (MS/MS) (Pollitt 1999; Therrell 2001; Fearing and Levy 2003). Duchenne muscular dystrophy (DMD) is an example of a condition for which there is some support for newborn screening even though it does not fulfill all of the Wilson and Jungner criteria (Bradley, Parsons, and Clarke 1993; Hildes et al. 1993; Drousiotou et al. 1998). In March 2004, the Centers for Disease Control and Prevention (2004) sponsored a one-day meeting to explore issues related to newborn screening for DMD. Following the meeting, the National Center on Birth Defects and Developmental Disabilities at the Centers for Disease Control announced that funds were available for research on screening of newborns and of infants (beyond the first month of life through 23 months), and grants were awarded to Columbus Children's Research Institute and Emory University, respectively (Centers for Disease Control and Prevention 2005).

Duchenne muscular dystrophy is an X-linked degenerative disease of skeletal muscle that affects approximately 1 in 3500 males. Because it is X-linked, girls are rarely affected. Symptoms of muscle degeneration in boys begin in early childhood. The condition is characterized by progressive loss of muscle strength leading to loss of ambulation and wheelchair dependency by adolescence. The two leading causes of death are respiratory and cardiac failure. The use of ventilators has extended life expectancy for those with respiratory insufficiency but not for those with cardiomyopathy (Miller, Colbert, and Schock 1988; Jeppesen et al. 2003). More recently, some women with a mutation in the dystrophin gene have been found to develop cardiomyopathies that are similar to those of males with DMD (Politano et al. 1996; Hoogerwaard et al. 1999).

Screening for DMD in newborns is done by measuring creatine phosphokinase (CPK; also known as creatine kinase, or CK). CPK can be measured from a bloodspot collected on the Guthrie card (Zellweger and Antonik 1975; Orfanos and Naylor 1984; Scheuerbrandt et al. 1986). Both affected boys and carrier girls have elevated levels of CPK in the newborn period. On average, the levels are much higher in affected boys than carrier girls, and the levels in girls may decrease to the normal range during infancy (Moser and Vogt 1974; Nicholson et al. 1979; Sumita et al. 1998). Screening for mutations in the dystrophin gene itself is possible, although the number of mutations (Muntoni, Torelli, and Ferlini 2003) and the size of the gene make testing difficult without an available affected proband (Hoffman et al. 1996; Alcantara et al.

2001). Identification of dystrophin mutations or muscle biopsies, or both, are used to confirm the diagnosis.

Newborn screening for DMD has been piloted in parts of the United States, Puerto Rico, Brazil, Cyprus, New Zealand, and France (Drummond and Veale 1978; Skinner et al. 1982; Plauchu et al. 1987; Naylor et al. 1992; Drousiotou et al. 1998). Currently, there are newborn screening programs in Wales (Bradley and Parsons 1998) and Manitoba, Canada (Greenberg et al. 1991). Germany offers testing between one month and one year of age (van Ommen and Scheuerbrandt 1993). There are no universal prenatal screening programs, although carrier testing of women with an affected male relative is available in many countries (targeted prenatal testing).

This chapter examines the pros and cons of screening newborns (and infants) for DMD. The analysis requires an examination of four overlapping policy and ethical issues. First, what are the risks and benefits of expanding newborn screening to include DMD? Second, if newborn screening were to expand to include DMD, should it require informed consent? Third, should newborn screening for DMD be limited to boys? Why or why not? Fourth, when is the ideal timing for screening (prenatal, newborn, or later in infancy) and what factors influence this determination?

Expanding Newborn Screening to Include Duchenne Muscular Dystrophy

The ethical and policy issues on expanding newborn screening to include DMD must begin with an examination of the public health nature of newborn screening (Khoury 1996; Holtzman 1997; Carlson 2004). With an incidence of 1 in 3500 boys, DMD is more common than PKU, the first condition for which universal newborn screening was implemented. CPK testing on Guthrie cards is a simple and accurate screen, and genetic confirmation and muscle biopsy are reliable confirmatory diagnostic tests. The natural history of the condition is understood. However, the main concern is whether early diagnosis improves prognosis. Although many treating neurologists use corticosteroids to prolong patients' ambulation (Wong and Christopher 2002; Bushby et al. 2004), when to start therapy is not clear (Moxley et al. 2005). The reason is that steroids are not without their own problems: they cause a decrease in bone density, worsen obesity, which can also curtail ambulation, and can lead to early development of cataracts or glaucoma. Moxley et al. (2005) reviewed all of the published clinical trials. They found scant data supporting use of steroids before the age of five years, an age by which most children with DMD will have been diagnosed even without newborn screening. Thus, if the recommendation is to begin steroids in the school-age child, there may not be a clinical need to diagnose the child's DMD predictively.

If one accepts the Wilson and Jungner (1968) criteria, then newborn screening for DMD can only be justified if it offers some therapeutic benefit to the child. Steroids are not standard of care for presymptomatic boys with DMD, and many who prescribe steroids wait until the child is older. Physiotherapy may be useful to younger boys, particularly those who are delayed in walking (Bradley and Parsons 1998), and respiratory muscle training has been suggested to reduce lung infections and delay respiratory failure, but the long-term benefits of these exercise programs are equivocal or modest at best (Eagle 2002).

Some argue that even without treatment, diagnosis promotes the child's best interest because it avoids the "diagnostic odyssey." Data show that it takes approximately two years from the time a mother first complains of her son's symptoms until a diagnosis is made (Crisp, Ziter, and Bray 1982; O'Brien, Sibert, and Harper 1983; Marshall and Galasko 1995; Bushby, Hill, and Steele 1999). One question is whether there is another way to shorten the diagnostic delay that avoids predictive testing. The obvious answer is to improve pediatricians' ability to recognize the early signs and symptoms of DMD. Early symptomatic diagnosis rather than diagnosis through the newborn screening program avoids labeling a child for future medical problems, while still leaving open the opportunities to pursue early experimental treatments. It avoids the problems of insurance discrimination because of a "preexisting condition" (Kaback 1994; Kass 1997). It also avoids the potential negative psychological reactions of parents to an early diagnosis (Clarke 1994; Institute of Medicine 1994; American Society of Human Genetics and American College of Medical Genetics 1995; American Academy of Pediatrics 2001). The problem is that the delay in diagnosing DMD has not improved over time (Crisp, Ziter, and Bray 1982; O'Brien, Sibert, and Harper 1983; Marshall and Galasko 1995; Bushby, Hill, and Steele 1999), and some data show that proposed strategies to improve diagnosis will be ineffective for a significant percentage of affected children (Parsons, Clarke, and Bradley 2004). This means that if avoidance of the diagnostic odyssey is an important goal, presymptomatic screening may be the only way to achieve it.

Another potential benefit of early diagnosis is parents' gain of reproductive knowledge, although professional consensus statements reject this as a reason for newborn screening (Institute of Medicine 1994; American Academy of Pediatrics 2001). If reproductive knowledge is a valid goal—and it is clear that many physicians and parents believe that it is (Zellweger and Antonik 1975; Scheuerbrandt et al. 1986; Bradley and Parsons 1998)—the question remains as to what is or ought to be the goal of reproductive knowledge. Although some physicians argue that screening needs to occur in the newborn period to provide adequate time for families to use this information in their family planning decisions, the data about whether the information is useful or used are equivocal. While the data from Wales show that most families take advantage of genetic counseling and prenatal testing (Bradley and Parsons 1998), the Manitoba group found that most families did not (Hildes et al. 1993) and the Lyon program found that the acceptability of prenatal genetic counseling and testing depended on religious and ethnic identification (Robert 1990). Fifty percent of at-risk women and couples accepted counseling in the German program, but only after repeated offers (Scheuerbrandt et al. 1986).

Another controversial matter is what should count as success in prenatal counseling (Rowley 1984; Chadwick 1993). A consensus statement by the European Neuromuscular Center in 1993 concluded that "the goal of neonatal DMD screening should not be stated in terms of prevention of new DMD cases" (van Ommen and Scheuerbrandt 1993, p. 234). Rather, the authors argued that success should be understood in terms of promoting reproductive choice. There are nonmedical practical benefits that can accrue from an early diagnosis. Families may use this information for life planning (e.g., buying a ranch house rather than a walk-up). It also permits families to adjust to the diagnosis and respects parents' right to know their child's genetic makeup (Michie et al. 1996; Patenaude et al. 1996; Bradley and Parsons 1998). Many parents of children with serious and life-threatening conditions state that they want this information as early as possible, even if treatments are not available (Scheuerbrandt 1980; Malkin et al. 1996; Patenaude et al. 1996; Parsons et al. 2002).

But this benefit must be weighed against the harms of diagnosing a child with a fatal disease months before he would be diagnosed clinically. One major concern is the impact, if any, on parent-child bonding. The data to date do not find that this information disrupts parent-child bonding, although it can cause a transient increase in anxiety (Parsons et al. 2002). There are also the concerns that parents may misuse the information and seek out alternative and potentially dangerous treatments (Campbell and Ross 2005).

False positives are another risk of screening. Although Parsons et al. (2002) did not find long-term negative psychosocial sequelae in the parents of boys with false positive screening results, other screening programs have found short-term and long-term anxiety and psychological distress (J. M. Green et al. 2004).

Overall, including DMD in newborn screening has potential benefits and risks, and individual couples and families may decide differently on whether or not the benefit-to-risk ratio is positive. But even for those who support screening, the question that remains is whether offering DMD screening as an add-on to newborn screening minimizes risks (Ross 2003) or whether an alternative screening time (later in infancy) might provide the same benefits at lower risk. I will return to this concern later.

Consent for Duchenne Muscular Dystrophy in Newborn Screening Programs

If one believes that it is reasonable for some parents to choose newborn screening for DMD and for other parents to refuse to test their children, then screening for DMD ought to be voluntary. To be voluntary, it requires the informed consent of the infant's parent(s). Most newborn screening programs for DMD seek explicit consent, although some permit an informed dissent or an opt-out program (van Ommen and Scheuerbrandt 1993; Clarke 1997). In Wales, where informed consent is required, the participation rate is approximately 94 percent when screening is done in the newborn period (Clarke 1997).

Why do so many parents consent to such screening if the benefit-to-risk ratio is equivocal? It is interesting to note that approximately 94 percent of parents also consent to newborn screening for type 1 diabetes when it is offered in the research context, even though a positive result from this newborn screening confirms only a 4 to 10 percent risk of developing diabetes (Flanders, Graves, and Rewers 1999; Kimpimaki et al. 2001). In part, the high uptake can be explained by our culture's unequivocal support for testing generally (Nelkin and Tancredi 1989; Wertz 2002), despite warnings to the contrary (Croyle 1995; Malm 1999; Ewart 2000; Raffle 2001; Marteau and Kinmonth 2002).

The high uptake may also be explainable, in part, by how the test is offered. Data show that uptake is highest when requested in person and when testing can be done immediately (Bekker et al. 1993). One way to promote informed decision making, then, would be to require more active parental involvement. To this end, Clarke and colleagues implemented a pilot project in England to determine the feasibility of providing newborn screening for DMD in a way that made the optional nature of the test explicit (Parsons et al. 2000). Health visitors sought consent from parents for traditional newborn screening samples and to screen for DMD. If the parents consented to the latter, the health visitor procured two Guthrie cards. Parents were given the second card and told to mail the card in a few days if they were still interested in knowing whether their son was at risk for DMD. The result was an uptake of 78 percent, significantly lower than the 94 percent uptake in Wales, where consent for DMD screening is obtained such that CPK testing can be done at the same time as screening for other conditions and using the same bloodspot. Clarke had earlier argued that a lower uptake rate for DMD screening was desirable: "To suggest that a lower uptake rate for a screening test would be preferable, that we should set a threshold of motivation so that infants are not screened unless their parents actively choose it, is certainly unusual but is perfectly appropriate in the context of an untreatable disease" (Clarke 1997, p. 115). One problem is that it is not clear that boys' parents who did not mail the second Guthrie card were refusing screening for them; rather, it may be that their parents simply forgot to mail in the card or did not understand the instructions.

DMD screening in Germany is done between 1 and 12 months of age and the uptake is much lower (approximately 5%) (van Ommen and Scheuerbrandt 1993). Whether the lower uptake reflects improved decision making because families have more time to consider the risks and benefits is indeterminable because other differences make direct comparisons useless. In Germany, DMD screening is offered in the practitioner's office and costs 15 euros. There are no data to show that all practitioners are offering the testing or that they are offering it in a way that promotes informed choice. Still, there are reasons to believe that uptake would be lower if the test were offered beyond the newborn period, even if it were free and even if it were being promoted by practitioners. Consider, for example, how difficult it is to get parents to comply with other pediatric public health programs such as immunizations (Mell et al. 2005).

Clarke's concern that 94 percent uptake is too high is supported by the low uptake by adults of testing for untreatable conditions such as Huntington disease (Chapman 1992; Laccone et al. 1999). The analogy is not perfect because the decision to test for Huntington disease is made by the adult at risk, whereas the decision to test for DMD is made by a parent. If anything, parents should be more circumspect in seeking predictive information about their children than about themselves (Ross 2002).

Delaying the mailing in of the bloodspot, as noted above, led to a modest decrease in DMD testing of newborns. Another possible method to decrease uptake would be to provide opportunities for prospective parents and pregnant women and couples to consider the risks and benefits of screening in a peer group setting, so that they can make a more informed decision after the birth of their children. Campbell and Ross (2003) conducted focus groups with parents in Illinois and found much less hypothetical interest in screening for DMD than currently expressed in Wales. The focus group participants supported greater discussion of newborn screening options in the prenatal period as a way to give them greater opportunity to make an informed decision (Campbell and Ross 2003, 2004). Whether the authors' data would translate into lower uptake in the clinical setting remains to be tested.

The ideal uptake for predictive testing of DMD is unknown. It depends, in part, on the goals of screening. The informed consent process can help clarify the benefits and risks for individual children and families and help ensure that the uptake reflects voluntary choice.

Whether to Test Boys Only or All Children

If the purpose of screening for DMD is to promote medical benefit—to provide the opportunity for early interventions and to avoid a diagnostic odyssey—then DMD screening should be restricted to young boys. There are several arguments, however, to include young girls. First, although it is rare for girls to develop symptoms of musculoskeletal degeneration, some girls do (Grain et al. 2001). Most have mild symptoms, but some girls are more severely affected (Shigihara-Yasuda et al. 1992; Romero et al. 2001). Second, another important benefit of newborn screening is reproductive information for families. The diagnosis of female carriers could alert families to their risk before the birth of an affected male. Third, although rarely symptomatic in childhood (Nolan et al. 2003), 10 to 20 percent of female carriers may have cardiac problems as adults (Politano et al. 1996; Grain et al. 2001).

These benefits raise an ethical problem in the screening of girls, because this leads to the diagnosis of individuals who are rarely affected in childhood but who have a 10 to 20 percent risk of developing cardiac abnormalities in adulthood and are at risk for having an affected child. The consensus statements are clear that carrier testing and screening for adult-onset conditions should be delayed until adulthood (Clarke 1994; American Society of Human Genetics and American College of Medical Genetics 1995; American Academy of Pediatrics 2001), although some parents and parental advocacy groups support testing of children (Dalby 1995; Campbell and Ross 2003, 2005). The concerns are the potential negative impact of information about being a carrier on self-esteem and the child's relationships with family and other third parties (Clarke 1994; American Society of Human Genetics and American College of Medical Genetics 1995). There are limited empirical studies to assess this claim. Preliminary data from Jarvinen and Kaariainen (1998) did not reveal any obvious psychological harm, but clearly more long-term follow-up data are needed.

One of the risks of CPK screening of infant girls is that the test is less sensitive in carrier girls than in affected boys. The decreased sensitivity means that the testing of girls may provide false reassurance (Petticrew et al. 2000). It also means that a negative test result could increase the delay in diagnosis of mildly affected girls (manifesting carriers) and increase distrust in the health care system (O'Brien, Sibert, and Harper 1983; Bushby, Hill, and Steele 1999). A second risk of CPK screening in girls is that the diagnosis of carrier girls does not distinguish between those who will be manifesting carriers, those who may develop symptoms as adults, and those who will be healthy and have only the reproductive risks associated with their carrier status. This could lead to increased anxiety on the part of parents and result in the "vulnerable child syndrome" (M. Green and Solnit 1964).

So the question of whether to screen only boys or both boys and girls depends on what the goals of screening are. If the goal is solely to detect children who will become symptomatic in the next decade and for whom early or experimental treatment may need to begin before symptoms develop, then one could argue for screening only boys, acknowledging that a rare manifesting carrier girl will be missed. If the goal of screening is to detect at-risk families, then boys and girls should be screened, but this raises the question of why screen in the newborn period (or beyond) rather than screen prenatally. If both goals are important, then it may be necessary to recommend screening of women prenatally and children postnatally, as is currently done for sickle cell anemia (Whitten and Whitten-Shurney 2001) and cystic fibrosis (Murray et al. 1999).

Timing of Screening

As suggested above, if the primary goal of DMD screening is to provide reproductive information and counseling to women at risk, why not screen all women prenatally? If the goal is reproductive knowledge, one can argue that newborn screening is too late because it detects affected probands only after they are born. One practical argument against prenatal screening is that many women do not seek prenatal care until they have conceived. A more serious practical problem is that there is no simple screening test to identify carrier women in the general population. Measuring CPK is not an accurate screen in adult women. Prenatal screening of adult women would have to involve genetic testing or biopsy. The genetic mutations for DMD are numerous, and the available tests are currently expensive and inaccurate in the general, low-risk population. Biopsies are too invasive for a screening test. Likewise, one could test the fetus in utero, but unless such testing were targeted to the fetuses of carrier women, it would require much invasive testing—which is not recommended in low-risk pregnancies.

Even if prenatal screening of adult women were feasible, one must ask whether it achieves the full benefits of screening. Only two-thirds of infants with DMD are born to women with a mutation. This means that one-third of affected boys will be missed because they have de novo mutations. If early diagnosis and avoiding the diagnostic odyssey are important, then prenatal screening of women alone is inadequate because it would miss at least one-third of clinical cases.

If the clinical benefits of early diagnosis and avoiding the diagnostic odyssey are the primary goals of screening, it is critical to test children before they become symptomatic. And if the goal is to avoid the odyssey, one may want to screen infant boys and girls so as not to miss the mildly affected girl (i.e., a manifesting carrier). Case reports reveal that there may be diagnostic delays or misdiagnoses of girls and adult women who are manifesting carriers (Kinoshita et al. 1995; Hoffman et al. 1996).

If presymptomatic screening of children is justifiable, the question remains whether screening should be in the newborn period or later in the first year of life. The benefit of delaying the screening is that it avoids confusing the public health nature of newborn screening for conditions in which early treatment minimizes morbidity and mortality with the benefits of predictive screening. One problem with delaying the testing is that CPK normalizes in many carrier girls by one year of age (Moser and Vogt, 1974; Nicholson et al. 1979; Sumita et al. 1998). A second problem is that it requires a separate blood draw, and parents and pediatricians do not want a second "heel stick" (Campbell and Ross 2003; Acharya, Ackerman, and Ross 2005). This problem can be minimized by bundling the screening with other blood screening (e.g., for lead or hemoglobin) that is recommended around 9 to 12 months of age. A third problem is that the delay separates the screening from the highly effective system already in place for testing, counseling, and follow-up in newborn screening programs (Newborn Screening Task Force 2000). Problems in follow-up and counseling may be more likely if screening is performed in individual physicians' offices without the support of the public health system.

In 1976, Gilboa and Swanson argued that DMD screening should be postponed beyond the immediate newborn period to avoid practical problems. Screening beyond the newborn period sidesteps the problem of CPK inconsistencies due to birth trauma, mode of delivery, and other nonspecific causes of CPK elevations that occur around the time of birth but revert to normal in days to weeks. There is also an ethical argument to delay DMD screening. Separating the sample and the time of testing helps distinguish predictive testing from conventional newborn screening programs designed as public health programs. It may also be easier to maintain the voluntary nature of the DMD screening program when the test is offered beyond the immediate newborn period.

Whether or Not to Screen for DMD

The discussions about which populations should be screened and the ideal timing of such screening assume that we should screen. But this is a policy decision that should be made only after extensive discourse in the public and professional communities, because it reflects a change in our traditional public health screening model. Whereas the traditional model focused on the detection of conditions for which early medical and dietary treatment could minimize serious morbidity or mortality, the newer programs seek to use a broader notion of benefit (Bailey, Skinner, and Warren 2005).

Like virtually all screening programs, screening for DMD has benefits and risks. Although many parents support screening for early detection, numerous consensus statements argue against predictive testing and screening of children (Clarke 1994; American Society of Human Genetics and American College of Medical Genetics 1995; American Academy of Pediatrics 2001). Elsewhere I have shown that the consensus statements fail to distinguish between predictive screening for early-onset conditions and adult-onset conditions (Ross 2002). It is reasonable and within the moral realm for parents to decide that the benefits of predictive screening for childhood-onset conditions such as DMD outweigh the harms. I argued in favor of supporting parental decisions, emphasizing that these programs should not be mandatory but should require a robust informed consent process. It would also be reasonable and within the moral realm to support adult women who seek such screening prenatally, although there is no valid prenatal screening test at present.

Given the risks and benefits of predictive screening, and given that DMD screening does not fulfill the Wilson and Jungner criteria, the focus of a screening program for DMD should seek to ensure that parental decision making is informed and should not be designed to maximize uptake. This would mean that if children are to be screened, screening should be offered beyond the newborn period. But whether to recommend screening for boys only or for all infants will depend on the goals of screening.

Policy Implications

Part of the debate on whether and when to screen for DMD should consider funding issues. Traditional newborn screening is paid for in a variety of ways, depending on the state in which the child is born (Association of State and Territorial Health Officials 2005). Funding and access for prenatal testing is more decentralized, with great disparities, and the accessibility and affordability of abortion even more so.

The main justification for state funding of DMD screening of infants is to ensure equity. In fact, equity concerns would also support screening in the newborn period using the Guthrie card, because disparities in pediatric care begin shortly after discharge from the newborn nursery (Olson, Tang, and Newacheck 2005).

Arguments for equity are powerful when the condition is one for which early treatment reduces morbidity and mortality. When the condition fails to meet the Wilson and Jungner criteria, however, one must consider the opportunity costs that such screening entails. Screening for DMD would have to compete with other public health programs that vie for state funding. Alternatively, such programs could be offered for a fee, but this would lead to disparities in access. Whether differential access is a problem, however, depends on what is being offered and what benefits it provides. In the case of DMD screening in infancy, early diagnosis provides predictive genetic information that may result in some clinical, psychosocial, and reproductive benefits as well as harms. Currently, such screening will not reduce serious morbidity or mortality of affected individuals. Given the ambiguity in benefit-to-harm ratio at this time, state funding is not morally obligatory and screening beyond the nursery to permit greater voluntariness in the informed consent process would be morally preferable.

One Caveat

Policy decisions about whether and when to offer screening for DMD and how to fund it should not be understood as an exceptional issue. There are other conditions that do not meet the traditional Wilson and Jungner criteria for which infant screening and prenatal screening programs are being developed (e.g., fragile X syndrome, predisposition for type 1 diabetes). Our policy decisions about when, how, and whom to screen ought to reflect a balance between maximizing uptake and diagnosis and maximizing autonomy and choice with respect to genetic information. While I have argued that screening for DMD in infancy is a valid moral option, I reject incorporating such a program into the mandatory newborn screening program. Rather, I propose that screening for DMD should be offered, on a voluntary basis, beyond the newborn period. Whether these programs are state-subsidized should depend on how the benefit-to-harm ratio compares with that of other, competing public health programs.

ACKNOWLEDGMENTS

An earlier version of this chapter was previously published in *American Journal of Medical Genetics* 140 (8): 914–22, copyright © 2006 AJMG, and is used with permission of Wiley-Liss, Inc., a subsidiary of John Wiley & Sons, Inc.

This work was supported by a grant from the National Institute of Child Health and Human

Development (NICHD) Newborn Genetic Screening: For Whose Benefit. An earlier draft of this manuscript was presented at the Hastings Center, Garrison, New York, in June 2005. I thank Paul Fernhoff, Ben Wilfond, Andrea Bonnicksen, Nancy Green, Ellen Wright Clayton, Scott Grosse, and two anonymous reviewers for thoughtful written comments on earlier drafts.

REFERENCES

Acharya, K., Ackerman, P. D., and Ross, L. F. 2005. Pediatricians' attitudes toward expanding newborn screening. *Pediatrics* 116 (4): e476–84 (available at http://pediatrics.aappubli cations.org/cgi/reprint/116/4/e476).

Alcantara, M. A., Garcia-Cavazos, R., Hernandez, U. E., Gonzalez-del Angel, A., Carnevale, A., and Orozco, L. 2001. Carrier detection and prenatal molecular diagnosis in a Duchenne muscular dystrophy family without any affected relative available. *Ann Genet* 44 (3): 149–53.

American Academy of Pediatrics, Committee on Bioethics. 2001. Ethical issues with genetic testing in pediatrics. *Pediatrics* 107 (6): 1451–55.

American Society of Human Genetics and American College of Medical Genetics. 1995. Points to consider: ethical, legal, and psychosocial implications of genetic testing in children and adolescents. *Am J Hum Genet* 57 (5): 1233–41.

Association of State and Territorial Health Officials. 2005. Financing state newborn screening systems in an era of change. www.astho.org/pubs/newbornscreening(3).pdf.

Bailey, D. B. Jr., Skinner, D., and Warren, S. F. 2005. Newborn screening for developmental disabilities: reframing presumptive benefit. *Am J Public Health* 95 (11): 1889–93.

Bekker, H., Modell, M., Denniss, G., Bobrow, M., and Marteau, T. 1993. Uptake of cystic fibrosis testing in primary care: supply push or demand pull? *BMJ* 306 (6892): 1584–86.

Bradley, D., and Parsons, E. 1998. Newborn screening for Duchenne muscular dystrophy. *Semin Neonatol* 3 (1): 27–34.

Bradley, D. M., Parsons, E. P., and Clarke, A. J. 1993. Experience with screening newborns for Duchenne muscular dystrophy in Wales. *BMJ* 306 (6874): 357–60.

Bushby, K. M. D., Hill, A., and Steele, J. G. 1999. Failure of early diagnosis in symptomatic Duchenne muscular dystrophy. *Lancet* 353 (9152): 557–58.

Bushby, K., Muntoni, F., Urtizberea, A., Hughes, R., and Griggs, R. 2004. Treatment of Duchenne muscular dystrophy: defining the gold standards of management in the use of corticosteroids. Report on the 124th ENMC (European Neuromuscular Center) International Workshop, 2–4 April 2004, Naarden, The Netherlands. *Neuromuscul Disord* 14 (8–9): 526–34.

Campbell, E., and Ross, L. F. 2003. Parental attitudes regarding newborn screening of PKU and DMD. *Am J Med Genet A* 120A (2): 209–14.

———. 2004. Incorporating newborn screening into prenatal care. *Am J Obstet Gynecol* 190 (4): 876–77.

———. 2005. Parental attitudes and beliefs regarding the genetic testing of children. *Community Genet* 8 (2): 94–102.

Carlson, M. D. 2004. Recent advances in newborn screening for neurometabolic disorders. *Curr Opin Neurol* 17 (2): 133–38.

Centers for Disease Control and Prevention. 2004. Newborn screening for Duchenne muscular dystrophy workgroup: lay report (of a meeting held March 2004). www.cdc.gov/ncbddd/duchenne/documents/NBS_Lay_Report.pdf.

———. 2005. Duchenne and Becker muscular dystrophy: activities update 2005. www.cdc.gov/ncbddd/duchenne/documents/CDCActivites2005.pdf.

Chadwick, R. F. 1993. What counts as success in genetic counselling? *J Med Ethics* 19 (1): 43–46.

Chapman, M. A. 1992. Canadian experience with predictive testing for Huntington disease: lessons for genetic testing centers and policymakers. *Am J Med Genet* 42 (4): 491–98.

Clarke, A. 1994. The genetic testing of children. Working Party of the Clinical Genetics Society (U.K.). *J Med Genet* 31 (10): 785–97.

———.1997. Newborn screening. In *Genetics, Society and Clinical Practice*, ed. P. S. Harper and A. J. Clarke, pp. 107–17. Oxford: BIOS Scientific.

Committee for the Study of Inborn Errors of Metabolism, Division of Medical Sciences, Assembly of Life Sciences, National Research Council. 1975. *Genetic Screening: Programs, Principles, and Research*. Washington DC: National Academy of Sciences.

Crisp, D. E., Ziter, F. A., and Bray, P. F. 1982. Diagnostic delay in Duchenne's muscular dystrophy. *JAMA* 247 (4): 478–80.

Croyle, R. T., ed. 1995. *Psychosocial Effects of Screening for Disease Prevention and Detection*. New York: Oxford University Press.

Dalby, S. 1995. GIG (Genetic Interest Group) response to the UK Clinical Genetics Society report "The genetic testing of children." *J Med Genet* 32 (6): 490–92.

Drousiotou, A., Ioannou, P., Georgiou, T., Mavrikiou, E., Christopoulos, G., Kyriakides, T., Voyasianos, M., Argyriou, A., and Middleton, L. 1998. A novel semiquantitative application of the bioluminescence test for creatine kinase in a pilot national program in Cyprus. *Genet Test* 2 (1): 55–60.

Drummond, L. M., and Veale, A. M. 1978. Muscular dystrophy screening. *Lancet* 1 (8076): 1258–59.

Eagle, M. 2002. Report on the muscular dystrophy campaign workshop: exercise in neuromuscular diseases. Newcastle, January 2002. *Neuromuscul Disord* 12 (10): 975–83.

Ewart, R. M. 2000. Primum non nocere and the quality of evidence: rethinking the ethics of screening. *J Am Board Fam Pract* 13 (3): 188–96.

Fearing, M. K, and Levy, H. L. 2003. Expanded newborn screening using tandem mass spectrometry. *Adv Pediatr* 50:81–111.

Flanders, G., Graves, P., and Rewers, M. 1999. Prevention of type 1 diabetes from laboratory to public health. *Autoimmunity* 29 (3): 235–46.

Gilboa, N., and Swanson, J.R. 1976. Serum creatine phosphokinase in normal newborns. *Arch Dis Child* 51 (4): 283–85.

Grain, L., Cortina-Borja, M., Forfar, C., Hilton-Jones, D., Hopkin, J., and Burch, M. 2001. Cardiac abnormalities and skeletal muscle weakness in carriers of Duchenne and Becker muscular dystrophies and controls. *Neuromuscul Disord* 11 (2): 186–91.

Green, J. M., Hewison, J., Bekker, H. L., Bryant, L. D., and Cuckle H. S. 2004. Psychosocial aspects of genetic screening of pregnant women and newborns: a systematic review. *Health Technol Assess* 8 (33): iii, ix–x, 1–109.

Green, M., and Solnit, A. A. 1964. Reactions to the threatened loss of a child: a vulnerable child syndrome. Pediatric management of the dying child, part III. *Pediatrics* 34:58–66.

Greenberg, C. R., Jacobs, H. K., Halliday, W., and Wrogemann K. 1991. Three years' experience with neonatal screening for Duchenne/Becker muscular dystrophy: gene analysis, gene expression, and phenotype prediction. *Am J Med Genet* 39 (1): 68–75.

Hildes, E., Jacobs, H. K., Cameron, A., Seshia, S. S., Booth, F., Evans, J. A., Wrogemann, K., and Greenberg, C. R. 1993. Impact of genetic counseling after neonatal screening for Duchenne muscular dystrophy. *J Med Genet* 30 (8): 670–74.

Hoffman, E. P., Pegoraro, E., Scacheri, P., Burns, R. G., Taber, J. W., Weiss, L., Spiro, A., and Blattner, P. 1996. Genetic counseling of isolated carriers of Duchenne muscular dystrophy. *Am J Med Genet* 63 (4): 573–80.

Holtzman, N. A. 1997. Genetic screening and public health. *Am J Public Health* 87 (8): 1275–77.

Hoogerwaard, E. M., Bakker, E., Ippel, P. F., Oosterwijk, J. C., Majoor-Krakauer, D. F., Leschot, N. J., Van Essen, A. J., Brunner, H. G., van der Wouw, P. A., Wilde, A. A., and de Visser, M. 1999. Signs and symptoms of Duchenne muscular dystrophy and Becker muscular dystrophy among carriers in The Netherlands: a cohort study. *Lancet* 353 (9170): 2116–19.

Institute of Medicine, Division of Health Sciences Policy, Committee on Assessing Genetic Risks. 1994. *Assessing Genetic Risks: Implications for Heath and Social Policy.* Washington DC: National Academy of Sciences.

Jarvinen, O., and Kaariainen, H. 1998. A retrospective study of genetic carrier testing in childhood. In *The Genetic Testing of Children*, ed. A. J. Clark, pp. 91–96. Oxford: BIOS Scientific.

Jeppesen, J., Green, A., Steffensen, B. F., and Rahbek, J. 2003. The Duchenne muscular dystrophy population in Denmark, 1977–2001: prevalence, incidence and survival in relation to the introduction of ventilator use. *Neuromuscul Disord* 13 (10): 804–12.

Kaback, M. M. 1994. Perspectives in genetic screening: principles and implications. *Int J Technol Assess Health Care* 10 (4): 592–603.

Kass, N.E. 1997. The implications of genetic testing for health and life insurance. In *Genetic Secrets: Protecting Privacy and Confidentiality in the Genetic Era*, ed. M. A. Rothstein, pp. 299–316. New Haven: Yale University Press.

Khoury, M. J. 1996. From genes to public health: the applications of genetic technology in disease prevention. Genetics Working Group. *Am J Public Health* 86 (12): 1717–22.

Kimpimaki, T., Kupila, A., Hamalainen, A. M., Kukko, M., Kulmala, P., Savola, K., Simell, T., Keskinen, P., Ilonen, J., Simell, O., and Knip, M. 2001. The first signs of B-cell autoimmunity appear in infancy in genetically susceptible children from the general population: the Finnish type I diabetes prediction and prevention study. *J Clinic Endocrinol Metab* 86 (10): 4782–86.

Kinoshita, H., Goto, Y., Ishikawa, M., Uemura, T., Matsumoto, K., Hayashi, Y. K., Arahata, K., and Nonaka, I. 1995. A carrier of Duchenne muscular dystrophy with dilated cardiomyopathy but no skeletal muscle symptom. *Brain Dev* 17 (3): 202–5.

Laccone, F., Engel, U., Holinski-Feder, E., Weigell-Weber, M., Marczinek, K., Nolte, D., Morris-Rosendahl, D. J., Zuhlke, C., Fuchs, K., Weirich-Schwaiger, H., Schluter, G., von Beust, G., Vieira-Saecker, A. M., Weber, B. H., and Riess, O. 1999. DNA analysis of Huntington's disease: five years of experience in Germany, Austria, and Switzerland. *Neurology* 53 (4): 801–6.

Malkin, D., Australie, K., Shuman, C., Barrera, M., and Weksberg, R. 1996. Parental attitudes to genetic counseling and predictive testing for childhood cancer. *Am J Hum Genet* 59 (4): A7.

Malm, H. M. 1999. Medical screening and the value of early detection: when unwarranted faith leads to unethical recommendations. *Hastings Center Rep* 29 (1): 26–37.

Marshall, P. D., and Galasko, C. S. B. 1995. No improvement in delay of diagnosis of Duchenne muscular dystrophy. *Lancet* 345 (8949): 590–91.

Marteau, T. M., and Kinmonth, A. L. 2002. Screening for cardiovascular risk: public health imperative or matter for individual informed choice? *BMJ* 325 (7355): 78–80.

Mell, L. K., Ogren, D. S., Davis, R. L., Mullooly, J. P., Black, S. B., Shinefield, H. R., Zangwill, K. M., Ward, J. I., Marcy, S. M., Chen, R. T., for the Centers for Disease Control and Prevention Vaccine Safety Datalink Project. 2005. Compliance with national immunization guidelines for children younger than 2 years, 1996–1999. *Pediatrics* 115 (2): 461–67.

Michie, S., McDonald, V., Bobrow, M., McKeown, C., and Marteau, T. 1996. Parents' responses to predictive genetic testing in their children: report of a single case study. *J Med Genet* 33 (4): 313–18.

Miller, J. R., Colbert, A. P., and Schock, N. C. 1988. Ventilator use in progressive neuromuscular disease: impact on patients and their families. *Dev Med Child Neurol* 30 (2): 200–207.

Moser, H., and Vogt, J. 1974. Follow up study of serum creatine-kinase in carriers of Duchenne muscular dystrophy. *Lancet* 2 (7881): 661–62.

Moxley, R.T. III, Ashwal, S., Pandya, S., Connolly, A., Florence, J., Mathews, K., Baumbach, L., McDonald, C., Sussman, M., Wade, C., for the Quality Standards Subcommittee of the American Academy of Neurology and Practice Committee of the Child Neurology Society. 2005. Practice parameter: corticosteroid treatment of Duchenne dystrophy. Report of the Quality Standards Subcommittee of the American Academy of Neurology and the Practice Committee of the Child Neurology Society. *Neurology* 64 (1): 13–20.

Muntoni, F., Torelli, S., and Ferlini, A. 2003. Dystrophin and mutations: one gene, several proteins, multiple phenotypes. *Lancet Neurol* 2 (12): 731–40.

Murray, J., Cuckle, H., Taylor, G., Littlewood, J., and Hewison, J. 1999. Screening for cystic fibrosis. *Health Technol Assess* 3 (8): i–iv, 1–104.

National Screening Committee. 1998. *First Report*. London: Department of Health (available at www.nsc.nhs.uk/pdfs/nsc_firstreport.pdf).

Naylor, E. W., Hoffman, E. P., Paulus-Thomas, J., Wessel, H. B., Reid, K. S., Mitchell, B., and Schmidt, B. J. 1992. Neonatal screening for Duchenne/Becker muscular dystrophy: reconsideration based on molecular diagnosis and potential therapeutics. *Screening* 1:99–113.

Nelkin, D., and Tancredi, L. 1989. *Dangerous Diagnostics: The Social Power of Biological Information*. New York: Basic Books.

Newborn Screening Task Force. 2000. Serving the family from birth to the medical home: a report from the Newborn Screening Task Force convened in Washington DC, May 10–11, 1999. *Pediatrics* 106 (2 Pt 2): 383–427.

Nicholson, G. A., Gardner-Medwin, D., Pennington, R. J. T., and Walton, J. N. 1979. Carrier detection in Duchenne muscular dystrophy: assessment of the effect of age on detection-rate with serum creatine-kinase activity. *Lancet* 1 (8118): 692–94.

Nolan, M. A., Jones, O. D., Pedersen, R. L., and Johnston, H. M. 2003. Cardiac assessment in childhood carriers of Duchenne and Becker muscular dystrophies. *Neuromuscul Disord* 13 (2): 129–32.

O'Brien, T., Sibert, J. R., and Harper, P. S. 1983. Implications of diagnostic delay in Duchenne muscular dystrophy. *BMJ* 287 (6399): 1106–7.

Olson, L. M., Tang, S. F., and Newacheck, P. W. 2005. Children in the United States with discontinuous health insurance coverage. *N Engl J Med* 353 (4): 382–91.

Orfanos, A. P., and Naylor, E. W. 1984. A rapid screening test for Duchenne muscular dystrophy using dried blood samples. *Clin Chim Acta* 138 (3): 267–74.

Parsons, E. P., Clarke, A. J., and Bradley, D. M. 2004. Developmental progress in Duchenne muscular dystrophy: lessons for earlier detection. *Eur J Paediatr Neurol* 8 (3): 145–53.

Parsons, E. P., Clarke, A. J., Hood, K., and Bradley, D. M. 2000. Feasibility of a change in service delivery: the case of optional newborn screening for Duchenne muscular dystrophy. *Community Genet* 3 (1): 17–123.

Parsons, E. P., Clarke, A. J., Hood, K., Lycett, E., and Bradley, D. M. 2002. Newborn screening for Duchenne muscular dystrophy: a psychosocial study. *Arch Dis Child Fetal Neonatal Ed* 86 (2): F91–95.

Patenaude, A. F., Basili, L., Fairclough, D. L., and Li, F. P. 1996. Attitudes of 47 mothers of pediatric oncology patients toward genetic testing for cancer predisposition. *J Clin Oncol* 14 (2): 415–21.

Petticrew, M. P., Sowden, A. J., Lister-Sharp, D., and Wright, K. 2000. False-negative results in screening programmes: systematic review of impact and implications. *Health Technol Assess* 4 (5): 1–120.

Plauchu, H., Cordier, M. P., Carrier, H. N., Dellamonica, C., Dorche, C., Guibaud, P., Lauras, B., Cotte, J., and Robert, J. M. 1987. Systematic neonatal detection of Duchenne's muscular dystrophy: results after 10 years' of experience in Lyons (France) [in French]. *J Genet Hum* 35 (4): 217–30.

Politano, L., Nigro, V., Nigro, G., Petretta, V. R., Passamano, L., Papparella, S., Di Somma, S., and Comi, L. I. 1996. Development of cardiomyopathy in female carriers of Duchenne and Becker muscular dystrophies. *JAMA* 275 (17): 1335–38.

Pollitt, R. J. 1999. Principles and performance: assessing the evidence. *Acta Paediatr Suppl* 88 (12): 110–14.

Raffle, A. E. 2001. Information about screening: is it to achieve high uptake or to ensure informed choice? *Health Expect* 4 (2): 92–98.

Reilly, P. 1977. *Genetics, Law, and Social Policy.* Cambridge: Harvard University Press.

Robert, J. M. 1990. The Lyon experience in neonatal screening for muscular dystrophy: the attenuation of critics. In *Genetic Screening from Newborns to DNA Typing* (Proceedings of the Workshop on Genetic Screening Held at La Sapiniere, Quebec, October 13–15, 1989), ed. B. M. Knoppers and C. M. Laberge, pp. 115–16. New York: Excerpta Medica.

Romero, N. B, DeLonlay, P., Llense, S., Leturcq, F., Touati, G., Urtizberea, J. A., Saudubray, J. M., Munnich, A., Kaplan, J. C., and Recan, D. 2001. Pseudo-metabolic presentation in a Duchenne muscular dystrophy symptomatic carrier with "de novo" duplication of dystrophin gene. *Neuromuscul Disord* 11 (5): 494–98.

Ross, L. F. 2002. Predictive genetic testing for conditions that present in childhood. *Kennedy Inst Ethics J* 12 (3): 225–244.

————. 2003. Minimizing risks: the ethics of predictive diabetes screening research in newborns. *Arch Pediatr Adolesc Med* 157 (1): 89–95.

Rowley, P. T. 1984. Genetic screening: marvel or menace. *Science* 225 (4658): 138–44.

Scheuerbrandt, G. 1980. Screening for early detection of Duchenne muscular dystrophy. In *Muscular Dystrophy Research: Advances and New Trends* (Proceedings of an International Symposium on Muscular Dystrophy Research, Venice, Italy, April 10–12, 1980), ed. C. Angelini, pp. 157–66. Amsterdam: Excerpta Medica.

Scheuerbrandt, G., Lundin, A., Lovgren, T., and Mortier, W. 1986. Screening for Duchenne muscular dystrophy: an improved screening test for creatine kinase and its application in an infant screening program. *Muscle Nerve* 9 (1): 11–23.

Shigihara-Yasuda, K., Tonoki, H., Goto, Y., Arahata, K., Ishikawa, N., Kajii, N., and Fujieda, K. 1992. A symptomatic female patient with Duchenne muscular dystrophy diagnosed by dystrophin-staining: a case report. *Eur J Pediatr* 151 (1): 66–68.

Skinner, R., Emery, A. E., Scheuerbrandt, G., and Syme, J. 1982. Feasibility of neonatal screening for Duchenne muscular dystrophy. *J Med Genet* 19 (1): 1–3.

Sumita, D. R., Vainzof, M., Campiotto, S., Cerqueira, A. M., Canovas, M., Otto, P. A., Passos-Bueno, M. R., and Zatz, M. 1998. Absence of correlation between skewed X inactivation in blood and serum creatine-kinase levels in Duchenne/Becker female carriers. *Am J Med Genet* 80 (4): 356–61.

Therrell, B. L. Jr. 2001. US newborn screening policy dilemmas for the twenty-first century. *Mol Genet Metab* 74 (1–2): 64–74.

van Ommen, G. J., and Scheuerbrandt, G. 1993. Workshop report: neonatal screening for muscular dystrophy. Consensus recommendation of the 14th workshop sponsored by the European Neuromuscular Center (ENMC). *Neuromuscul Disord* 3 (3): 231–39.

Wertz, D. 2002. Testing children and adolescents. In *A Companion to Genethics*, J. Burley and J. Harris, pp. 92–113. Oxford: Blackwell.

Whitten, C. F., and Whitten-Shurney, W. 2001. Sickle cell. *Clin Perinatol* 28 (2): 435–48.

Wilson, J. M. G., and Jungner, F. 1968. *Principles and Practice of Screening for Disease.* Geneva: World Health Organization.

Wong, B. L., and Christopher, C. 2002. Corticosteroids in Duchene muscular dystrophy: a reappraisal. *J Child Neurol* 17 (3): 183–90.

Zellweger, H., and Antonik, A. 1975. Newborn screening for Duchenne muscular dystrophy. *Pediatrics* 55 (1): 30–34.

CHAPTER 6

Lessons to Be Learned from the Move toward Expanded Newborn Screening

ELLEN WRIGHT CLAYTON, M.D., M.S., J.D.

State-run newborn screening programs were born in politics. When physicians were slow to incorporate screening for phenylketonuria (PKU) into clinical care, parents and physician advocates went to their state legislatures to urge them to require that this screening be performed. Once these programs were in place, political action by physicians and patient advocates continued to play a role, in some states resulting in new legislative mandates, in others bringing pressure to bear on state health departments. As a result, other disorders were added to the screening panel. Most of these, including congenital hypothyroidism, hemoglobinopathies, galactosemia, and congenital adrenal hyperplasia, had the potential for identification and treatment to avert serious disability and even death. Until recently, the most powerful brake on expansion of newborn screening was the reality that each test required a different method, forcing state departments of health to weigh the potential benefits of screening for an additional disorder against limited resources and competing priorities.

This focus on severe, treatable disorders has begun to change, not with the dramatic increases in our understanding of genetics, as many had prophesied, but with the advent of a new technology, tandem mass spectrometry

(MS/MS), which is capable of measuring dozens and even hundreds of metabolites at one time. This technology is the optimal approach for identifying certain disorders, such as PKU and medium-chain acyl-CoA dehydrogenase deficiency (MCAD), for which early intervention can dramatically improve health outcomes. The power of MS/MS, however, creates new challenges. Some of the metabolic derangements that can be detected cause serious diseases for which treatment is at best only partially effective. Other detectable variations only sometimes, if ever, seem to be associated with clinical disease. A decision to detect only some of the metabolites, such as those associated with PKU and MCAD, raises concerns that not all available information is being provided to parents and providers.

Tennessee, which has adopted the use of MS/MS for newborn screening, chose to report all the detectable metabolites, as have several other states that are using this technology. In this chapter, I review the events that led to this decision, relying on the public minutes of the state's genetics advisory committee, of which I am a member, and then reflect on the implications of these developments for newborn screening programs more generally.

Slouching toward Expanded Screening with Tandem Mass Spectrometry

Tennessee has a population of just under six million, with 75,000 to 80,000 births per year. For many years, Tennessee's state-run newborn screening program has had a genetics advisory committee (GAC), composed of relevant specialists, one to two generalists, and parent advocates. During the early to mid-1990s, the committee spent most of its time attempting to ensure access to medical foods, refining methods for already existing tests, developing parent information brochures, discussing criteria for adding new tests, addressing the problem of unsatisfactory samples, dealing with managed care organizations about follow-up testing (a problem that became acute after the advent of TennCare), and ensuring appropriate emergency follow-up. What evolved during this period was a system of care in which children with abnormal screening results are followed up until a diagnosis is made or excluded, and those affected are directed to appropriate specialists for care.

The question of screening for MCAD arose early. In 1992, a study using leftover bloodspots from newborns showed a mutation-carrier frequency of 1 in 249 in Tennessee. This meant that direct mutation analysis could detect one child with MCAD in every 62,000 newborns tested, or about one child a year in Tennessee. Looking for a single mutation, however, fails to detect a substantial number of affected infants, because several different mutations can cause this disease. The following year, an autopsy study of infants who died from sudden infant death syndrome was undertaken to assess the contribution of MCAD to these deaths. On both occasions, the GAC concluded that the data were not sufficient to warrant newborn screening for this disorder. The question arose again in 1998, when a prominent state senator forwarded to the committee a letter urging Tennessee to adopt MS/MS, written by parents of a child with MCAD whose disorder had been detected in another state. The GAC at that time recommended against adoption of this technology, reasoning that while reporting of only some results would be politically unacceptable, "several of the diseases detected [by MS/MS] have no known treatment." As a result, MS/MS did not meet the committee's criteria for screening, which had been informed by numerous documents emphasizing that newborn screening was justified only if early detection is required to avert serious harm. At the same time, the committee recommended screening for congenital adrenal hyperplasia and biotinidase deficiency, reasoning that the test characteristics and benefits of early intervention were more compelling for those disorders.

Two years later, the topic of MS/MS came up again. Initially the GAC continued to express concerns about the lack of effective treatment for many of the disorders detectable by this technique, issues of cost-effectiveness, and the lack of funds for follow-up. The committee also wanted to see the results of the pilot studies in progress in other states, most notably Massachusetts (Comeau, Larson, and Eaton 2004; Comeau et al. 2004). Later that year, however, the committee recommended adding MCAD, maple syrup urine disease (MSUD), and homocystinuria to the newborn screening panel, largely in response to the new recommendations issued by the March of Dimes (Marshall 2001).

A year later, Tennessee's Department of Health decided to adopt MS/MS at least for screening for MCAD, deferring for the moment the question of whether to report other results. At approximately the same time, a bill was introduced and ultimately passed in Mississippi's legislature, driven by the advocacy of Vince and Robin Haygood, that required all parents be offered screening of their children by MS/MS for 30 disorders (House Bill 986; codified as Miss. Code §41-21-203). This law was just one example of the political impact of parents who increasingly were insisting on expanded screening (Guthrie 2001, 2003, 2004; Hannon et al. 2001; Kritz and Mazel 2002; Cheng 2004), despite the limited evidence of efficacy of treatment. Previously,

Tennessee had been providing newborn screening for Mississippi, but this had to stop in the light of Mississippi's new requirements.

Tennessee's cautious approach to expanding newborn screening suddenly changed in 2003 with the introduction of Senate Bill 0056 in the state legislature, which provided, in part, that (emphasis added):

> (c) Regulations promulgated by the department pursuant to this section *shall not preclude the use of private laboratories, as an alternative to state government operated laboratories*, to conduct the analysis required by subdivision (a)(1) so long as such laboratory meets the following requirements.
>
> (1) The laboratory must be certified according to the federal Clinical Laboratory Improvement Amendments of 1998, 42 U.S.C. Section 263(a), and must be licensed to perform screening testing of newborn infants in the state in which the laboratory is located and such license must be in good standing.
>
> (2) The laboratory must provide screening for at least the following:
> (A) Phenylketonuria;
> (B) Galactosemia;
> (C) Hypothyroidism;
> (D) Sickle Cell Anemia and other hemoglobinopathies;
> (E) Cystic Fibrosis;
> (F) Congenital Adrenal Hyperplasia;
> (G) Maple Syrup Urine Disease;
> (H) Homocystinuria;
> (I) Biotinidase Deficiency; and
> (J) Medium Chain Acyl-CoA Dehydrogenase Deficiency.
>
> (3) The laboratory must agree to provide the division of maternal and child health with prompt reports and data to ensure that the patient has confirmatory testing, diagnosis and treatment.

The driving force behind the bill was Dr. Rick Rader, the medical director of the Orange Grove Center, in Chattanooga, Tennessee, and editor-in-chief of *Exceptional Parent* magazine, who was concerned that Tennessee was not expanding its newborn screening program quickly enough.

This bill, which ultimately was not enacted, was remarkable in two respects. First, unlike other states (including Mississippi) that simply mandated the offering of additional or supplemental screening in addition to the state's program, this bill would have permitted physicians to opt out of sending samples to the state-run newborn screening program. The fees for those samples would go to the commercial company that performed the initial screening. The responsibility for follow-up, however, would remain with the state program, suddenly becoming a new unfunded mandate that threatened the viability of the whole program. Second, although the disorders listed above are the ones on which there is general consensus about the desirability of newborn screening (with the possible exceptions of cystic fibrosis and homocystinuria), no company has ever offered this limited panel. NeoGen, which was later acquired by Pediatrix—the only entity that screens for all these disorders and the only one that complied with the bill's requirements—screens for more than 50 metabolic disorders at one time, only some of which, by the company's own admission, are treatable.[1] Notably, Pediatrix, which in 2005 ran more than 220 neonatal intensive care units in the United States, already had a substantial presence in Chattanooga at the time the bill was introduced.[2]

Two things happened in response to the introduction of Tennessee's Senate Bill 0056. Metabolic geneticists went to the legislature to talk about the state's newborn screening *system* and the importance of follow-up. In addition, the GAC, which had previously decided to adopt screening by MS/MS, at least initially, for only three disorders, decided to report all the analytes detectable by this technology so as to approach the commercially available panel. Screening using MS/MS began in January 2004, initially for MCAD, MSUD, and homocystinuria, expanding to full reporting by the summer of that year. The bill ultimately was tabled in response to the efforts to educate the legislators and the decision to expand the newborn screening panel dramatically.

Discussion

Since the early 1970s, virtually every policy group that has considered the question has urged that newborns should be screened only for serious disorders with effects that can be significantly ameliorated by early intervention, which usually must be instituted before the onset of clinical symptoms (Newborn screening for metabolic disorders 1973; President's Commission for the Study of Ethical Problems in Medicine and Biomedical and Behavioral Research 1983; Andrews 1994; New York State Task Force on Life and the Law 2000). These recommendations are based on several normative conclusions.

At the most basic level, health policy favors interventions that improve clinical outcomes. This can be seen throughout the move toward evidence-based practice. On an individual level, this means that clinicians typically pursue screening or testing only when they believe that the knowledge gained will alter management. Pediatricians and other child health care providers, who typically espouse a strong commitment to promoting the interests of their child patients, have been particularly reluctant to perform genetic tests on children unless the results will be used to alter management in the short term. Most scholars and professional groups who have addressed the issue have argued that it is inappropriate to test a child to provide information about predispositions for diseases that will occur, if at all, only in adulthood or to provide reproductive risk information for either the child or the parents (Harper and Clarke 1990; Clarke 1994; Wertz, Fanos, and Reilly 1994; American Society of Human Genetics and American College of Medical Genetics 1995; Clayton 1995; Nelson et al. 2001). These commentators frequently urge that because many adults choose not to get genetic tests for themselves, in part due to widespread concerns about genetic privacy, it is inappropriate to take that choice away from the adults that children will become, by testing them as children—unless there is some overwhelming medical reason to do it earlier. Identifying incompletely penetrant disorders or variants that have unclear clinical significance falls outside these guidelines as well.

Furthermore, finding unsuspected disorders in newborns may not be altogether benign for families, particularly if the abnormalities either are not treatable or are incompletely penetrant. Some families will value this information, but others will not. Had they been given a choice, some of the latter probably would have rejected screening in the first place. One thing that has been clearly demonstrated in the many studies of genetic testing, and in health care more generally, is that people differ widely in their preferences for information. And, of course, the overwhelming majority of abnormal results on newborn screening are false positives, raising the specter of illness for children who are, in fact, healthy.

Thus, it is of consequence that newborn screening programs are virtually unique in public health and medical care in almost always being mandatory, certainly as a practical matter and usually as a matter of law. Until recently, in fact, relatively little attention was paid even to educating parents about these tests. Bypassing parents was thought to be justified by the great benefit to be gained by early detection and treatment. Proponents of screening argued in essence that no parent would, or should be allowed to, refuse a test that would prevent a child's death or serious morbidity. Setting aside the legal and ethical appropriateness of such an assertion (Clayton 1992), this calculus is altered if screening is undertaken for minor disorders or for disorders with a course that cannot be significantly altered by treatment. (See chapters 2, 4, 5, 10, and 15 for varying perspectives on consent to newborn screening.)

So why has newborn screening expanded so broadly in the face of policies that would limit screening to those disorders for which early detection and treatment produce dramatically improved outcomes? The answer lies once again in political advocacy (Hannon et al. 2001). Some of the advocates have been clinicians, convinced of the value of early diagnosis. Parents often share this conviction as well, as is evidenced by the many testimonials about the need to detect disorders such as trifunctional protein deficiency and 3-methylcrotonyl-CoA carboxylase deficiency.[3] Their arguments, however, are sometimes broader than beliefs that early intervention improves outcome (see chapter 3). Many parents urge that they have a right to know about any conditions that could affect their children now or in the future and that they are in the best position to decide how to help their children prepare for what lies ahead, a view also held by many parents on the predictive genetic testing of children for predisposition to cancer (Patenaude 1996; Benkendorf et al. 1997; Hamann et al. 2000). These parents also cite the desirability of avoiding "diagnostic odysseys" (Grosse et al. 2004), their desire to inform their own reproductive decisions,[4] and benefits to their families more generally. They reject the notion that it is ever appropriate to withhold testing against parents' wishes; if technology can provide them with more information about their child, then they are entitled to it.[5] These arguments often receive sympathetic responses from legislators.[6] A growing number of scholars also urge that parents' desires merit at least some consideration (Pelias and Blanton 1996; Ross 1998; Robertson and Savelescu 2001). And hovering in the background is the threat of litigation if tests are not performed or test results are not reported (Hehmeyer 2001), even when the scientific and legal foundations for such claims are shaky.

The clash between clinicians and policymakers, on one side, and advocates on the other is by no means new, but it is particularly stark in the context of newborn screening. The adoption of expanded screening with MS/MS flies in the face of previously articulated criteria informed by ethical analysis. What, then, should be done? Is it appropriate simply to accede to parental demands and commercial pressures, as heard in the political process? Does it matter that parents who receive results they wish they had not received are probably less likely to express their concerns to their legislators?

The fundamental reality that has to be taken into account is the mandatory nature of newborn screening. Although efforts are finally being made to educate prospective parents about newborn screening during the prenatal period (American College of Obstetricians and Gynecologists 2003), it remains unlikely that parents will know or have much choice about whether or not to proceed with screening. "Naming," or knowledge for its own sake, is important and deserves more weight than it currently receives in health policy analysis. But parents (and patients) differ widely in their preferences for knowing what is coming, and recent experience with genetic testing reveals that even those who intend to get tested often change their minds when the opportunity actually arises. As a result, it would be better to reserve screening conducted primarily for these reasons to the setting that has more opportunity for choice—namely, the clinician-patient/parent relationship. Communication in this setting is less than optimal, but clinicians have an incentive to say *something* when offering a test or must face the consequences of failing to do so—namely, the unhappiness of parents who are taken by surprise. The drawback of locating interventions in the clinical setting, of course, is that clinicians will vary in what they do and payers will vary in what they reimburse. To some extent, clinician behavior can be dealt with by peer pressure, parental demand, and, yes, the threat of litigation. The problem of addressing the inequities that attend variable reimbursement is more difficult to resolve in the light of ERISA (Employee Retirement Income Security Act), which largely precludes states from regulating self-insured health plans, but much can be achieved by requiring that tests be reimbursed by state programs and by non-ERISA plans.

State programs should steadfastly insist on screening only for serious, treatable disorders. Just because technology such as MS/MS can detect disorders that do not meet this criterion, those results should not necessarily be reported in a mandatory public health program. Some states may choose to rely on private companies to provide the state-mandated screening, but the state programs should insist that the private companies develop limited panels that fit these criteria.

Maintaining a focus on serious, treatable disorders will require state programs to be vigilant to be aware of what is happening in the legislature (Kunk 1998). At times, clinicians and others may need to take part in the political process—educating senators, representatives, and their staffs about the harms that can attend receiving unwanted news that one's child has a serious disorder for which no treatment is possible, or learning about and having to live with the sword of Damocles of an incompletely penetrant disorder. Until the day comes when parents truly have choices about newborn screening, these programs must not be expanded beyond highly penetrant, treatable, serious disorders.

NOTES

1. Pediatrix Screening, "Step One Supplemental Newborn Screening" (http://pediatrixu .com/bookstore/pss_prod.asp?category=meta_scrn; accessed 2004). Two other entities, the Mayo Clinic and Baylor Medical Center Institute of Metabolic Disease, provide supplemental screening using MS/MS only, and so did not qualify as alternate laboratories under the Tennessee bill (http://genes-r-us.uthscsa.edu/resources/newborn/commercial.htm).

2. Pediatrix, "About Pediatrix" (www.pediatrix.com/body.cfm?id=48&oTopID=517; accessed 2005).

3. Save Babies through Screening Foundation, "Family Stories: Fatty Oxidation Disorders" (www.savebabies.org/familystories/2FattyAcidOxidationDisorders.php; accessed 2005).

4. Many studies demonstrate that parents of children with a Mendelian disorder often have more children, and many of them do not use prenatal diagnosis or assisted reproductive technologies to avoid having more affected children (Varekamp et al. 1990, 1992; Mischler et al. 1998).

5. A symposium addressing the appropriateness of newborn screening for nontreatable disorders is to be published in *Health Matrix* in early 2009. My current analysis, "Ten Fingers, Ten Toes: Newborn Screening for Untreatable Disorders," will appear in that volume.

6. National Conference of State Legislatures, "Newborn Genetic and Metabolic Screening" (www.ncsl.org/programs/health/genetics/newborn.htm; accessed 2005). Legislatures in several states have adopted MS/MS in their newborn screening programs; these include California, Illinois, Indiana, Kentucky, Missouri, and New Jersey.

REFERENCES

American College of Obstetricians and Gynecologists. 2003. ACOG committee opinion number 287, October 2003: newborn screening. *Obstet Gynecol* 102 (4): 887–89.

American Society of Human Genetics and American College of Medical Genetics. 1995. Points to consider: ethical, legal, and psychosocial implications of genetic testing in children and adolescents. *Am J Hum Genet* 57 (5): 1233–41.

Andrews, L. B. 1994. *Assessing Genetic Risks: Implications for Health and Social Policy*. Washington, DC: National Academy Press.

Benkendorf, J. L., Reutenauer, J. E., Hughes, C. A., Eads, N., Willison, J., Powers, M., and Lerman, C. 1997. Patients' attitudes about autonomy and confidentiality in genetic testing for breast-ovarian cancer susceptibility. *Am J Med Genet* 73 (3): 296–303.

Cheng, V. 2004. Newborn screening becomes crusade: a mother whose son suffers a rare genetic disorder pushes to get every child tested. *News and Observer*, August 5.

Clarke, A. 1994. The genetic testing of children. Working Party of the Clinical Genetics Society (U.K.). *J Med Genet* 31 (10): 785–97.

Clayton, E. W. 1992. Screening and treatment of newborns. *Houst Law Rev* 29 (1): 85–148.

———. 1995. Removing the shadow of the law from the debate about genetic testing of children. *Am J Med Genet* 57 (4): 630–34.

Comeau, A. M., Larson, C., and Eaton, R. B. 2004. Integration of new genetic diseases into state-wide newborn screening: New England experience. *Am J Med Genet C Semin Med Genet* 125 (1): 35–41.

Comeau, A. M., Parad, R. B., Dorkin, H. L., Dovey, M., Gerstle, R., Haver, K., Lapey, A., O'Sullivan, B. P., Waltz, D. A., Zwerdling, R. G., and Eaton, R. B. 2004. Population-based newborn screening for genetic disorders when multiple mutation DNA testing is incorporated: a cystic fibrosis newborn screening model demonstrating increased sensitivity but more carrier detections. *Pediatrics* 113 (6): 1573–81.

Grosse, S. D., Boyle, C. A., Botkin, J. R., Comeau, A. M., Kharrazi, M., Rosenfeld, M., and Wilfond, B. S. 2004. Newborn screening for cystic fibrosis: evaluation of benefits and risks and recommendations for state newborn screening programs. *MMWR Recomm Rep* 53 (RR-13): 1–36.

Guthrie, P. 2001. Georgia upgrades newborn screening. *Atlanta Journal-Constitution*, April 28.

———. 2003. Newborns at risk: couple who lost infant son take up my father's cause. *Atlanta Journal-Constitution*, February 2.

———. 2004. Georgia to expand testing on newborns. *Atlanta Journal-Constitution*, July 1.

Hamann, H. A., Croyle, R. T., Venne, V. L., Baty, B. J., Smith, K. R., and Botkin, J. R. 2000. Attitudes toward the genetic testing of children among adults in a Utah-based kindred tested for a BRCA1 mutation. *Am J Med Genet* 92 (1): 25–32.

Hannon, W. H., Becker, W. J., Chace, D. H., Cunningham, G., Grady, G. F., Hoffman, G. L., Mann, M. Y., Muenzer, J., Mulvihill, J. J., and Panny, S. R. 2001. *Using Tandem Mass Spectrometry for Metabolic Disease Screening among Newborns*. Report of a work group. Atlanta: Centers for Disease Control and Prevention.

Harper, P. S., and Clarke, A. 1990. Should we test children for "adult" genetic diseases? *Lancet* 335 (8699): 1205–6.

Hehmeyer, C. P. 2001. The case for universal newborn screening. *Exceptional Parent* 31 (8): 88–93.

Kritz, F. L., and Mazel, S. 2002. Too much for too little? Costly newborn test fuels debate on value. *Washington Post*, February 2.

Kunk, R. M. 1998. Expanding the newborn screen: terrific or troubling? *MCN Am J Matern Child Nurs* 23 (5): 266–71.

Marshall, E. 2001. Fast technology drives new world of newborn screening. *Science* 294 (5550): 2272–74.

Mischler, E. H., Wilfond, B. S., Fost, N., Laxova, A., Reiser, C., Sauer, C. M., Makholm, L. M., Shen, G., Feenan, L., McCarthy, C., and Farrell, P. M. 1998. Cystic fibrosis newborn screening: impact on reproductive behavior and implications for genetic counseling. *Pediatrics* 102 (1 Pt 1): 44–52.

Nelson, R. M., Botkin, J. R., Kodish, E. D., Levetown, M., Truman, J. T., Wilfond, B. S., Harrison, C. E., Kazura, A., Krug, E. III, Schwartz, P. A., Donovan, G. K., Fallat, M., Porter, I. H., and Steinberg, D. 2001. Ethical issues with genetic testing in pediatrics. *Pediatrics* 107 (6): 1451–55.

New York State Task Force on Life and the Law. 2000. *Genetic Testing and Screening in the Age of Genomic Medicine.* New York: New York State Task Force on Life and the Law.

Newborn screening for metabolic disorders. 1973. *N Engl J Med* 288 (24): 1299–1300.

Patenaude, A. F. 1996. The genetic testing of children for cancer susceptibility: ethical, legal, and social issues. *Behav Sci Law* 14 (4): 393–410.

Pelias, M. Z., and Blanton, S. H. 1996. Genetic testing in children and adolescents: parental authority, the rights of children, and duties of geneticists. *Univ Chic Law Sch Roundtable* 3 (2): 525–43.

President's Commission for the Study of Ethical Problems in Medicine and Biomedical and Behavioral Research. 1983. *Screening and Counseling for Genetic Conditions: A Report on the Ethical, Social, and Legal Implications of Genetic Screening, Counseling, and Education Programs.* Washington, DC: Government Printing Office.

Robertson, S., and Savelescu, J. 2001. Is there a case in favour of predictive genetic testing in young children? *Bioethics* 15 (1): 26–49.

Ross, L. F. 1998. *Children, Families, and Health Care Decision Making.* Oxford: Clarendon Press.

Varekamp, I., Suurmeijer, T., Brocker-Vriends, A., and Rosendaal, F. R. 1992. Hemophilia and the use of genetic counseling and carrier testing within family networks. *Birth Defects Orig Artic Ser* 28 (1): 139–48.

Varekamp, I., Suurmeijer, T. P., Brocker-Vriends, A. H., van Dijck, H., Smit, C., Rosendaal, F. R., and Briet, E. 1990. Carrier testing and prenatal diagnosis for hemophilia: experiences and attitudes of 549 potential and obligate carriers. *Am J Med Genet* 37 (1): 147–54.

Wertz, D. C., Fanos, J. H., and Reilly, P. R. 1994. Genetic testing for children and adolescents: who decides? *JAMA* 272 (11): 875–81.

CHAPTER 7

State Newborn Screening Advisory Committees

How Programs Introduce Public Participation into Decision Making

BRUCE JENNINGS, M.A.

ANDREA BONNICKSEN, PH.D.

As newborn screening programs have developed within state health departments during the past 30 years, various groups have repeatedly recommended the creation of newborn screening advisory committees (NBSACs) as part of the overall newborn screening policymaking process. These groups have argued that NBSACs will provide representation for the broader community, contribute to grassroots participation in the newborn screening policy process, and promote fair procedures in decision making in newborn screening programs.

States differ in the substance of their newborn screening policies and in the procedures for developing those policies (Hiller, Landenburger, and Natowicz 1997; Stoddard and Farrell 1997; U.S. General Accounting Office 2003). Likewise, the role and impact of NBSACs vary among the states. While some variation in the process of policymaking is to be expected, given that newborn screening programs are governed by states and there are no uniform federal standards to which such programs must adhere, this variation can be troublesome nonetheless. It leads to differences in the tests offered and conditions screened for, and in the public health effectiveness of the programs. In addition, the differences can reflect discrepancies in fairness and justice among newborn screening programs nationwide.

Newborn screening advisory committees constitute only part of the overall newborn screening policymaking process. As the name implies, their role is more often advisory than determinative, but prevailing political conditions and outside pressures on state legislators and health policymakers are often such that a failure to accept a recommendation made by an NBSAC could cause controversy or adverse publicity. Hence, the effective influence of the committees can be more substantial than their de jure authority might suggest. Moreover, much of the ethical and democratic justification for and legitimacy of newborn screening policies and programs has been invested in the advisory committee mechanism. Although the NBSAC is only one segment of the policy process, then, it is emblematic of a broader range of fairness issues. Convened by virtually all of the states, NBSACs touch on issues related to the nature of representation, the value placed on consumer involvement, and the meaning of public participation.

In theory, NBSACs help legitimize newborn screening programs, first, by virtue of the credentials of the specific individuals who comprise them. As multidisciplinary committees, they contribute different perspectives that provide a comprehensive look at facts and issues. Medical, scientific, and public health members with reputation, expertise, experience, and stature help ensure accountability and assure the public that the oversight of the newborn screening program is in capable and trustworthy hands. Citizen or consumer members of the committee contribute a voice of experience from families who are the clients of newborn screening programs.

The NBSACs also lend credibility to newborn screening programs by offering substantive advice and direction to policymakers. Ideally, their members will be sensitive to the ethical as well as scientific, practical, administrative, and financial issues faced by the program. As advisors, they keep the program oriented to the needs, interests, and concerns of the families at the grassroots level. They keep the program oriented toward the "common good," and their members are attentive to issues of individual rights, dignity, privacy, equality, and justice in the distribution of burdens and benefits within a program.

In practice, however, the ideals of citizen representation are not necessarily met. The appointment of members to NBSACs on the basis of their interest and experience can create a bias in perception and perceived decision-making role. Professional members may be oriented to the particular disorder or screening technology in which they specialize, and family members may be oriented to the disorder with which they have personal experience. They thus become advocates for a particular viewpoint or policy, which differs from the ideals described above. In addition, NBSACs are not well situated to evaluate newborn screening policies and activities in relation to the public health arena more generally.

Some of these difficulties are illustrated by decision making at the federal level during the past few years in an attempt to develop a uniform national newborn screening panel. Newborn screening is a dynamic field, and innovations in testing technology have led to the ability to test for a growing range of conditions. At present there is considerable variation among the states in the number of conditions tested for. In 2000, several professional, government, and advocacy groups called for the development of a national panel that would have access to the best available scientific information. This would, it was argued, improve both the rationality and the equity of newborn screening throughout the country. This effort did not take the politics out of the newborn screening arena, however, as seen by the ensuing developments, which proved highly contentious.

The American College of Medical Genetics (ACMG), acting on behalf of the Health Resources and Services Administration (HRSA), conducted a study as part of the effort to develop this national panel. The study used a methodology that was subsequently criticized. For this and other reasons, the findings and recommendations posed difficult problems for the Department of Health and Human Services and the HRSA Advisory Committee on Heritable Disorders and Genetic Diseases in Newborns and Children (U.S. Department of Health and Human Services 2005), which faced considerable pressure from advocates for broader screening—both inside and outside the government—to approve the recommendations of the ACMG study. These recommendations would significantly expand the range of disorders tested for by state newborn screening programs. The advisory committee did eventually approve the recommendations, but, arguably, committee members had not had sufficient time or background to digest the report. Moreover, sufficient technical assistance had not been given to assess the report critically and thoroughly. When the advisory committee formally approved the ACMG's report, the document had not yet been publicly released for broader comment. (See chapters 2 and 10 for further discussion of the ACMG study.)

If there is likely to be a gap between the expectations of accountability placed on NBSACs and their ability to serve as representative bodies, this prompts one to explore further the role of these committees in decision making and the implications of the gap for the fair allocation of resources. It is, to say the least, not clear that the NBSAC experience in general and citizen involvement in particular have lived up to the initial rationale for the committees. Several questions come to mind. First, how closely do the committees meet the expectations of legitimacy, credibility, and orientation to a common good? Second, are the expectations reasonable? Third, what representational roles do advisory committees see for themselves? Fourth, what can be done to improve the democratic function of NBSACs, especially for citizen members of the committees?

To assess the processes by which newborn screening programs introduce public participation into decision making, this chapter focuses on NBSACs as one element of newborn screening systems. In so doing, it analyzes the normative goals of representation, participation, and accountability that have been loosely and rhetorically associated with the structure and functioning of NBSACs from the beginning. We use theories of representation as a benchmark for assessing the role of NBSACs in framing newborn screening policy. We conclude with suggestions for bringing greater congruence between the theory and practice of citizen involvement in NBSACs.

The Origins of Newborn Screening Advisory Committees

Recommendations by policy advisory groups and government commissions to set up NBSACs with public representation date from the 1960s. A background paper for the 1968 World Health Organization Scientific Group on Screening for Inborn Errors of Metabolism recommended that advisory bodies, representing both "medical and non-medical expertise," be set up to promote deliberative and coherent decision making (Therrell 2001, pp. 68–69). Five years later, the Maryland legislature demonstrated a respect for consumer participation when it set up the Maryland Commission on Hereditary Disorders and stipulated that it would have a "substantial consumer representation" (Holtzman 1980, p. 253; Hiller, Landenburger, and Natowicz 1997, p. 1285). This evolved into a requirement that 5 of the 11 voting members be other than health care professionals.

Two years after Maryland's experience, the National Academy of Sciences reiterated the principle of public participation with its recommendation that "parents and consumers must be involved in policymaking and program implementation" and that newborn screening programs should develop "strategies to inform and involve families and the general public" in the overall program (Therrell 2001, pp. 70–71). In 1994, the Institute of Medicine (Andrews et al. 1994) recommended that states form independent advisory bodies that included members of the public and families affected by newborn screening (Newborn Screening Task Force 2000, pp. 409, 411). In 1997, the Task Force on Genetic Testing (Holtzman and Watson 1997) recommended consumer involvement in policy regarding "the adoption, introduction, and use of new, predictive genetic tests" (quoted in Newborn Screening Task Force 2000, p. 409). The Council of Regional Networks for Genetic Services also recommended that each state have at least one advisory committee with consumer representation (Newborn Screening Task Force 2000, p. 409).

The American Academy of Pediatrics (AAP) in 2000, through its Newborn Screening Task Force, clearly endorsed public participation by recommending that each state set up an NBSAC that would include a "broad range of public advisors representing parents, health professionals, third-party payers, appropriate government agencies, and other concerned citizens" (Newborn Screening Task Force 2000, p. 411). Parents and consumers in particular were to be "involved in all parts of the policy-making and implementation process" in a partnership of professionals and consumers (p. 395). The AAP also spoke more generally of the need for a national policy on the selection of screening tests and guidelines for programs. It recommended the establishment of a standing advisory body on national newborn screening, and it urged the development of model state regulations to guide newborn screening policy (p. 395).

Newborn Screening Advisory Committees as Vehicles of Community Representation

Although each of the groups mentioned above had its particular reasons for recommending NBSACs, it is possible to discern common threads and theoretical orientations behind these recommendations. In general, recommendations for community and consumer representation and participation are made on both philosophical and practical grounds.

The philosophical case for including citizen representatives—and thereby grassroots perspectives—in the policymaking process, discussed more thoroughly below, is not unique to the area of newborn screening. The idea can be traced at least as far back as important government programs during the New Deal era. For example, the Tennessee Valley Authority (TVA) set an important early precedent in its Depression-era public works and rural electrification projects.

The idea of "maximum feasible participation" enjoyed a resurgence during the 1960s and 1970s in many Great Society programs and, later, in many health and environmental planning programs. While the primary ideal may be to promote democratic participation, a secondary effect is pragmatic, if integrating those with a stake in the outcome lessens their opposition. Political scientist Philip Selznick ([1949] 1984) coined the term *co-optation* to describe how opposition to TVA projects was neutralized by inviting representatives of critical groups into the planning process and giving them a vested interest in the projects' success. Similarly, the Office of Economic Opportunity incorporated community members into the governing boards of local community action programs in efforts to foster economic development during the War on Poverty (Marris and Rein 1967). Participation by nonprofessionals was also important in health planning in the 1970s, through state-based health systems agencies and regulatory processes, for major capital development in health care services and facilities (Morone and Marmor 1981).

The creation of the first newborn screening programs reflected the same climate of opinion that inspired these earlier experiments in supplementing the usual structures of representative democracy. In the usual framework of representative democracy, those who make policy and wield government authority are kept both responsive and accountable to citizens because they are supervised by appointed officials, ultimately accountable to a popularly elected executive and legislature, and occasionally and ultimately are constrained by courts interpreting both constitutional and statutory law. What, then, brings about a call for citizen involvement on advisory committees to supplement representative government with experiments in a different kind of representation and participatory democracy?

For one thing, contemporary notions of justice presuppose that groups affected by policy have a right to a voice and a place at the policy table. Affected citizens are thought to have not only a right to the opportunity to participate but also a right to have a participatory process in place. Further, the sheer magnitude, size, and impersonality of official government, even at the state level, create the perception that a participatory mechanism is needed. This perception is accompanied by a widespread feeling that the normal mechanisms of responsiveness and accountability are not working well in government bureaucracies and by a distrust of expertise and professional knowledge. Experts, representatives of special interests, and other "insiders" have so captured the levers of influence in the legislative and policymaking process that citizens perceive the interests and common sense of ordinary people as not being presented or heard. Requiring citizen representatives to be present at the table during policy discussions and oversight activities has been offered as one practical way to counterbalance elite dominance, without going to more inclusive, open participatory forums such as town hall meetings or ballot referenda that might go too far afield from the professional expertise and specialized knowledge needed for newborn screening policy. (See table 7.1 for a summary of these rationales.)

On the practical level, it is thought that public participation on NBSACs will result in better policy outcomes. It can help educate both the public members themselves and public health personnel (Therrell 2001, p. 67). Parents of children affected by genetic diseases can bring a helpful perspective to committee members who have not been exposed to living with children with the disorders. Those whose lives have been directly touched by serious disease have a special authenticity in policymaking. They can contribute stories that help "ground" practitioners in the lived experiences of patients and families, and they can balance the committee so it is not so heavily made up of medical personnel (see chapter 4). Further, consumers help identify the need for education and can help prepare materials for public engagement and information. If the idea of consumer members is occasionally criticized because educating these members about the technologies and their ramifications takes extra time, this is revealing. If a community member does not understand that it takes more than a few dollars to add another disease to the screening list, this is a sign of a broader misperception and an indication of the need for education in general. Moreover, being called to explain technologies in terms understandable to nonmedical individuals is not, from a public-spirited point of view, a liability. Ideally, citizen members will bring common sense to the meetings as an antidote to special interests' influence and lobbying. Families also contribute to critiques of follow-up studies and oversight in that they can identify needs and point out policy deficiencies (Hiller, Landenburger, and Natowicz 1997, p. 1286).

Advisory committees are interdisciplinary units that can expose members to different points of view and provide the state's Department of Public Health with feedback. An NBSAC can help tie together the screening, follow-up, di-

TABLE 7.1
Rationales for Citizen Involvement

- Affected groups have a right to a voice and a place at the policy table.
- Citizens have a right of opportunity to participate and to have a participatory process in place.
- Citizen involvement counterbalances special interests' influence and lobbying.
- Citizens affected by genetic disease have a special authenticity to contribute to policymaking.

agnosis, treatment, and other components of a newborn screening program; provide reviews of programs and statistics; and act as a vehicle for telling the Department of Public Health what is working well and what is not. Ideally, an NBSAC is a resource to assist the state in running its program. In some states, NBSAC members are encouraged to be advocates for the program and to motivate legislators, in contrast to the neutrality of public health personnel.

On the other hand, NBSACs can be viewed as problematic by public health personnel if the committees draw unwanted attention from legislators interested in saving money or recommend discontinuing a screening program. In addition, legally mandated NBSACs can become unwieldy if the law lists the categories of individuals to be represented, and can also be expensive to maintain in a context of limited resources. NBSACs may be perceived as powerless in the overall political process in which essential decision-making authority lies in the state legislature. Even superior reports and recommendations by NBSACs are meaningless if newborn screening is not a top legislative priority. And having NBSACs in each state can be inefficient; regional NBSACs, as seen in the New England states and in the northwest, might be a viable alternative (Stoddard and Farrell 1997, p. 563).

In many aspects, today's newborn screening decision-making process is extemporaneous, with questions about adding to the list of screened disorders energized in response to pressure by highly organized interests. Advocacy by business and patient groups, among others, may divert attention from the Wilson and Jungner (1968) and other evidence-based criteria as a basis for expanding the list of screened disorders. This also contributes to a weakened power base for NBSACs, at least at the stage of expanding newborn screening. It is possible that NBSACs are more effective in contributing to newborn screening policies on education and other decisions made after decisions on program expansion. Another difficulty of NBSACs is that they are oriented to newborn screening programs and are not equipped (or even expected) to consider how the money would be spent by public health personnel if it were not spent on these screening programs. The committees offer advice on spending money for newborn screening programs rather than on public health in general. Moreover, citizen members may themselves be indebted to special interests, which reduces their ability to be dispassionate policy advisors (Fischer 2003).

The differing styles and outcomes of citizen participation and community representation point to a need to examine what the experience is meant to accomplish and how it should be evaluated. To judge the success and effectiveness of citizen representatives in the advisory process of newborn screening (or any other public policy programs), it is necessary to clarify the democratic values and rationales at work.

Modes of Democratic Representation and Participation

The democratic foundations of public participation on NBSACs can be more clearly understood by distinguishing between the concept of representation and the concept of participation, and by making a parallel distinction between the orientation of an interested consumer and that of a more civic- or community-oriented citizen. These concepts are summarized in table 7.2.

To represent is to make present something that is physically absent. Thus, a painting or photograph may represent a person who is far away or no longer living, or an imaginary person who exists only in the mind of the painter. Language and other semiotic systems have the capacity to represent ideas or objects in the same way. Applied to human interactions, this capacity to make that which is absent present in a symbolic sense makes possible a whole range of transactions that would not be undertaken if the physical presence of all parties were required (Pitkin 1967).

For centuries, political theorists have recognized that the institution of representation holds the key to practical and morally legitimate governance, particularly from a democratic point of view. Governance by the direct participation of all affected parties is generally impossible, undesirable, or both. It is impossible because direct participatory assemblies—ancient Athens, the Swiss canton, the New England town meeting—are workable only on a small scale (Dahl and Tufte 1973).[1] Plebiscite arrangements, which permit direct participation of large numbers of citizens, are undesirable because they reflect

TABLE 7.2
Concepts of Democratic Decision Making

Activity Orientation	Representation	Participation
Consumer	Act on the basis of the personal self-interest(s) of the represented: 1 As the constituents define their interests—delegate style of representation 2 As the representative defines the constituents' interests—trustee style of consumer-oriented representation	Act on the basis of one's own personal self-interest
Civic	Act to promote the common good of the community of the represented: 1 As the community members define their common good—delegate style of representation 2 As the representative defines the common good—trustee style of civic-oriented representation	Act to promote the common good of the community of which one is a member

choices and judgments uninformed by the process of face-to-face deliberation and debate that is possible in small direct assemblies or in larger representational ones. Therefore, under the conditions of the modern nation-state, the institution of representation allows for governance of all the people by only a few of the people (Bachrach 1967; Pennock 1979, pp. 309–62; Dahl 1982).

For our purposes in this chapter, the most important dimensions of democratic theory have to do with contrasting forms of activity, contrasting styles of representation, and contrasting orientations that one can take toward the activities of democratic involvement and decision making.

Representation and Participation

The first distinction is that between *representation* and *participation.* By and large, democratic participation is limited for most people to periodic voting, and a smaller number may become actively involved in campaigning, make financial donations to candidates, parties, or causes they favor, and the like. When individuals (via election or appointment) are cast in a government decision-making or advisory role, as are members of NBSACs, their democratic participation takes on a special form and becomes a kind of representation.[2] Representation and participation, while theoretically distinguishable, are not opposed or antithetical (Fleck 1992, 1994). Representation is simply one important kind of participation, which carries with it various special responsibilities and various ways (styles) of fulfilling those responsibilities.

Delegate and Trustee

A second distinction pertains to the way the representative perceives his or her representational role. This is the distinction between the *delegate* and the *trustee*. In the delegate style of representation, the person endeavors to find out the opinions, preferences, and positions of his or her constituents (those he or she is representing) and to then serve as the advocate for these positions in the legislative or governing process. In the trustee style of representation, the representative relies on his or her own thinking and judgment about what is in the best interests of the constituents (or in the best interests of the community as a whole) and acts accordingly. Made famous in the writings of British political theorist and politician Edmund Burke in the eighteenth century, the conception of trustee holds that the representative is not obligated to convey only the particular opinions and views of the constituents (Burke [1774] 1960). Contemporary surveys of legislative representatives indicate that they combine delegate and trustee roles and attempt to balance knowledge of constituents' interests (the delegate role) with their own judgment about positions that would be best for those represented (the trustee role) (Fenno 1978).

These conceptions of representation are useful in indicating the complexity of representation and highlighting models to guide representatives as they carry out their duties. However, these notions give only broad indications of real-world practices, where the complexities of decision making make it difficult to adhere to ideal democratic models—which are of limited utility in the context of citizen representation on NBSACs. Because members of NBSACs are appointed rather than elected, the distinction between direct and virtual representation is not pertinent. On the distinction between delegate and trustee roles, it is difficult for citizen members of the NBSAC to act as delegates, because they may not have regular links or direct lines of communication with the individuals or groups that the newborn screening program serves. Thus, it is not clear how the NBSAC member can be a delegate if he or she does not know what messages to carry and what positions and preferences to represent. If the delegate role is to be embraced, therefore, such lines of communication must be opened for the citizen representative and for all advisory committee members as well.

Open lines of communication are also necessary if the more paternalistic trustee role is to be embraced. This type of representation also presupposes communication with and working knowledge of the lives and experiences of outside groups so that the trustee can make judgments about their best interests. The trustee-style representative can no more afford to be aloof and disconnected from the constituency in question than can a delegate-style representative. The balance between the two styles requires that all members listen to what people who are directly affected by newborn screening policies have to say and that members are able to exercise a measure of independent and reasonable judgment about what is just and best for all concerned.

Consumer and Civic Orientations

The third distinction has less to do with the activity or style of democratic involvement than with the perspective or, as we call it, the "orientation" of the individual who is acting democratically. Generally speaking, one can evaluate a political action or policy relative to its impact on the interests of an individual or individuals separately, or its impact on the interests of particular groups in society, or its impact on the common good or public interest of the affected community as a whole. When the private interests of individuals or groups make up the principal orientation of the political agent (whether acting as a representative of others or as an individual participating citizen), we refer to the orientation as "consumerist," or a *consumer orientation*. When the common good or the public interest is the touchstone, we call this a *civic orientation* or community orientation. In the context of NBSACs, a member with a consumer orientation would, for example, tend to reflect a focused perspective of families affected by genetic disease. The member considers the impact of various decisions as if he or she were directly affected (e.g., as if the person's child had a genetic condition or his or her professional practice would grow or diminish in response to a policy decision). As table 7.2 indicates, both the delegate and the trustee styles are compatible with either a consumer or a civic orientation.

Despite the positive features of a consumer orientation, in theories of democratic representation a civic- or community-oriented perspective is usually taken to be more sound from an ethical point of view. A representative with a civic orientation is more detached, impartial, and objective than a consumer-oriented representative. And certainly justice, impartiality, and generality are qualities to be prized in policymaking or policy advising. Public policy is made difficult by the often conflicting interests of various stakeholder groups affected by the policy in question. Such is the case in newborn screening programs, where disagreements arise over the reliability of screening tests and laboratory quality standards, the desirability of screening for conditions of very low incidence in a population but with severe impact on the individual, and the equitable allocation of limited resources among the epidemiological, counseling, medical, and long-term care needs implicated in the disorders with which newborn screening programs routinely deal. Given these complex empirical and normative disagreements, at some point an effective policymaking process must transcend the level of stakeholder debate and engage in a kind of moral deliberation sincerely aimed at achieving consensus on a course of action reasonably thought to be just and in the common good or the public interest.

In point of fact, though, all representatives, including NBSAC members, have to walk a fine line that includes both the consumer and the civic orientations. Representatives are elected or appointed to give voice to and to serve the interests of a particular constituency, and so must be faithful to that trust. On the other hand, advisors (and lawmakers) are making decisions that affect the whole community, not just one group or constituency. Hence, they have a responsibility to be mindful of the common good or public interest as well. It should be added that all members of the committee could be evaluated on their consumer and civic orientations. The greater the ability of all to transcend stakeholder interests, while at the same time preserving the dedication that comes with having a particular interest in an issue, the more the ideals of justice will be maintained. Thus we argue that a combined consumer and civic or community perspective is the desideratum for members of NBSACs, lay (or ordinary citizen) members and expert members alike.

Now, taking this one step further, we should remember that these roles and orientations are not necessarily fully formed when individuals first join a body such as an NBSAC. People do not necessarily join with a particular perspective, but more typically are open to numerous styles and ways of playing their appointed role. They watch other members, they get orientation and advice from old hands, and, perhaps most interesting and important for our purposes here, their representational role is shaped and developed through the process of participatory deliberation itself. The activity of deliberation encourages people to have "public-spirited perspectives" on issues, which is essential to a well-functioning policy process within a democracy as well as to democracy as a whole (Gutmann and Thompson 1997, p. 39; Forester 2001; Fischer 2003; Hajer and Wagenaar 2003). In this way, deliberative participation contributes to fair process as well as fair substance (see chapter 2) and helps promote the "legitimacy of collective decisions" (Gutmann and Thompson 1997, p. 39). It is often said that decisions about newborn screening programs are more than technical matters; they also reflect social values (Hiller, Landenburger, and Natowicz 1997, p. 1280). These concepts of democratic decision making, role, and style allow one to analyze more precisely when, where, and how in the decision-making process "social values" play an important role in policy.

Thus far we have discussed the orientations and the ethical considerations that inform the activities and deliberations of members of NBSACs. It is also important to consider the qualities or virtues that one should look for in the individuals who serve on these committees. There are no formal mechanisms of accountability that will guide a given member to play this role of representation. The impulse comes from the conscience, awareness, and commitment of the individual NBSAC member. Our intention is not to suggest that these requirements are actually put into practice in real-world NBSACs, nor even to argue that they can or should be, but rather to develop a benchmark against which the performance and composition of an NBSAC membership can be assessed. Three general qualities of representatives are important to consider: (1) their personal attributes, (2) their social identity, and (3) their commitment to fair democratic process.

By *personal attributes* we mean those special characteristics that a given individual brings to the position of member of an NBSAC. These include intelligence; expertise; ability to articulate views and arguments; skills in group dynamics; ability to see the interrelation between scientific, economic, clinical, and psychosocial components of newborn screening programs—all attributes that enhance a member's effectiveness no matter what his or her perspective.

A second feature is *social identity*, by which we mean the way in which an individual—for reasons of ancestry, race, ethnicity, religious practice, linguistic competency, or personal or family medical history, or in other ways— sees himself or herself and is seen by others to represent a particular social or cultural group. In what sense is this a kind of representation, and why should it be pertinent to democratic representation? Given these personal characteristics, it may be thought that the individual is a representative because he or she shares similar experiences (e.g., being the victim of discrimination or bigotry) with the represented group. This may or may not be the case, of course, depending on the life history of the individual in question. But another sense of representation is also at work here, and that is the notion that a person is an appropriate representative if (and, some would argue, only if) he or she resembles or reflects the socially salient characteristics of a particular group. To be truly representative, it might be argued, a body such as an NBSAC should not only promote the interests of constituents and serve the public interest, but also, in the composition of its membership, resemble and reflect the racial, ethnic, and other diversity of the community as a whole (see chapter 8).

A third characteristic that should be taken into account in assessing the adequacy of representation is what we call *commitment to fair process*. By this we mean that individuals who are representatives should be able to take effective part in achieving consensus, building trust, balancing conflicting interests, and combining consumer and civic perspectives. Although individuals appointed to serve on NBSACs are often persons who have been active in advocacy groups or are parents of a child affected by one of the disorders screened for by the program, this background alone does not necessarily guarantee that a person will function well and effectively as a member of an NBSAC.

A new citizen member of an NBSAC sometimes, but not always, assumes his or her position in at least a partial political vacuum. Personal conflicts of interest aside (e.g., stock ownership in a genetic testing company), this is an ideal situation for a democratic representative, because the lack of ties and obligations may permit the individual to have a genuinely objective orientation. There is a risk, however, that the member is so committed to his or her own agenda of a particular disease or screening that he or she is primarily a consumer and does not take on the community role. That NBSAC members are stakeholders should not be surprising, given that many are appointed precisely because they do have an orientation and are thus not necessarily objective. At the least, commitment to fair procedure ought to be a key characteristic of any prospective NBSAC member.

Before moving on, we should say something more about the social identity criterion of representation, both because it seems to have such a potent political appeal and because it is problematic in both theory and practice. This notion of what is required of a good or legitimate representative frequently arises in the context of policy domains, like newborn screening, that are marked by high degrees of ethnic and racial diversity. It is often assumed that a committee can be representative of the community it serves only if it has a racial or ethnic composition that reflects that of the community. This seems to indicate that a committee member with the same ethnic or racial background as certain members of the community automatically is a representative of that group.

There are difficulties with the identity concept of representation, however. It does not follow that the racial or ethnic identity of an NBSAC member necessarily makes that member a representative of his or her ethnic or racial background. On the contrary, the assumption of automatic identity would point the representative's attention in the wrong direction by suggesting that his or her representational skills and capacities lie solely within his or her own experiences rather than in a willingness to turn outward to the constituency in question, to listen to and learn from them. Similarly, it would be wrong to assume that committee members affected by a particular genetic disease will be a delegate for all families affected by that disease. In our view, the skills of representation lie more with outward orientations to the greater constituency than with the social identities and symbols the individual may reflect.

Nonetheless, one must tread carefully here. Arguments of this kind do not mean that selection of NBSAC members should never be based on adding ethnic, racial, gender, or health diversity to a committee. It is possible that having the same traditions as a particular group assists the person in communicating with and having empathy for other members of that group. There are times when this is wise and has salutatory effects, such as lending a new tone and dynamic to interpersonal relations on the committee. It may make an important symbolic statement by the newborn screening program and the state government to a particular minority community and thereby help to restore trust. In the final analysis, however, we question the notion that having the composition of the NBSAC mirror the composition of the surrounding community makes the committee more representative or, more precisely, makes it a more effective and ethical representational institution.

Newborn Screening Advisory Committees in Practice

Against this theoretical background, it is helpful to examine the workings of NBSACs in the United States today. Although systematic empirical information about the committees is limited, the published case studies and surveys that do exist illuminate some dimensions of the committees' role in decision making. Virtually all of the states have NBSACs, and informal interviews with personnel affiliated with the committees reveal a respect for and reliance on the committees' contributions to policymaking. While an understanding of variations in the structure of individual state committees is informative in its own right—among other things, to provide models for other states—it also provides a basis for examining the context in which experiments in civic representation and participation are carried out.

One case study that illustrates a commitment to public participation in newborn screening programs comes from Massachusetts, where the state's Department of Public Health formed a temporary NBSAC in 1997 to assist it in deciding whether to expand the number of diseases for mandatory screening (Grosse and Gwinn 2001, p. 169). The committee's 17 members, including a parent/consumer representative, worked in a framework that encouraged public participation (Atkinson et al. 2001, p. 124). It also had a "broad charge" that enabled it to produce interrelated recommendations with guiding criteria and a rationale (p. 129). It held a public meeting for which it solicited input, and then it met 12 times before developing criteria for mandatory screening and producing a report with recommendations.

The Massachusetts NBSAC reviewed issues related to informed consent, quality control, and other factors. It had input from citizens, parents, and experts during the entire process, and its members reached agreement on numerous issues over the six months in which it met. Arguably, "public involvement in and access to" the NBSAC was key in developing a stable and legitimate policy (Atkinson et al. 2001, p. 129). The committee's recommendations were translated into regulations in 1998 (p. 127). The outcome was to add disorders for screening through tandem mass spectrometry (MS/MS) in a pilot program subject to Institutional Review Board (IRB) approval. The committee recommended a permanent NBSAC to review the results of the pilot program and to provide ongoing advice to the commissioner of public health on "new developments in the field of newborn screening" (p. 126). This recommendation was acted on by the Department of Public Health, which established a permanent NBSAC (p. 128).

In a second state, Wisconsin, the Department of Health and Social Services created an NBSAC in 1990 to make periodic reviews of the state program and offer recommendations to the legislature (Stoddard and Farrell 1997). The state's newborn screening advisory group is made up of 17 individuals representing "experts in newborn care, technical experts in screening tests and technology, metabolic and genetic disease specialists, ethicists, parents of affected children, and representatives of medical societies" from around the state (Stoddard and Farrell 1997, p. 563). It is funded in part by a fee attached to each test and charged to third-party payers. The NBSAC meets twice a year, with subcommittees meeting more frequently. Two observers of the committee, Stoddard and Farrell, conclude that the systematic method of recommendations by the committee contributes to a "policy-making process that is relatively insulated from extraneous political considerations" and is "driven by objectivity over ideology" (p. 564).

Three surveys give data about the number and structure of NBSACs in the United States today. The U.S. General Accounting Office (GAO) reported in 2003 that most states (44 states and Washington, DC) had NBSACs as part of their newborn screening programs. This was an improvement over 1995, when, as Hiller, Landenburger, and Natowicz (1997) reported, 33 jurisdictions had NBSACs for their newborn screening programs and 3 more were setting them up. In addition, 8 states set up NBSACs as needed, and 5 used consultants instead of NBSACs (p. 1283). Two states did not have NBSACs and 15 had IRB involvement. Most jurisdictions set up their NBSACs voluntarily without statutory mandate. The GAO also found that most states did not require NBSACs by law or regulation (U.S. General Accounting Office 2003, p. 11).

According to the GAO, in 2003 only 35 states had parents of children or individuals with disorders as NBSAC members. The number of states with other categories of members are: physician specialists (44), laboratory specialists (41), pediatricians and primary providers (40), health department staff (38), ethicists (16), and other, such as dieticians and representatives of the state March of Dimes and hospital associations (28) (U.S. General Accounting Office 2003, p. 12). The number of states with consumer members increased between 1995 and 2003; according to Hiller, Landenburger, and Natowicz (1997), in 1995 only 26 of the states had consumer members. Stoddard and Farrell (1997) identified 37 states with NBSACs in 1997.

Advisory committees vary significantly across the states. Some are formed by public health personnel on a voluntary and ad hoc basis when decisions, such as expansion of screening to cover additional disorders, need to be made, and the committees are then disbanded after the decisions are made. Other voluntary committees function more or less as permanent institutions, even though they are not required by law. Some committees meet only once or twice a year, while others meet up to six times a year. Members generally include laboratory personnel, geneticists, nutritionists, and others with expertise related to the issue under discussion. They may or may not include a parent or citizen representative. Committees may or may not have a written charter or policies that define the committee's authority, roles and responsibilities, membership guidelines, and operating procedures. In their survey of all state newborn screening programs, Stoddard and Farrell (1997) found that advisory committees in 6 states had policymaking authority. Committees in 16 states needed regulatory action to implement their recommendations, and committees in 4 states needed statutory action. The authors noted that states reported a variety of other models too, thereby indicating "multitiered approaches to policy formulation" (p. 562).

Implementing Advisory Committees

Different methods exist to integrate the public into NBSACs, and these are motivated in part by different perceptions of "public" and "participation." The effectiveness of an NBSAC depends on a range of factors, including commitment by newborn screening personnel, the value placed on public participation in genetics policy in the state as a whole, and funding available for the NBSACs. In the absence of a national model for state procedures, states vary in the format and functioning of their NBSACs (Therrell 2001, p. 67). Among other things, the committees differ in authorization (statutory or administrative discretion), duration (ad hoc or standing), and composition (e.g., citizen involvement). Issues relating to membership and representational model are of particular interest.

To promote fairness, it helps to have some precision about who is on the committee and what role the members are expected to play. The need for some expert members, such as a neonatologist or endocrinologist, may be self-evident, but there may be more ambiguity when one moves to the ideal of public participation. A "parent/consumer" can mean an individual or family member affected by a heritable disease, and a "public" member might include nonmedical experts who are independent of the newborn screening program. As members are added beyond the core medical personnel, one shifts from a model of consumer representation to one of public representation. The latter would include persons representing the public more generally, such as a social worker, medical ethicist, or representatives from the insurance industry, hospital administration, government, and professional medical or nursing associations.

The membership of Massachusetts's temporary NBSAC included two pediatricians, a parent/consumer, a neonatologist, a researcher, a medical ethicist, and representatives from the Massachusetts Hospital Association, Department of Public Health, and U.S. Centers for Disease Control and Prevention. Its permanent NBSAC has four parent members (Atkinson et al. 2001, p. 129).

In California, Senate Bill 231, had it passed, would have created an expectation that its NBSAC would have a rotating membership to include individuals or parents affected by a genetic disorder and experts in clinical genetics, pediatrics, cytogenetics, biochemical genetics, obstetrics/gynecology, genetic counseling, and bioethics. The bill also listed as possible members representatives of hospital administration, professional organizations, the insurance industry, and persons reflecting maternal and child issues.

Selecting NBSAC members is not always a systematic process. Some potential members approach the director or committee chair and others are known to committee personnel. Having the discretion to appoint members who are known to the NBSAC might lead to a more effective and tightly run committee. But it can introduce an element of arbitrariness into the process. It also runs the risk of hand-selecting consumer members who may not necessarily be selected for their assertive participation. Written policies on membership can minimize arbitrary selection, improve accountability, and give additional legitimacy to the idea of consumer involvement.

Consumer and public involvement can also be encouraged through methods other than committee membership. Consumers can be used as consultants and guest presenters at meetings in which issues of relevance to them are discussed. For example, representatives from the Cystic Fibrosis Foundation and families affected by cystic fibrosis should participate in deliberations about adding this disease to the mandatory screening program. The same effort should be made for issues related to informed consent, public education, follow-up procedures, and other stages in the newborn screening program. A systematic method of and commitment to ensuring public participation contributes to a mindset that welcomes innovative ways of inviting public input.

Public input can also be organized through public notices of proposed rulemaking, in which citizens can send comments and attend hearings. A disadvantage is that this process is usually not known to the general public, so one hears only from those with an intense stake in the outcome. Also, the information may be technical and not directly related to broader ethical issues. A third form of participation is consumer advocacy and influence on legislators (Therrell 2001, pp. 65, 71–72). The power of advocacy groups is illustrated by efforts of such groups in the 1960s to mobilize support and succeed in getting screening for phenylketonuria mandated in most states (Newborn Screening Task Force 2000). Also, consumer advocacy was behind the Massachusetts expansion to include MS/MS in its screening program (Grosse and Gwinn 2001, p. 169). Here again, though, what is advantageous for some groups is not necessarily advantageous for others, and reliance on advocacy can lead to decision making based on something other than objective data.

Perhaps more important than the technicalities of membership is an expectation that public participation will be part of the full newborn screening system. As the AAP observed in 1999, the system "should be clinically, socially, and ethically acceptable to the public and health professions" (Newborn Screening Task Force 2000, p. 395). Obviously a single member cannot accomplish this, and NBSACs need to be part of a broader ethic of parent/consumer involvement in all stages of policymaking. As one commentator put it, "consumer participation [in genetic policymaking] is critically influenced by professional attitudes toward it" (Holtzman 1980, p. 253).

Developing written policies, if they are not part of a legislative mandate, also serves to clarify representational roles and encourage other ways of maximizing public participation through consultancies, focus groups, and consumer committees. Written policies can include voting procedures, if any; duties and responsibilities of the committee and its members; and a mission statement to help members understand their roles and the expectations of them (see chapter 2).

Conclusion

Procedural inclusiveness should be a core element of newborn screening programs in general and of newborn screening advisory committees in particular. Although inclusiveness can be achieved in various ways, a state of mind that expects public participation is critical.

It is not surprising that we see differences between democratic theory and practice in the performance of NBSACs. Virtually all other attempts to institutionalize deliberative community participation in public policy have encountered similar problems and have only partly realized representational ideals. Our analysis does not provide a blueprint for whether and how NBSACs ought to be modified, but it does provide some general guidelines for conveying representational ideals to new citizen members.

1 Procedural inconsistency across states poses serious issues of equity and fairness, not only in the services offered by newborn screening programs but also in the way NBSACs are used and allowed to function.

- We do not recommend the creation of federal rules or standards on NBSACs at this time, but the federal government may play an important role in developing guides, educational manuals, and other practical resource materials on the conduct and operations of NBSACs.
- The practices of the most active and successful state NBSACs should be recorded and shared as examples of best practices.

2 The orientation and training of NBSAC members could be improved.

- Clear mission statements and other planning documents should be developed, not only for their finished product but also for the educational value of the discussion entailed.
- The complex task of being an effective representative and engaging in deliberation leading to advice and recommendations to policymakers is not immediately apparent to individuals recruited to or serving on NBSACs. Efforts should be undertaken to make NBSAC service more reflective and self-conscious.
- All committee members should have a clear understanding of their role and responsibilities. They should have a sense of their obligations and the expectations that are placed on them by the policy process. They should be attentive to the need to balance or minimize their own interests in a public-spirited manner.
- Newborn screening program leaders should promote the sense that service on an NBSAC is an opportunity to contribute to a vital area of public health and health policy that can substantially promote the health of children and their families.

3 Creative links for consumer involvement should be developed throughout the program, and NBSACs should undertake efforts to open multiple access points to the public. The NBSAC can be effective only if it engages in meaningful and respectful community outreach and communication. Policy advisors must be able to listen as well as give advice. This is true of all NBSAC members.

4 Additional complex issues will arise in the future for newborn screening programs, including risk factor testing, DNA diagnostics, and screening for rare disorders, all of which will expand the base of families affected by newborn screening. Systematic avenues of public participation are vital and can set the stage for more effective mechanisms in the future.

NOTES

1. For a contrasting perspective, see Barber 1984.

2. More widespread forms of citizen participation could supplement the workings of an NBSAC within a state's newborn screening program, such as public hearings, focus group studies, and discussions sponsored by local hospitals, libraries, churches, or other civic groups on the topic of genetics and health and newborn screening (Fleck 1996, 1997). But alternative avenues for participation are not our concern in this chapter. We are more interested here in how to make the most of the opportunity for public participation in NBSACs.

REFERENCES

Atkinson, K., Zuckerman, B., Sharfstein, J. M., Levin, D., Blatt, R. J., and Koh, H. K. 2001. A public health response to emerging technology: expansion of the Massachusetts newborn screening program. *Public Health Rep* 116 (2): 122–31.

Bachrach, P. 1967. *The Theory of Democratic Elitism: A Critique.* Boston: Little, Brown.

Barber, B. R. 1984. *Strong Democracy: Participatory Politics for a New Age.* Berkeley: University of California Press.

Burke, E. [1774] 1960. Speech to the electors of Bristol. In *Selected Writings*, ed. W. J. Bate. New York: Modern Library.

Dahl, R. A. 1982. *Dilemmas of Pluralistic Democracy.* New Haven: Yale University Press.

Dahl, R. A., and Tufte, E. R. 1973. *Size and Democracy.* Stanford: Stanford University Press.

Fenno, R. F. 1978. *Home Style: House Members in Their Districts.* Boston: Little, Brown.

Fischer, F. 2003. *Reframing Public Policy: Discursive Politics and Deliberative Practices.* Oxford: Oxford University Press.

Fleck, L. M. 1992. Just health care rationing: a democratic decisionmaking approach. *Univ Pa Law Rev* 140 (5): 1597–1636.

———. 1994. Just caring: Oregon, health care rationing, and informed democratic deliberation. *J Med Philos* 19 (4): 367–88.

———. 1996. *Genome Technology and Reproduction: Values and Public Policy. A Report on the Fall Community Dialogues.* East Lansing: Michigan State University.

———. 1997. *Genome Technology and Reproduction: Values and Public Policy. A Report on the Spring Community Dialogues.* East Lansing: Michigan State University.

Forester, J. F. 2001. *The Deliberative Practitioner: Encouraging Participatory Planning Processes.* Cambridge, MA: MIT Press.

Grosse, S., and Gwinn, M. 2001. Assisting states in assessing newborn screening options. *Public Health Rep* 116 (2): 169–72.

Gutmann, A., and Thompson, D. 1997. Deliberating about bioethics. *Hastings Cent Rep* 27 (3): 38–41.

Hajer, M. A., and Wagenaar, H. 2003. *Deliberative Policy Analysis: Understanding Governance in the Network Society.* Cambridge: Cambridge University Press.

Hiller, E. H., Landenburger, G., and Natowicz, M. R. 1997. Public participation in medical policy-making and the status of consumer autonomy: the example of newborn screening programs in the United States. *Am J Public Health* 87 (8): 1280–88.

Holtzman, N. A. 1980. Public participation in genetic policymaking: the Maryland Commission on Hereditary Disorders. In *Genetics and the Law II*, ed. A. Milunsky and G. Annas, pp. 247–58. New York: Plenum Press.

Holtzman, N. A., and Watson, M. S. 1997. *Promoting Safe and Effective Genetic Testing in the United States: Final Report of the Task Force on Genetic Testing*. Bethesda, MD: National Institutes of Health.

Marris, P., and Rein, M. 1967. *Dilemmas of Social Reform*. New York: Atherton Press.

Morone, J. A., and Marmor, T. R. 1981. Representing consumer interests: the case of American health planning. *Ethics* 91 (3): 431–50.

Newborn Screening Task Force. 2000. Serving the family from birth to the medical home: a report from the Newborn Screening Task Force convened in Washington DC, May 10–11, 1999. *Pediatrics* 106 (2 Pt 2): 383–427.

Pennock, J. R. 1979. *Democratic Political Theory*. Princeton, NJ: Princeton University Press.

Pitkin, H. F. 1967. *The Concept of Representation*. Berkeley: University of California Press.

Selznick, P. [1949] 1984. *TVA and the Grass Roots: A Study in the Sociology of Formal Organization*. Berkeley: University of California Press.

Stoddard, J. J., and Farrell, P. M. 1997. State-to-state variations in newborn screening policies. *Arch Pediatr Adolesc Med* 151 (6): 561–64.

Therrell, B. L. 2001. U.S. newborn screening policy dilemmas for the twenty-first century. *Mol Genet Metab* 74 (1–2): 64–74.

U.S. Department of Health and Human Services. 2005. Advisory Committee on Heritable Disorders and Genetic Diseases in Newborns and Children: meeting transcripts 2004–2005. http://mchb.hrsa.gov/programs/genetics/committe/2ndmeeting.htm.

U.S. General Accounting Office. 2003. Newborn screening characteristics of state programs. www.gao.gov/new.items/d03449.pdf.

Wilson, J. M. G., and Jungner, G. 1968. *Principles and Practice of Screening for Disease*. Geneva: World Health Organization.

CHAPTER 8

Racial/Ethnic Communities and Newborn Screening Policies

TOBY CITRIN, J.D.
STEPHEN M. MODELL, M.D., M.S.

There are epidemiological, historical, and sociological reasons why it is important to consider racial and ethnic populations, their self-identities, characteristics, and perspectives, when developing policies to guide newborn screening programs. In this chapter, we identify these reasons and consider why we should and how we can develop educational programs cognizant of racial and ethnic groups' needs and identities, how we can engage these populations in shaping newborn screening policies and participating in screening programs, and what role community-based organizations might play in achieving these objectives. We occasionally draw on the opinions and recommendations of the Communities of Color and Genetics Policy project (CCGP), which engaged 170 African American and 90 Latino community members in six Michigan cities and Tuskegee, Alabama, in dialogues about genetics, issues of concern, and suggested policies to maximize benefits and minimize harms (Fleck et al. 2001). While the problems described have a basis in U.S. history and culture, common ground exists with other countries, particularly in the policy approaches suggested.

Epidemiological Reasons for Considering Race and Ethnicity

The reported prevalence of particular genetic variants in specific racial and ethnic populations continues to suggest the importance of adequate attention to these groups when conducting screening for particular conditions. Gaucher disease, for example, has a high carrier frequency (~1 in 13) in the Ashkenazi Jewish population; sickle cell disease (SCD) has a high frequency in African Americans (~1 in 12) and African Caribbeans (~1 in 10), among other groups. Both are multiorgan conditions, are associated in particular individuals with bone or joint pain and a characteristic anemia, and can reduce life expectancy. Reflecting these associations, some university-based programs and diagnostic companies maintain Ashkenazi Jewish genetic screening panels that include Tay-Sachs disease and Gaucher disease, which are principally assessed via adult carrier and prenatal testing. Several of the newborn screens facilitated by tandem mass spectrometry (MS/MS) and DNA-based assays, and currently being implemented as part of expanded state newborn screening programs (Atkinson et al. 2001; American College of Medical Genetics 2005), also tend to detect conditions with a higher relative prevalence in particular groups. Cases of citrullinemia are reported more often in Japanese infants than in any other group, and, indeed, citrullinemia type II is found almost exclusively in Japan. HMG-CoA lyase deficiency causes up to 16 percent of inherited metabolic disease in Saudi Arabia and may be particularly severe in Saudi patients (Ozand, Devol, and Gascon 1992). These conditions can lead to organ failure, mental retardation, and death. In U.S. states where newborn screening for a condition is not mandated, health care providers whose clients include members of the groups predominantly affected should be aware of the risks to infants and should offer testing and whatever dietary measures are needed to avoid the stark consequences of these disorders.

Assurance of screening in the clinical context is not synonymous with the broader question of what shape a population screening program should take, however. Awareness of a particular group's needs sets a minimum on who should be screened. In the case of SCD, an earlier focus on screening a specific racial group (Bowman 1991; Avard, Kharaboyan, and Knoppers 2006) gave way to universal screening in the United States and United Kingdom as more evidence disclosed a large number of unscreened newborns with SCD and the prevalence of the mutation among diverse populations (Leary 1993; Olney 2000), and in the United States as African Americans were increasingly subjected to harms resulting from stigmatization and discrimination (Markel 1992). These harms were across the board, causing loss of jobs in the public and private sectors and unnecessary increases in life insurance rates for carriers, who are not at risk for SCD (Fost 1992). Many other conditions traditionally screened for (phenylketonuria [PKU], maple syrup urine disease, homocystinuria) and additional conditions now screened for in many state programs (argininemia, glutaric acidemia, medium-chain acyl-CoA dehydrogenase deficiency) broadly affect sociodemographic groups.

As we learn more about genetic variations among racial and ethnic populations, public health professionals responsible for newborn screening programs will be challenged to balance the benefits and harms of targeting specific racial and ethnic groups. Targeting such groups may be a cost-effective way to promote acceptance of newborn screening and provide education, counseling, assurance of access, and availability of therapeutic responses to positive tests. However, targeted screening programs may result in stigmatization of and discrimination against the targeted groups and may deprive other populations of the full measure of health benefits resulting from newborn screening. In contrast to a policy of broad inclusiveness, targeting of particular groups for genetic screening should not be undertaken without clear substantiation of individual and group benefit, and of the extent and limits of the benefits (see also chapter 2).

African American and Latino dialogue groups participating in the CCGP project concluded that newborn screening programs and, for that matter, any other genetic testing programs should not be limited to specific racial or ethnic populations unless the benefits of such targeting clearly exceed the risks of harm (Fleck et al. 2001). Benefits such as early identification of risk for a serious genetic condition and institution of preventive or therapeutic measures would need to be counterbalanced by the existence of suitable privacy protections and policies that ensure the avoidance of harms associated with group discrimination. While targeted screening was used for SCD before its universalization was recommended by the former Agency for Health Care Policy and Research, and has been employed in other genetic testing arenas (Kaback 2001)—sometimes not without controversy—its use for newborn screening since the advent of MS/MS is unsubstantiated. Epidemiological rationales for the consideration of race and ethnicity point toward greater inclusiveness in all forms of neonatal testing and the preservation of group protections (see chapter 3).

Historical Reasons for Considering Race and Ethnicity

The history of the impact of genetic programs on minority racial and ethnic groups suggests further reasons why race and ethnicity need to be taken into account in the design and implementation of newborn screening programs. The experience of the U.S. Public Health Service syphilis study at Tuskegee, the events during the early years of implementation of SCD screening programs, and the history of eugenics in the United States have all influenced the attitudes of various racial and ethnic groups toward any genetic screening program.

The Tuskegee syphilis story does not involve genetics, but it does illustrate reasons for the lack of trust among members of the African American community toward public health agencies and researchers seeking to conduct studies or medical tests with populations of color. In 1972, Jean Heller, an Associated Press reporter, wrote the newspaper article that shocked the public with the story of a 40-year study in which the U.S. Public Health Service exploited 399 African American men in Tuskegee, Alabama. The syphilis study sought information on the nature and progression of the disease, and the research subjects, African American men, were not told of their disease and were denied effective treatment (Jones 1993). Published medical reports suggest that between 28 and 100 participants died as a result of syphilis; some of these deaths could probably have been prevented by treatments that were developed, but not used for the research subjects, during the course of the study (Tuskegee Syphilis Study Legacy Committee 1996). Trust in the beneficent nature of the physician-patient relationship, in physicians' willingness to disclose the risks involved in medical procedures, and in the ability of the medical establishment to treat people of color as primary beneficiaries rather than in an instrumental fashion was deeply eroded (Corbie-Smith et al. 1999).

The syphilis study has become a symbol in the African American community of the exploitation of that community by government and by the medical and research communities to carry out research that benefits mostly other populations—generally more affluent and often nonminority (Gamble 1997; Thomas and Curran 1999). While the syphilis study ended shortly after the public disclosure in 1972, the U.S. government did not apologize for the study until 25 years later, in 1997. As demonstrated by the constant references to the Tuskegee study by the CCGP participants (Fleck et al. 2001), any discussion of genetic testing or screening among African American groups today evokes references to Tuskegee and expressions of distrust of the government agencies responsible for implementing screening programs. Participants suggested vigilance: "What we have to do is have people in all aspects of this who are community minded people that make sure we don't get taken advantage of and who are looking out for people in African, Hispanic, Latino people in the community. That we aren't taken advantage of again, like we did in the 30, 40 years ago in the Tuskegee syphilis study" (Communities of Color and Genetics Policy Project 1999, p. 7).

The history of SCD screening in the United States demonstrates how genetic testing can harm targeted groups. Lack of sufficient education for the groups tested, coupled with misunderstanding of the implications of a positive test result for sickle cell hemoglobin in the earlier, solubility-based testing, led to discriminatory practices and to internal group perceptions of implied inferiority (Bradby 1996). The story of SCD screening, particularly among African Americans, provides lessons on the need for education of both test subjects' families and the general public on the implications of positive results of newborn screening tests.

The history of eugenics in the United States is another reason why communities of color and other minorities are sensitive to genetic testing. In the early part of the twentieth century, Southern public health practitioners viewed syphilis as a problem of the black community. Public health officials drew polarized images of African Americans as lawless and infectious and of white folk, particularly women, as invaded and infected by disease from the "other" (Hirschbein 1997). Public health officials embraced eugenics, including its assumptions that some racial and ethnic groups had inherited characteristics that made them more susceptible to disease than other groups (Pernick 1997). The public health "interventions" resulting from these beliefs included sterilization and restrictions on immigration through race-based quotas (Garver and Garver 1991; Markel 1992). Racial antimiscegenation laws prohibited mixed racial marriages. Passed in 30 U.S. states, Germany, and elsewhere, these laws were not repealed until after World War II (Proctor 1992).

The repercussion of these events in the present is that many people of color are leery of government programs—recent examples being anti-HIV needle-exchange efforts in drug-ridden communities (Thomas and Quinn 1993) and Norplant promotion for welfare recipients (King 1992)—that would directly or indirectly fall more heavily on racial and ethnic minorities. While newborn screening is not currently motivated by a desire to stigmatize minority groups and is not associated with government policies inimical to such groups, communities of color may still feel that any such screening might disclose genetic information that could be used to discriminate or to reinforce stereotypical notions of group inferiority.

Societal Reasons for Considering Race and Ethnicity

The combination of historical reasons discussed above with the broader history of race and ethnicity in U.S. society results in a number of societal reasons for viewing newborn screening programs from the perspective of racial and ethnic groups. Racialization of genetics and lack of trust in the public health and medical care systems are aspects of these minority group perspectives (Dula 1994; Ikemoto 1997).

The current racialization of genetics has a precedent. Western societies used concepts of race to name and organize populations that they subjugated in the process of building empires. Since colonial times, race has taken on a range of meanings, mixing social and biological components in varying degrees (Cooper 2003). Given the plasticity of racial designations—varying with host country, with shifting political climate and census reclassifications, and even in hospital records—many authorities have come to view conceptions of race and ethnicity as strictly social and cultural constructs (Lee, Mountain, and Koenig 2001; Krieger 2003; Shields et al. 2005; Smedley and Smedley 2005). The opposing view is that race categories are genetically informative (Risch et al. 2002), that they can serve as proxies for social and environmental variables and as facilitators of medical treatment and enrollment in studies (Shields et al. 2005). Racial and ethnic categories do serve to highlight where racism and differential treatment have affected individual and group health (Krieger 2003; Smedley and Smedley 2005).

Scholars have pointed out the dangers of carrying out genetics research and imposing genetic policies in an American society inclined to view human variation in terms of racial and ethnic group differences (Duster 1994; Smedley and Smedley 2005). Group concerns over the potential harms of genetic research are likely to translate into unwillingness to use genetic services (Furr 2002; Laskey et al. 2003; Thompson et al. 2003). Using racial or ethnic categories in implementing newborn screening programs or reporting on their results could lead to the further racialization of genetics (Lee, Mountain, and Koenig 2001). And if the marketing of newborn screening programs leads to more widespread belief in genetic determinism, those who seek to spread beliefs in the inherent inferiority of minority groups will find powerful ammunition for their argument (Duster 1994; Ikemoto 1997).

The overriding theme of African American and Latino dialogues in the CCGP was distrust of those in government, health care organizations, insurers, employers, and "powerful interests" who direct and determine the path of genetics research and its applications (Fleck et al. 2001). The inability of government to balance special interests with community interests and to adequately regulate private industry were points of concern. Participants feared that government-sponsored research, like the syphilis study in Tuskegee, would once again take advantage of poorer, more vulnerable citizens who are members of minority groups.

One apprehension relating to researchers was that they might be too eager to complete research projects, thus exposing participants to excessive risk. This concern spilled over into discussion of medical practice. One participant disclosed her belief that a pregnancy-related HIV test she had refused was nonetheless performed on her; she was wary of this happening with genetic testing.

As is well known, those who are in leadership positions shaping U.S. policies on genetics research and practice are disproportionately European Americans. Only 1.1 percent of the members of the American Society of Human Genetics are black (Lin-Fu and Lloyd-Puryear 2000). Only 1 percent of members of the National Society of Genetic Counselors are African American, and an equal percentage are of Hispanic origin. Newborn screening programs designed and implemented by those not representative of the communities expected to participate in them are likely to elicit distrust and suspicion among communities of color.

Given the potential of newborn screening programs to cause harm to racial and ethnic minorities, the perception of these potential harms among communities of color, and the possibility that these perceptions might have an adverse effect on the participation of these communities in pilot, expanded screening programs, we need to consider strategies to protect against these harms and ensure that the benefits of screening programs are fully enjoyed by these groups. The strategies are of two types, relating to substance and to process.

Substantive Strategies

The ultimate test of whether newborn screening programs are designed with sufficient concern for the interests of racial and ethnic minorities should be whether the programs are likely to have a positive or negative impact on health disparities. This "health disparities impact" test suggests that attention must be paid to several aspects of screening programs likely to have positive or negative effects.

1. *Is the program designed with attention to characteristics of the diverse cultures represented in the population to be screened?* The misunderstandings in the early SCD programs are likely to increase with expanded newborn screening if appropriate steps are not taken. Cystic fibrosis (CF) testing has long achieved the 90 percent carrier detection rate recommended by the American Society of Human Genetics and National Institutes of Health working groups established in the early 1990s (National Institutes of Health 1997). However, carrier detection rates are below the 90 percent standard for particular groups. For African Americans, the standard 25-mutation CF test battery detects 69 percent of true gene carriers. Sensitivity plummets to 57 percent (pooled data) for Latino Americans (Langfelder-Schwind 2003). There is no reason to believe these figures for adult CF testing, which generate the possibility for false negatives, would be any different for newborns (newborn screening for CF had expanded to a required test in 39 states by the end of 2007; see table 1.1). Thus, from a purely technical point of view, race and ethnicity should be borne in mind and clarified by definition for conditions with significant differences in frequency between groups. In multiethnic California, where 50 percent of the screening population is Latino, newborn screening is based on normal values derived for a population with more than 16 different ethnic groups (Marshall 2001). While multitiered and multistandard testing alternatives, like other strategies, present their own complexities (Comeau et al. 2004), this example illustrates the possibility of more nuanced thought in screening of different racial and ethnic groups.

As with other public health programs, educational materials, materials promoting participation in the program, information related to informed consent, and explanations of positive and negative test results all must be designed to be understood by members of diverse cultures. The future of newborn screening may well revolve around a series of mandated core tests and noncompulsory elective tests. Presentational format and the language used make a difference in the acceptability of genetic testing to different groups and in how they use the information (Faden et al. 1982; Grody et al. 1997; Lerman et al. 1999; Singer et al. 2001; Thompson et al. 2003). Translated materials, focus groups, and representation of multicultural groups in the design and testing of informational materials, such as those handed out at prenatal visits, can ensure that these messages are clearly understood. It is unacceptable that only half of current newborn screening programs provide multilingual educational materials or translation services (Hiller, Landenburger, and Natowicz 1997).

2. *Do the educational aspects of the screening program help reduce and not expand health disparities?* Newborn screening programs need to be accompanied by education for the parents and families of the infants screened, the health care professionals and government employees involved in the programs, and the public at large. Education should make clear the reasons for the tests, the implications of negative and positive test results, and the extent to which factors other than genetics might affect the conditions to which the tests relate. The Human Genome Project has demonstrated a largely shared DNA sequence for humankind, with the health-influencing variations differing more within racial and ethnic groups than between them. Education on newborn screening programs should be shaped as part of the broader educational strategy for using genetics to further the understanding that individual variation is the hallmark of being human, that we all have genetic mutations, that more than 99 percent of our genetic makeup is identical to that of all other humans, and that race and ethnicity are subject to social definition rather than being mechanistically determined by genetic characteristics (McInerney 2002; Keita et al. 2004).

3. *Is there equal access to screening and follow-up services for all groups?* As with other public health programs, access needs to be measured by the "5 A's" test—whether screening is affordable, available, accessible, accommodating, and acceptable to all groups for whom it is intended (Penchansky and Thomas 1981). The "5 A's" test needs to be applied not only to the screening itself but also to the follow-up services that are appropriate when a test result is positive. To the extent that screening or follow-up services are less accessible to a group because of expense, location, lack of cultural sensitivity, or lack of cultural competence of service providers, the screening program may result in a widening of health disparities (Gurney and Simon 1993; Nickens 1996; Geiger 2001).

The literature clearly documents lower rates of health insurance coverage for racial and ethnic minorities, including coverage for prenatal care and newborn screening (Streetly et al. 1994; Davidson et al. 2000; Lin-Fu and Lloyd-Puryear 2000; United Health Foundation 2004). Payment of an $8 newborn specimen screening charge or a $2000 metabolic clinic management fee for PKU follow-up often depends on public assistance, either Medicaid or a State Children's Health Insurance Program. One CCGP participant stated: "I'm very concerned about what that does in terms of financing if there's a certain disease, like cystic fibrosis, that is not one primarily held by African Americans—what funding follows that one as opposed to sickle cell." Similar sentiments have emerged from Latino community groups in the genome policy project, with members noting how the universal-donor type O blood that is so abundant in the Latino community is welcomed by blood banks, yet many individuals lack ready access to clinical services. As Medicaid and other programs funding health services for the uninsured become subject to increasing budget constraints, access to screening and follow-up services may shrink for groups disproportionately uninsured or relying on Medicaid (Newborn Screening Task Force 2000; Centers for Disease Control and Prevention 2002a).

Concerns about disproportionate access to newborn screening are not limited to publicly funded programs. To the extent that parents are faced with options to pay for newborn genetic tests beyond those provided at public expense, the result might be a widening of health disparities. This issue of disproportionate access to genetic services is part of the broader issue of whether genetics is likely to lead to a new "genetic underclass," as more-affluent parents are able to use genetic technologies to minimize the risk of disease, disability, and deformity in ways not accessible to those with lesser means (Paul 1992).

4. *Is the cost of the program justified in relation to the need for other health services?* Some CCGP participants asked whether we were spending too much money on genetic research when basic health services are still inaccessible to groups disproportionately poor and uninsured. A parallel question, open to deliberation, might be whether the cost of a newborn screening program, especially that portion of the cost covering screening for diseases rarely found in the population screened, is justifiable when other fundamental public health services are being denied funding and when disparities in some diseases are not shrinking (Clayton and Byrd 2001; CDC 2002b; American Heart Association 2005; see also chapter 2).

Process Strategies

While attention to the *substance* of newborn screening programs is essential to addressing the interests and concerns of racial and ethnic groups, the *process* by which such programs are designed and implemented is at least as important and can ensure that sufficient attention is paid to the substantive features. The process goal of screening programs should be to enable the full participation of racial and ethnic minorities in the design and implementation of the programs, so that these programs are not perceived as being conducted by "them" on "us."

In seeking participation, it is important to distinguish "advice" from "engagement" and "participation." In communities most sensitive about harms from genetically related tests and distrustful of those who are seen to be the decision makers, fear and distrust will not be allayed simply because community members are asked for their opinions. Those participating in the CCGP strongly recommended that decision-making bodies be constituted so that they either represent the diversity of the U.S. population or can be monitored by "watchdog" groups reflecting this diversity (Fleck et al. 2001). These groups can have an umbrella role (e.g., March of Dimes, the National Organization of Rare Disorders, the Genetic Alliance) or a more specialized role (e.g., the Sickle Cell Disease Association of America, the National Urea Cycle Disorders Foundation). Past experience—one example being the Hadassah Jewish women's organization in the case of BRCA1 and 2 screening—has shown that consumer organizations can be helpful in raising critical questions and promoting programs shown to be scientifically and ethically justified (Rothenberg and Rutkin 1998). A synergistic effect is to be expected when responsible individuals within the organization come from the very communities they represent.

The value of a participatory approach in newborn screening policymaking has been underscored in screening frameworks emerging from the United Kingdom (Brameld 2006). In the United States, the American College of Medical Genetics Uniform Screening Panel expert group contained consumer participants (American College of Medical Genetics 2005). In Australia, teams in New South Wales have held community consultations with different stakeholder groups, recognizing differing bloodspot policies among the states (Muchamore, Morphett, and Barlow-Stewart 2006).

The number of U.S. states having newborn screening advisory committees has gradually increased, from 36 states in a 1997 survey by Hiller, Landenburger, and Natowicz to 48 states in a 2005 survey by the National Newborn Screening and Genetics Resource Center, a change due in part to the changing survey methodology and in part to actual increases. While "consumer" representation on these committees is mandated in some states, the majority do not have such requirements. Further, racial and ethnic representation is not usually a mandated characteristic (Hiller, Landenburger, and Natowicz 1997). The authors of the 1997 survey found, in a question item not revisited elsewhere, that in 17 states the public played no role in deciding which conditions should be covered by newborn screening programs. Moreover, the representation of "consumers," where such representation is mandated in state law, is usually satisfied by appointing an active member of a group that is representative of those experiencing a particular genetic condition. As a result, while groups with an interest related to a specific condition are represented in advisory bodies, the general public—and, more specifically, the racial and ethnic diversity of the general public—is usually not represented. Because newborn screening affects the entire population and, as this chapter suggests, poses special risks for racial and ethnic minorities, it is essential that efforts be made to adequately represent these groups on advisory bodies and that issues of concern to broad societal constituencies, including racial and ethnic minorities, be part of the agenda (see also chapter 7).

While representation of racial and ethnic minorities on newborn screening advisory bodies would be a step forward, it would still not address the need for full participation of these groups in policy and program development and implementation. The attitude of those shaping these programs often reflects a view that the programs must be determined by professional "experts," while the role of the public is to provide advice. This attitude ignores the nature of public health programs generally, and genetics programs specifically. Programs developed on this basis inevitably raise issues of values and priorities as well as technical issues related to program validity and utility.

The 1988 Institute of Medicine report on public health defined "policy development" as "the means by which problem identification, technical knowledge of possible solutions, and societal values join to set a course of action" (p. 114). The increased emphasis on evidentiary policymaking to optimize the cost-effectiveness of screening programs also calls for a union of empirical (clinical and epidemiological) evidence with evaluation of underlying normative values (Wilfond 1995; Wilfond and Thomson 2003). Consideration of normative values is a significant ingredient in ensuring program acceptability, a mainstay of the Wilson and Jungner criteria incorporated into the World Health Organization framework for implementing screening programs (Shickle 1999). Decisions on what conditions to include in newborn screening programs, whether these programs should be mandatory or voluntary and how elective tests should be structured, whether inclusion of a test should be conditional on universal access to appropriate follow-up services—all require the consideration of societal values and priorities, along with technical knowledge of test validity and utility and cost-benefit comparisons of various program options. Just as the policy decisions require a consideration of technical issues and values issues, those bodies entrusted with power to develop newborn screening policies and to design screening programs should include technical experts along with representatives of the public in all its diversity.

Neither professionals nor members of the public can be expected to be in complete agreement on formative policies. In our CCGP groups, African American participants tended to mention the importance of research and care directed at SCD more frequently than our Latino members, whereas the latter often focused on diabetes (considered by the American College of Medical Genetics [2005] in its analysis of conditions for inclusion in newborn screening). We have conducted dialogue projects recruiting participants from vastly different geographic and socioeconomic backgrounds within the same city and state (e.g., participants from the Ozarks and from the southeastern tip of Missouri; groups in Lansing, Michigan, with mean household incomes differing by $45,000). The CCGP groups from these disparate backgrounds collectively valued addressing conditions that either have a high frequency or "cause more human suffering or threaten loss of life earlier in life" (Communities of Color and Genetics Policy Project 2001, p. 11). The community-based groups felt the advantages of newborn screening for a particular condition should be balanced against its potential for stigmatization. "Income levels should not be a consideration when providing treatment" following newborn screening.

Community-based organizations can play a significant role in ensuring the meaningful participation of racial and ethnic groups in newborn screening decision-making bodies. These organizations, representing the voluntary collective expression of communities bound by common values and characteristics, can serve as bridges connecting grassroots communities with government agencies. They can elicit engagement of their constituents in voicing concerns, discussing policy options, and developing policy recommendations and can articulate the collective voice of their constituents in government decision-making bodies, as well as joining other such groups in advocacy of policies essential to the interests of their constituent populations (Garland and Hasnain 1990). These organizations, having satisfied the requirement for meaningful participation in newborn screening policymaking, can also become valuable partners with public health agencies in promoting full participation in the screening programs with their constituencies.

Newborn screening programs have the potential for applying public health prevention strategies that will avoid a great deal of human suffering. Careful attention to the implications of these programs for racial and ethnic groups can ensure that the programs do not inadvertently widen health disparities, but instead become powerful tools to reduce disparities. To promote this result, we have here suggested several strategies for the substance of these programs and the process by which they can be developed and implemented.

REFERENCES

American College of Medical Genetics. 2005. Newborn screening: toward a uniform screening panel and system. http://mchb.hrsa.gov/screening.

American Heart Association. 2005. Heart disease and stroke statistics—2005 update. www .americanheart.org/presenter.jhtml?identifier=3000090.

Atkinson, K., Zuckerman, B., Sharfstein, J. M., Levin, D., Blatt, R. J., and Koh, H. K. 2001. A public health response to emerging technology: expansion of the Massachusetts newborn screening program. *Public Health Rep* 116 (2): 122–31.

Avard, D., Kharaboyan, L., and Knoppers, B. M. 2006. Newborn screening for sickle cell disease: socio-ethical implications. In *First Do No Harm: Law, Ethics and Healthcare*, ed. S. A. McLean, pp. 495–510. Aldershot, UK: Ashgate.

Bowman, J. E. 1991. Prenatal screening for hemoglobinopathies. *Am J Hum Genet* 48 (3): 433–38.

Bradby, H. 1996. Genetics and racism. In *The Troubled Helix: Social and Psychological Implications of the New Human Genetics*, ed. T. Marteau and M. Richards, pp. 187–210. Cambridge: Cambridge University Press.

Brameld, K. 2006. Framework for adding new tests for conditions within the newborn screening protocol. www.genomics.health.wa.gov.au/publications/docs/2006_07_Annual_Report_OPHG.pdf.

Centers for Disease Control and Prevention. 2002a. Barriers to dietary control among pregnant women with phenylketonuria—United States, 1998–2000. *MMWR Morb Mortal Wkly Rep* 51 (6): 117–20.

———. 2002b. Recent trends in mortality rates for four major cancers, by sex and race/ethnicity—United States, 1990–1998. *MMWR Morb Mortal Wkly Rep* 51 (3): 49–53.

Clayton, L. A., and Byrd, W. M. 2001. Race: a major health status and outcome variable 1980–1999. *J Natl Med Assoc* 93 (3 Suppl): 35–54S.

Comeau, A. M., Parad, R. B., Dorkin, H. L., Dovey, M., Gerstle, R., Haver, K., Lapey, A., O'Sullivan, B. P., Waltz, D. A., Zwerdling, R. G., and Eaton, R. B. 2004. Population-based newborn
screening for genetic disorders when multiple mutation DNA testing is incorporated: a cystic
fibrosis newborn screening model demonstrating increased sensitivity but more carrier detections. *Pediatrics* 113 (6): 1573–81.

Communities of Color and Genetics Policy Project. 1999. Focus group transcripts. Unpublished
report. Ann Arbor: University of Michigan School of Public Health.

———. 2001. Grid report. Unpublished report. Ann Arbor: University of Michigan School of
Public Health.

Cooper, R. S. 2003. Race and genomics. *N Engl J Med* 348 (12): 1166–70.

Corbie-Smith, G., Thomas, S. B., Williams, M. V., and Moody-Ayers, S. 1999. Attitudes and beliefs of African Americans toward participation in medical research. *J Gen Int Med* 14 (9):
537–46.

Davidson, M. E., David, K., Hsu, N., Pollin, T. I., Weiss, J. O., Wilker, N., and Wilson, M. A. 2000.
Consumer perspective on genetic testing: lessons learned. In *Genetics and Public Health in the
21st Century*, ed. M. J. Khoury and W. Burke, pp. 579–601. New York: Oxford University
Press.

Dula, A. 1994. African American suspicion of the healthcare system is justified: what do we do
about it? *Camb Q Healthc Ethics* 3 (3): 347–57.

Duster, T. 1994. Human genetics, evolutionary theory, and social stratification. In *The Genetic
Frontier: Ethics, Law and Policy*, ed. M. S. Frankel and A. H. Teich, pp. 131–53. Washington,
DC: American Academy for the Advancement of Science.

Faden, R., Chwalow, A. J., Holtzman, N. A., and Horn, S. D. 1982. A survey to evaluate parental
consent as public policy for neonatal screening. *Am J Public Health* 72 (12): 1347–52.

Fleck, L., Castillo, J., Krouse, F., Lewis, E. Y., Smith, S., Soza, D., and Sydnor, B. K. 2001. Communities of Color & Genetics Policy Project summary dialogue report. www.sph.umich.edu/
genpolicy/current/reports/summary_dialogue_report.pdf.

Fost, N. 1992. Ethical implications of screening asymptomatic individuals. *FASEB J* 6 (10):
2813–17.

Furr, L. A. 2002. Perceptions of genetics research as harmful to society: differences among
samples of African-Americans and European-Americans. *Genet Test* 6 (1): 25–30.

Gamble, V. N. 1997. Under the shadow of Tuskegee: African Americans and health care. *Am J
Public Health* 87 (11): 1773–78.

Garland, M. J., and Hasnain, R. 1990. Community responsibility and the development of Oregon's health care priorities. *Bus Prof Ethics J* 9 (3–4): 183–200.

Garver, K. L., and Garver, B. 1991. Eugenics: past, present, and the future. *Am J Hum Genet* 49
(5): 1109–18.

Geiger, H. J. 2001. Racial stereotyping and medicine: the need for cultural competence. *CMAJ*
164 (12): 1699–1700.

Grody, W. W., Dunkel-Schetter, C., Tatsugawa, Z. H., Fox, M. A., Fang, C. Y., Cantor, R. M., Novak,
J. M., Bass, H. N., and Crandall, B. F. 1997. PCR-based screening for cystic fibrosis carrier mutations in an ethnically diverse pregnant population. *Am J Hum Genet* 60 (4): 935–47.

Gurney, E. L., and Simon, P. 1993. Inner-city pediatrics: perspectives on access. *R I Med* 76 (4):
181–84.

Hiller, E. H., Landenburger, G., and Natowicz, M. R. 1997. Public participation in medical policy-making and the status of consumer autonomy: the example of newborn screening programs in the United States. *Am J Public Health* 87 (8): 1280–88.

Hirschbein, P. 1997. African-American and public health. In *Public Health: Past and Present*, pp. 5–23. Ann Arbor, MI: Resource for Public Health Policy and Management.

Ikemoto, L. C. 1997. The racialization of genomic knowledge. *Seton Hall Law Rev* 27 (3): 937–50.

Institute of Medicine, Committee for the Study of the Future of Public Health. 1988. *The Future of Public Health*. Washington, DC: National Academy of Sciences.

Jones, J. H. 1993. *Bad Blood: The Tuskegee Syphilis Experiment*. New York: Free Press.

Kaback, M. M. 2001. Screening and prevention in Tay-Sachs disease: origins, update, and impact. In *Tay-Sachs Disease*, ed. R. J. Desnick and M. M. Kaback, pp. 253–65. San Diego: Academic Press.

Keita, S. O., Kittles, R. A., Royal, C. D., Bonney, G. E., Furbert-Harris, P., Dunston, G. M., and Rotimi, C. N. 2004. Conceptualizing human variation. *Nat Genet* 36 (11 Suppl): S17–20.

King, P. 1992. The past as prologue: race, class, and gene discrimination. In *Gene Mapping: Using Law and Ethics as Guides*, ed. G. J. Annas and S. Elias, pp. 94–111. New York: Oxford University Press.

Krieger, N. 2003. Does racism harm health? Did child abuse exist before 1962? On explicit questions, critical science, and current controversies: an ecosocial perspective. *Am J Public Health* 93 (2): 194–99.

Langfelder-Schwind, E. 2003. Family history and ethnicity alter interpretation of cystic fibrosis carrier test. www.nchpeg.org/newsletter/newsletter.asp.

Laskey, S. L., Williams, J., Pierre-Louis, J., O'Riordan, M., Matthews, A., and Robin, N. H. 2003. Attitudes of African American premedical students toward genetic testing and screening. *Genet Med* 5 (1): 49–54.

Leary, W. E., 1993. Screening for all newborns urged for sickle cell disease. *New York Times*, April 28.

Lee, S. S., Mountain, J., and Koenig, B. A. 2001. The meanings of "race' in the new genomics: implications for health disparities research. *Yale J Health Policy Law Ethics* 1 (Spring 2001): 33–69.

Lerman, C., Hughes, C., Benkendorf, J. L., Biesecker, B., Kerner, J., Willison, J., Eads, N., Hadley, D., and Lynch, J. 1999. Racial differences in testing motivation and psychological distress following pretest education for BRCA1 gene testing. *Cancer Epidemiol Biomarkers Prev* 8 (4 Pt 2): 361–67.

Lin-Fu, J. S., and Lloyd-Puryear, M. 2000. Access to genetic services in the United States: a challenge to genetics in public health. In *Genetics and Public Health in the 21st Century*, ed. M. J. Khoury, W. Burke, and E. J. Thomson, pp. 273–89. New York: Oxford University Press.

Markel, H. 1992. The stigma of disease: implications of genetic screening. *Am J Med* 93 (2): 209–15.

Marshall, E. 2001. Medicine: fast technology drives new world of newborn screening. *Science* 294 (5550): 2272–74.

McInerney, J. D. 2002. Education in a genomic world. *J Med Philos* 27 (3): 369–90.

Muchamore, I., Morphett, L., and Barlow-Stewart, K. 2006. Exploring existing and deliberated community perspectives of newborn screening: informing the development of state and national policy standards in newborn screening and the use of dried blood spots. *Aust N Z Health Policy* 3 (14): 1–9.

National Institutes of Health. 1997. Genetic testing for cystic fibrosis: National Institutes of Health consensus development conference statement, April 14–16. http://consensus.nih .gov/1997/1997GeneticTestCysticFibrosis106html.htm.

National Newborn Screening and Genetics Resource Center. 2005. National newborn screening status report: US national screening status report. http://genes-r-us.uthscsa.edu/nbs disorders.pdf.

Newborn Screening Task Force. 2000. Serving the family from birth to the medical home: a report from the Newborn Screening Task Force convened in Washington DC, May 10–11, 1999. *Pediatrics* 106 (2 Pt 2): 383–427.

Nickens, H. 1996. The Genome Project and health services for minorities. In *The Human Genome Project and the Future of Health Care*, ed. T. H. Murray, M. A. Rothstein, and R. F. Murray, pp. 58–78. Indianapolis: Indiana University Press.

Olney, R. S. 2000. Newborn screening for sickle cell disease: public health impact and evaluation. In *Genetics and Public Health in the 21st Century*, ed. M. J. Khoury, W. Burke, and E. J. Thomson, pp. 431–47. New York: Oxford University Press.

Ozand, P. T., Devol, E. B., and Gascon, G. G. 1992. Neurometabolic diseases at a national referral center: five years experience at the King Faisal Specialist Hospital and Research Centre. *J Child Neurol* 7 (Suppl): S4–11.

Paul, D. B. 1992. Eugenic anxieties, social realities, and political choices. *Soc Res* 59 (3): 663–83.

Penchansky, R., and Thomas, J. W. 1981. The concept of access: definition and relationship to consumer satisfaction. *Med Care* 19 (2): 127–40.

Pernick, M. S. 1997. Eugenics and public health in American history. *Am J Public Health* 87 (11): 1767–72.

Proctor, R. N. 1992. Genomics and eugenics: how fair is the comparison? In *Gene Mapping: Using Law and Ethics as Guides*, ed. G. J. Annas and S. Elias, pp. 57–93. New York: Oxford University Press.

Risch, N., Burchard, E., Ziv, E., and Tang, H. 2002. Categorization of humans in biomedical research: genes, race and disease. *Genome Biol* 3 (7): 1–12.

Rothenberg, K. H., and Rutkin, A. B. 1998. Toward a framework of mutualism: the Jewish community in genetics research. *Community Genet* 1 (3): 148–53.

Shickle, D. 1999. The Wilson and Jungner principles of screening and genetic testing. In *The Ethics of Genetic Screening*, ed. R. Chadwick, D. Shickle, H. Ten Have, and U. Wiesing, pp. 1–34. Boston: Kluwer Academic.

Shields, A. E., Fortun, M., Hammonds, E. M., King, P. A., Lerman, C., Rapp, R., and Sullivan, P. F. 2005. The use of race variables in genetic studies of complex traits and the goal of reducing health disparities: a transdisciplinary perspective. *Am Psychol* 60 (1): 77–103.

Singer, E., Modell, S., Coe, S., Caldwell, C., Schulz, A., and Antonucci, T. 2001. Communities of Color and Genetics Policy Project evaluation of dialogue process. Unpublished report. Ann Arbor: University of Michigan School of Public Health.

Smedley, A., and Smedley, B. D. 2005. Race as biology is fiction, racism as a social problem is real:

anthropological and historical perspectives on the social construction of race. *Am Psychol* 60 (1): 16–26.

Streetly, A., Grant, C., Bickler, G., Eldridge, P., Bird, S., and Griffiths, W. 1994. Variation in coverage by ethnic group of neonatal (Guthrie) screening programme in south London. *BMJ* 309 (6951): 372–74.

Thomas, S. B., and Curran, J. W. 1999. Tuskegee: from science to conspiracy to metaphor. *Am J Med Sci* 317 (1): 1–4.

Thomas, S. B., and Quinn, S. C. 1993. The burdens of race and history on black Americans' attitudes toward needle exchange policy to prevent HIV disease. *J Public Health Policy* 14 (3): 320–47.

Thompson, H. S., Valdimarsdottir, H. B., Jandorf, L., and Redd, W. 2003. Perceived disadvantages and concerns about abuses of genetic testing for cancer risk: differences across African American, Latina and Caucasian women. *Patient Educ Couns* 51 (3): 217–27.

Tuskegee Syphilis Study Legacy Committee. 1996. Report of the Tuskegee Syphilis Study. www .med.virginia.edu/hs-library/historical/apology/report.html.

United Health Foundation. 2004. America's health: state health rankings, 2004 edition: health disparity within states. www.unitedhealthfoundation.org/shr2004/HealthDisparity.html.

Wilfond, B. S. 1995. Screening policy for cystic fibrosis: the role of evidence. *Hastings Cent Rep* 25 (3): S21–23.

Wilfond, B. S., and Thomson, E. 2003. Models of public health genetic policy development. In *Genetics and Public Health in the 21st Century*, ed. M. J. Khoury, W. Burke, and E. J. Thomson, pp. 61–81. New York: Oxford University Press.

CHAPTER 9

The Role of the Federal Government in Supporting State Newborn Screening Programs

MICHELE A. LLOYD-PURYEAR, M.D., PH.D.
BRADFORD L. THERRELL, PH.D.
MARIE Y. MANN, M.D., M.P.H.
JAMES R. ECKMAN, M.D.
JOSEPH TELFAIR, DR.P.H., M.S.W., M.P.H.

In the past few decades, the possibilities for genetic testing in both clinical and public health practice have expanded rapidly. Increased knowledge of the metabolic and molecular basis of disease, advances in testing technologies, and, of most importance, the potential for improved health outcomes stimulated a recent increased investment in newborn screening by government and the private sector. The multistep process of translating basic research into clinical and public health applications such as newborn screening is critical for expanding the field of genetic testing and extending the benefits to the public. To be effective, this translation process requires partnerships and interplay between government and public and private institutions.

However, there is often a tension in this translation process between the government, both federal and state, and the private sector, such as commercial interests and lay advocacy groups. The general public may expect rapid translation and implementation of new technologies, while government engages in a more cautious, deliberative process that seemingly delays implementation. State and federal government policymakers' role is to manage the health impact of new technologies. The general public and private sector often see this role as ponderous and slow. In the history of newborn screening, however, there are examples of partnerships between the government and private sector that have effectively and cooperatively translated research findings into improvements in newborn screening programs.

Using four examples, we describe how the federal government has engaged in the process of translating research into improvements in states' population-based newborn screening programs. We also present future roles for the federal government in expanding and improving newborn screening activities.

Background

One of the greatest accomplishments of preventive public health services over the past 40 years has been the development, implementation, and improvement of state-based public health newborn screening programs. Each day, more than 10,000 newborns across the country receive screening for genetic, infectious, and other congenital disorders that can threaten their life and health. Forty years ago, studies funded in part by the federal government (Children's Bureau) showed that population-based early newborn screening, detection, and treatment for inborn errors of metabolism could reduce or eliminate the adverse consequences of certain congenital disorders such as phenylketonuria (Guthrie 1992; Paul 1997). And, indeed, federal funding support was particularly critical in establishing public health newborn screening systems within the states.

Newborn screening programs and systems have continued to be influenced by federal funding. However, federal financial support is usually prescriptive, evidence-based, and designed to encourage orientation of these programs in a specific direction that provides for equity across the country.

Lay advocacy groups and developments in the private sector also have had an influence. Lay advocacy is often disorder-specific and may be more subjectively based. The examples presented here show that public advocacy can be powerful and that newborn screening would not be as significant a component of the public health system without the support of lay advocacy groups.

Technological developments in the private sector occasionally have led to newer or broader laboratory screening services. At times, this broadened screening capacity is not accompanied by essential system components, such as follow-up, education, and systems evaluation, that must accompany testing for it to be effective. Because commercial testing usually is profit-oriented, those who cannot pay may be excluded from the benefits of newborn screening services (Hoffman et al. 2005). On the other hand, commercial implementation of technological advances has contributed to reevaluation and improvement of public programs such as newborn screening.

In addition, health care, public health, and newborn screening professionals have developed professional (or practice-oriented) guidelines for the care, treatment, and management of specific screened disorders;[1] for quality assurance in the screening process, such as laboratory performance (Therrell and Hannon 2006), filter paper characteristics (Hannon et al. 2007), and so forth; and for selecting conditions for inclusion in newborn screening (Watson et al. 2006). This guidance has been essential in establishing successful, high-quality newborn screening systems.

The Federal Role

The federal government has long been active in newborn screening. Activities have focused primarily on developing infrastructure for: (1) research, (2) policy development, (3) service delivery, (4) program quality, and (5) education and training. Federal funding strategies (Title V of the Social Security Act or the Public Health Service Act) have also provided support for screening and testing, nutritional needs and services, professional training, and public education. With Title V funding, the manner in which these funds are used is left to the discretion of each state. Funding priorities are usually identified by the federal funding agency.

The bulk of federal support for basic and translational research is provided by the National Institutes of Health (NIH), followed by the Health Resources and Services Administration (HRSA), the Centers for Disease Control and Prevention (CDC), and the Agency for Healthcare Research and Quality (AHRQ). Because the level of support correlates with an agency's mission and budget, there are large differences in the amounts of funding from the various federal agencies. While NIH funding has supported the majority of basic scientific research projects, HRSA, CDC, and AHRQ have funded projects mainly related to secondary data analysis, information development and dissemination, education and training, implementation, and postdevelopment issues. For more than 30 years, CDC has maintained a national quality assurance and proficiency testing program (partially funded by HRSA from 1976 through 2001) to assist newborn screening laboratories in maintaining and enhancing the quality of test results (Therrell and Hannon 2006). Additionally, AHRQ, CDC, HRSA, and NIH have provided support for consensus conferences, workshops, task forces, and expert panels, all of which have helped to define and facilitate support for key research and implementation questions.

To better describe and understand the federal government's role in translation of new knowledge into public health programs for newborn screening, we describe four examples of federal activities: (1) newborn screening research (phenylketonuria), (2) newborn screening implementation (sickle cell disease), (3) newborn screening policy development (Newborn Screening Task Force and other federal advisory committees), and (4) newborn screening evaluation and quality assurance (newborn screening consultation and review team). These examples only partially document the role of federal support in advancing and translating genetics research into public health applications in newborn screening programs.

The history of newborn screening for phenylketonuria (PKU) and sickle cell disease (SCD) reveals a remarkable interconnection with the histories of the maternal and child health programs at HRSA and at NIH. The examples described focus on initiatives funded by NIH and HRSA's Maternal and Child Health Bureau (MCHB) or by federal maternal and child health programs that existed before the establishment of HRSA and the child health programs at NIH. Because the bulk of funding for implementing research findings in newborn screening programs and other relevant translational activities continues to be provided by HRSA, we focus primarily on HRSA activities.

Example 1. Research: Phenylketonuria

This example illustrates federal support for research that was key to the establishment of newborn screening programs.

Classical PKU is a rare genetic inborn error of metabolism with an incidence of about 1 in 19,000 births, based on data reported by state newborn screening programs from 1991 to 2000 (Therrell and Hannon 2006). Symptoms arise from a deficiency of a liver enzyme that catalyzes the conversion of phenylalanine to tyrosine, which is critical to brain development. In the absence of therapy, phenylalanine can accumulate at toxic levels in the blood, resulting in mental retardation (Kaye and Committee on Genetics 2006). Screening for PKU is required in all U.S. newborn screening programs.

The history of newborn screening for PKU is synonymous with the history of newborn screening in the early 1960s. Robert Guthrie began reporting the results of his research on PKU screening at scientific meetings (Guthrie 1962, 1964). His 1963 report of a simple blood-screening procedure and mechanism for transporting a blood sample opened the way for population-based newborn screening for PKU (Guthrie and Susi 1963). However, the concept of mass screening of all newborns for this condition was not without controversy. The scientific evidence for treatment benefits and incidence was lacking, and professionals' initial reactions to screening were less than enthusiastic (Guthrie 1992). The federal Children's Bureau funded a study to address questions and concerns about the efficacy of testing (Guthrie and Whitney 1964). In addition, in 1962 the Children's Bureau provided funding support for a voluntary newborn screening program at the Massachusetts Department of Health (Koch 1964).

At the outset, PKU screening was not a legislated public health activity and its application across the country was uneven. Guthrie and the National Association of Retarded Children (NARC) worked to develop model legislation for mandatory screening and, in so doing, gained the support of the Children's Bureau and many state public health departments. NARC promoted the idea that newborn screening for PKU and other conditions resulting in mental retardation would lead to early treatment and prevention of adverse sequelae.

This grassroots optimism was a major factor in the establishment in 1962 of the National Institute of Child Health and Human Development (NICHD) at NIH to lead research studies for PKU-like conditions and their treatment for possible inclusion in newborn screening programs (Public Law 87-838, Public Health Service Act, October 17, 1962). Through the combined efforts of public advocacy groups such as NARC and the March of Dimes, and federal funding support for program research and implementation, a majority of states mandated newborn screening for PKU by the end of the 1960s (Committee for the Study of Inborn Errors of Metabolism 1975; Guthrie 1992). Additional funding from HRSA in the 1970s eventually contributed to state policies making newborn screening a requirement in every state and some U.S. territories. State and territorial public health departments assumed the central role in implementing mandates for newborn screening.

Among the early research activities supported by NICHD and the Children's Bureau was an extended follow-up study of children with PKU diagnosed through newborn screening programs and treated with a restricted diet. This study provided important validation that early screening and dietary restriction could provide marked improvement in development and mental function for children with PKU. The results of the study further encouraged the adoption of newborn screening in states in which screening was not yet mandated (Azen et al. 1996). Over the years, NIH/NICHD has continued to engage in research relevant to PKU, such as an extended maternal PKU study (Koch et al. 1990; Rouse et al. 1997; American Academy of Pediatrics 2003). In 2000, a Consensus Development Conference on Phenylketonuria: Screening and Management was cosponsored by NIH and HRSA to develop consensus guidance for the care and treatment of children, adolescents, and adults with PKU (National Institutes of Health 2000).

Example 2. Newborn Screening for Sickle Cell Disease

This example illustrates the support of clinical research and the translation of clinical research findings into newborn screening program practice.

Sickle cell anemia was initially described by Herrick ([1910] 2001). Sickle cell disease is an autosomal recessive group of genetic disorders characterized by the presence of sickle hemoglobin (HbS) in red blood cells (www .scinfo.org). Heterozygotic individuals are carriers; carrier status is generally a benign, asymptomatic state. Homozygous and some compound heterozygotic individuals have symptomatic disease. Four genotypes—sickle cell anemia (Hb S/S), sickle-hemoglobin C disease (Hb S/C), and two types of sickle-β-thalassemia (S-β⁺-thalassemia and S-β°-thalassemia)—account for most SCD in the United States. Genes with mutations for SCD are common in persons of African, Mediterranean, Middle Eastern, and Indian ancestry and persons from the Caribbean and parts of Central and South America. Taken as a group, SCDs are the most prevalent group of disorders identified by newborn screening, with more than 1500 affected infants born in the United States each year.

In 1973, Garrick, Dembure, and Guthrie reported an electrophoresis technique for hemoglobin screening using filter paper bloodspots, opening the way for testing for hemoglobinopathies in newborn screening programs. Pilot testing, independently introduced by Pearson et al. (1974) and Serjeant et al. (1974), showed that newborn screening with cord blood was practical, and arguments were made that early diagnosis and appropriate health care could improve the outcome for infants with SCDs. At that time, the estimated median expected survival for individuals with SCD living in the United States was 20 years, in part because of high mortality in early life (Scott 1970; Diggs 1973).

In 1971, the African American community lobbied Congress and other policymakers to make SCD a scientific and health care priority. In response, the National Sickle Cell Anemia Control Act, establishing the National Sickle Cell Disease Program, was passed in May 1972. This was followed by passage of the National Genetic Disease Act in 1978, which provided funding for SCD activities.

Under the 1972 and 1978 legislative authorities, the National Heart, Lung and Blood Institute, responsible for implementing both acts, transferred funds to HRSA's genetic disease program (now the Genetic Services Branch, HRSA/MCHB) to develop community-based SCD education, screening, and counseling services. Under their authority, NIH funded SCD research projects and established comprehensive care centers. This funding resulted in: (1) development of 23 comprehensive SCD centers in 1978 (which were reduced to 10 federally funded study centers by 1986); and (2) establishment of screening and education clinics in 40 states and the District of Columbia by 1981.

Early newborn screening and education programs for SCD confirmed that early identification of sickle cell diseases combined with comprehensive care is effective in decreasing overall morbidity and mortality (Powars et al. 1981). Further, they provided valuable experience that defined the effectiveness and deficiencies of a variety of strategies for newborn screening (Grover et al. 1978; Grover 1989; Harris and Eckman 1989; Therrell, Simmank, and Wilborn 1989; Githens et al. 1990).

Despite the success of these programs, newborn screening for SCD was not universally accepted as a public health strategy for improving health outcomes, and some reports stressed the potential for harm. Haste and lack of education of the community, the general public, lawmakers and policymakers, and public health and heath care providers led initially to poor screening practices (Sinnette, Smith, and Smith 1974).

In addition, the African American community was split regarding the risks and benefits of screening, around the issues of the social and political consequences of screening and the merits of screening in the absence of adequate treatment, education, and follow-up. Controversies included: (1) the perception of population-based screening as a means to further shame and degrade African Americans; (2) African American leaders' advice to avoid screening because of the possible adverse effects of job loss and denial of insurance coverage; (3) legislation requiring SCD testing either on entering school or as part of premarital testing; and (4) the perception that screening programs were promoting genocide for African Americans.

Concurrent with the statewide education and counseling programs, the NIH-funded comprehensive centers encouraged the first coordinated efforts to study the natural history of SCD in the Cooperative Study of Sickle Cell Disease in 1978. This study prospectively defined the causes of the mortality and morbidity in newborns with SCD. A smaller study within the larger cooperative study was initiated in 1983 to assess the efficacy of using prophylactic penicillin to prevent pneumoccocal sepsis and meningitis, the major cause of death in children with SCD. The smaller study was terminated eight months before its scheduled end date when an 84 percent reduction in mortality and morbidity was observed in the group of infants identified and treated early. When the results of this study were published (Gaston et al. 1986), newborn SCD screening gained increased support as a useful public health program.

The 1987 Consensus Development Conference cosponsored by HRSA and NIH concluded that universal newborn SCD screening, combined with the administration of prophylactic penicillin in a medical setting that provides comprehensive care, produced compelling benefits, and SCD screening should therefore be included in newborn screening programs (National Institutes of Health, Consensus Conference 1987).

As a result of better-informed and organized efforts by the SCD community and to help implement consensus conference recommendations, federal funding specifically for newborn screening programs greatly increased during the late 1980s. NIH transferred significant funds to HRSA for implementation of the consensus conference recommendations, again through the genetic services program at HRSA. Over the seven years following publication of the SCD consensus guidelines, HRSA dedicated more than $30 million (much of this from NIH) to establishing and improving newborn screening programs for SCD (Therrell, Panny, and Davidson 1992). Funding earmarks included improved follow-up services, application of DNA technology to the diagnosis of SCD in newborns, development and dissemination of educational materials, and technical assistance for statewide SCD newborn screening programs. This funding provided a direct and necessary stimulus for rapidly expanding these newborn screening programs, as well as increasing the genetic service capacity of states.

In addition, Congress appropriated funds directly to HRSA to fund state genetic service programs in fiscal years 1987 to 1989. Twenty-nine states instituted programs for statewide SCD screening for newborns with this federal funding. In 1989, however, the federal government curtailed HRSA funding for genetic services and related health care programs, which included SCD screening programs. By 1990, 80 percent of the state programs mandated SCD screening, illustrating that federal support can stimulate and effect change in state programs. Because now *all* states mandate universal newborn screening, routine screening now identifies all newborns with SCD in the United States and many of its jurisdictions (Therrell, Johnson, and Williams 2006).

Example 3. Policy Development: Use of a Newborn Screening Task Force and Other Federal Advisory Groups

This example illustrates the engagement of the federal government in the policy or guideline development process and the effect of federal policy or guidelines on newborn screening programs.

One of the most important recent federal activities has been the HRSA-funded American Academy of Pediatrics Newborn Screening Task Force. In 1998, HRSA asked the academy to convene a task force to assess the issues affecting newborn screening programs and to make recommendations for subsequent actions. The process was both cosponsored and cofunded by NIH. Other cosponsors included CDC and AHRQ and various consumer, professional, and public health organizations. The task force, using multiple working groups, evaluated and reviewed state newborn screening programs and published its findings as a national agenda for action (Newborn Screening Task Force 2000). Actions and activities emphasized several areas:

- Public health infrastructure for newborn screening
- The roles of families and health professionals in newborn screening
- Oversight of newborn screening systems
- Research and surveillance activities related to newborn screening
- Finance mechanisms supporting newborn screening systems

The task force recommended specific actions for federal agencies. In particular, HRSA was asked to continue its support of public health infrastructure for newborn screening systems and genetic services, including: (1) developing integrated information systems; (2) reviewing (evaluating) newborn screening programs; (3) creating performance measures for evaluating newborn screening systems; (4) establishing a national resource center devoted to newborn screening and genetics; (5) developing training programs on using new technologies; (6) supporting projects for educating health care professionals, families, and individuals about informed decision-making processes (genetics, in general, and newborn screening, in particular); (7) evaluating the use of new and innovative tests and technologies in newborn screening; and (8) developing guidance and standards for the use of new genetic-based technologies. In response, HRSA initiated a number of contracts, grants, and cooperative agreements addressing these items. One project initiated was with the American College of Medical Genetics to evaluate the available scientific evidence for possible conditions currently available for screening consideration and recommend a uniform panel of conditions for which all states should screen, and to develop a model decision matrix for newborn screening programs to use in establishing screening panels (Watson et al. 2006).

Federal activities have also included policy development efforts and regulatory actions aimed at providing equitable health care services in genetics and newborn screening. As an example, the Secretary's Advisory Committee on Genetic Testing (SACGT), under the Department of Health and Human Services, was chartered in June 1998 in response to recommendations of two working groups commissioned jointly by NIH and the Human Genome Project for the Department of Energy. These groups identified the need for broad-based public policy development to help the nation address the benefits and challenges of genetic knowledge and genetic testing. SACGT management was assigned to NIH. The advisory committee was established with the goal of advising the government on all aspects of the development and use of genetic tests, including the complex medical, ethical, legal, and social issues raised by genetic testing. SACGT concluded that the oversight of genetic testing should be multifaceted to ensure that safe and valid tests are used for clinical and public health practice and that those tests are appropriately applied and interpreted. Although generally considered a part of genetic testing, newborn screening was only peripherally considered in the committee's actions.

SACGT also emphasized the importance of information disclosure in informed decision making. Based on the rapidly evolving nature of genetic tests, their anticipated widespread use, and concerns about their potential misuse, SACGT recommended additional testing oversight by the U.S. Food and Drug Administration. The agency was urged to develop oversight approaches focusing on analytical and clinical testing validity and clinical utility, without obstructing the development and availability of new genetic tests. SACGT also recommended that the Clinical Laboratory Improvement Act of 1988 (Public Law 100-578, §353 Public Health Service Act [42 U.S.C. 263a], October 31, 1988), regulating laboratory testing, should be augmented to include specific provisions to ensure the quality of laboratories conducting genetic tests. With expiration of its charter, SACGT was reconstituted in 2002 as the Secretary's Advisory Committee on Genetics, Health, and Society, with several roles: (1) to provide a forum for expert discussion and deliberation and the formulation of advice and recommendations on the range of complex and sensitive medical, ethical, legal, and social issues raised by new technological developments in human genetics; (2) to assist the secretary of the Department of Health and Human Services and, at the secretary's request, other federal agencies in exploring issues raised by the development and application of genetic technologies; and (3) to make recommendations to the secretary on how such issues should be addressed.

Another recently chartered federal advisory committee is the Secretary's Advisory Committee on Heritable Disorders and Genetic Diseases in Newborns and Children. This committee was authorized by Congress in 2000 and chartered in 2003 to provide advice and recommendations on grants and projects and technical information to the secretary of the Department of Health and Human Services. Specifically, the committee is to advise and guide the secretary regarding the most appropriate application of universal screening tests, technologies, policies, guidelines, and programs for effectively reducing morbidity and mortality in newborns and children having or at risk for heritable disorders. Congress envisioned that this committee and its associated grant programs will enhance the ability of state and local health agencies to provide for newborn and child screening and for counseling and health care services for newborns and children having or at risk for heritable disorders. The committee presents a deliberative advisory process that involves parents, scientists, public health and health professionals, and the federal government with the potential for bringing uniformity and national performance standards to state-based newborn screening programs. The committee has agreed on the following fundamental principles for the nomination and review process of conditions that would be added or deleted from newborn screening panels:[2]

1 The deliberative process will be rigorously evidence-based, even for relatively rare conditions.
2 The procedures for the creation of a deliberative system and the system itself will be transparent and accessible to the scientific and lay public.
3 The process will be consistent across the different phases of the review process and will be applied to all of the proposed conditions.

Example 4. Program Evaluation as a Part of Quality Assurance and Continuous Improvement

This example illustrates the role of the federal government in one aspect of quality assurance and the nature of the partnership between states and the federal government in the process of continuous improvement.

Following the first international newborn screening meeting in 1986, HRSA was requested by New Jersey state health officials to assist the state's Department of Health in improving its newborn screening program by providing an unbiased external program review using national expertise. Responding to this request, an expert review team with knowledge and experience in newborn screening program administration and financing, laboratory services, follow-up activities, medical management, and overall quality assurance was assembled, and a comprehensive three-day review of the state newborn screening program took place in June 1987. The report noted that "all DOH [Department of Health] staff involved in the review found it stimulating and educational," and many of the panel's recommendations were subsequently implemented (Rappaport 1989). Building on the success of this review in evaluating and assessing program needs, HRSA responded to requests for nine similar state reviews over the next two years, and the review activity became an important federal resource (Therrell, Tuerck, and McCabe 1992), which translated into the Newborn Screening Review Team.

Working through the Newborn Screening Committee of the Council of Regional Networks for Genetic Services, review team members were instrumental in developing and publishing guidelines for U.S. newborn screening programs. Not only were state programs experiencing similar successes, but their questions and challenges were often the same. Thus, general guidance provided a framework for establishing and evaluating the success of a newborn screening program (Therrell, Panny, and Davidson 1992). Although it was initially intended to be periodically updated, the careful thought process used in developing the initial guidance continues to provide a useful framework for programs 20 years later. Areas addressed by the guidelines include: (1) organization and administration, (2) selection and evaluation of disorders for screening, (3) communication, (4) quality assurance, (5) funding, (6) diagnosis, (7) program evaluation, and (8) liability.

Today, this expert Newborn Screening Review Team, which includes representation from CDC and HRSA, continues to conduct reviews at the invitation of state public health programs, as part of the activities of the National Newborn Screening and Genetics Resource Center (an HRSA-funded cooperative agreement at the University of Texas Health Science Center at San Antonio). Since 1987, more than 30 states and territories have requested and received reviews; several states have requested second reviews (Therrell and Hannon 2006). An external evaluation of the state review activity in May 2003 documented the states' favorable responses and the important role of the reviews in shaping the newborn screening programs that were surveyed. The written review reports have provided documented program successes and suggestions for improvement and have been useful as templates for continuous quality improvement throughout the systems surveyed.

Conclusion

The cited examples of the growth in newborn screening programs illustrate how public-private partnerships have positively affected the 40-year history of newborn screening in the translation of research into clinical and public health applications.

While the recent past shows the federal government's partnership with states and the private sector to ensure the strength of newborn screening programs, this partnering for the health and well-being of children was not always the case. The concept of a partnership between states and the federal government first appeared in 1912, when the Children's Bureau was established to promote the health and welfare of children with special needs. The first federal grant-in-aid program to the states was established with enactment of the Sheppard-Towner Act in 1921. The act was controversial and was labeled as radical. The American Medical Association, the Catholic Church, and the U.S. Public Health Service were opposed to giving grants to the states and were instrumental in having the act repealed eight years after its enactment, ending the federal-state partnerships. It was not until the 1930s that the Social Security Act provided for a growth of maternal and child health programs and the reemergence of programs that rested on a federal-state partnership.

The federal newborn screening activities described in this chapter demonstrate the usefulness and continued need for a federal-state partnership to ensure the success of newborn screening programs. The four examples provide evidence of the federal government's commitment to support and facilitate the appropriate introduction of newborn genetic testing into clinical and public health practice. Indeed, screening for sickle cell diseases, phenylketonuria, and other metabolic disorders would not have achieved widespread implementation in newborn screening programs without federal support and advocacy.

The examples also illustrate that federal funding provided the impetus for research, implementation of new ideas and technologies, development of policies and guidelines, and quality assessment and program improvement. Federal monies have also been used effectively for developing educational materials, supporting training and educational activities, and facilitating discussions, communication, and dissemination of critical and relevant findings (Therrell et al. 2007). Frequently, initial funding for various demonstration program activities has led to supplemental funding of more comprehensive program implementation.

To ensure equitable prevention activities in public health across the country, the federal government probably will be asked to provide additional support, and the prudent exercise of responsibility and leadership should continue. Inevitably tension may arise from federal efforts to achieve equity, either because of a perceived unfunded federal mandate or because of a state's inability to respond to a federal recommendation. It remains to be seen whether federal efforts will be appropriately responsive and adequately financed to ensure public health oversight of newborn screening programs, while encouraging innovation in the use of technology.

DISCLAIMER

Opinions stated herein are those of the authors and not necessarily of the Health Resources and Services Administration or the Department of Health and Human Services.

NOTES

1. "Newborn Screening Act Sheets and Confirmatory Algorithms" (www.acmg.net/resources/policies/ACT/condition-analyte-links.htm).

2. Health Resources and Services Administration, Maternal and Child Health, Advisory Committee on Heritable Disorders in Newborns and Children (http://www.hrsa.gov/heritable disorderscommittee).

REFERENCES

American Academy of Pediatrics. 2003. The Maternal Phenylketonuria Collaborative Study: new developments and the need for new strategies. *Pediatrics* 112 (Suppl): 1513–87.

Azen, C., Koch, R., Friedman, E., Wenz, E., and Fishler, K. 1996. Summary of findings from the United States Collaborative Study of children treated for phenylketonuria. *Eur J Pediatr* 155 (1): S29–32.

Committee for the Study of Inborn Errors of Metabolism, Division of Medical Sciences, Assembly of Life Sciences, National Research Council. 1975. *Genetic Screening Programs, Principles, and Research.* Washington, DC: National Academy of Sciences.

Diggs, L. W. 1973. Sickle cell disease diagnosis, management, education, and research. In *Sickle Cell Disease: Diagnosis, Management, Education, and Research*, ed. J. F. Bertles and D. L. Wethers, pp. 189–219. Saint Louis, MO: Mosby.

Garrick, M. D., Dembure, P., and Guthrie, R. 1973. Sickle-cell anemia and other hemoglobin-opathies: procedures and strategy for screening employing spots of blood on filter paper as specimens. *N Engl J Med* 288 (24): 1265–68.

Gaston, M. H., Verter, J. I., Woods, G., Pegelow, C., Kelleher, J., Presbury, G., Zarkowsky, H., Vi-chinsky, E., Iyer, R., and Lobel, J. S. 1986. Prophylaxis with oral penicillin in children with sickle cell anemia: a randomized trial. *N Engl J Med* 314 (25): 1593–99.

Githens, J. H., Lane, P. A., McCurdy, R. S., Houston, M. L., McKinna, J. D., and Cole, D. M. 1990. Newborn screening for hemoglobinopathies in Colorado: the first 10 years. *Am J Dis Child* 144 (4): 466–70.

Grover, R. 1989. Newborn screening for sickle cell disease and other hemoglobinopathies: newborn screening in New York City. *Pediatrics* 83 (5 Pt 2): 819–22.

Grover, R., Wethers, D., Shahidi, S., Grossi, M., Goldberg, D., and Davidow, B. 1978. Evaluation of the expanded newborn screening program in New York City. *Pediatrics* 61 (5): 740–49.

Guthrie, R. 1962. Screening for inborn errors of metabolism in the newborn infant: a multiple test program. *Birth Defects* 4:92–98.

———. 1964. Routine screening for inborn errors in the newborn: "inhibition assays," "instant bacteria" and multiple tests. In *Proceedings of the International Congress on the Scientific Study of Mental Retardation, Copenhagen*, pp. 495–99. Copenhagen: Statens Andssvage Forsong.

———. 1992. The origin of newborn screening. *Screening* 1:5–15.

Guthrie, R., and Susi, A. 1963. A simple phenylalanine method for detecting phenylketonuria in large populations of newborn infants. *Pediatrics* 32 (3): 338–43.

Guthrie, R., and Whitney, S. 1964. *Phenylketonuria: Detection in the Newborn Infant as a Routine Hospital Procedure.* Children's Bureau Publ. No. 419. Washington, DC: U.S. Department of Health, Education and Welfare.

Hannon, W. H., Whitley, R. J., Davin, B., Fernhoff, P., Halonen, T., Lavochkin, M., Miller, J., and Therrell, B. L. Jr. 2007. *Blood Collection on Filter Paper for Newborn Screening Programs—Fifth Edition: Approved Standard.* CLSI Document LA4–A5. Wayne, PA: Clinical Laboratories Standards Institute.

Harris, M. S., and Eckman, J. R. 1989. Georgia's experience with newborn screening, 1981 to 1985. *Pediatrics* 83 (5 Pt 2): 858–60.

Herrick, J. B. [1910] 2001. Peculiar elongated and sickle-shaped red blood corpuscles in a case of severe anemia. *Yale J Biol Med* 74 (3): 179–84.

Hoffman, T. L., Simon, E. M., and Ficicioglu, C. 2005. Biotinidase deficiency: the importance of adequate follow-up for an inconclusive newborn screening result. *Eur J Pediatr* 164 (5): 298–301.

Kaye, C. I., and the Committee on Genetics. 2006. Newborn screening fact sheets. *Pediatrics* 118 (3): e934–963 (available at http://aappolicy.aappublications.org/cgi/content/abstract/ pediatrics;98/3/473).

Koch, R. 1964. *Pediatric Aspects of Phenylketonuria.* Washington, DC: Children's Bureau, U.S. Department of Health, Education and Welfare, US Government Printing Office.

Koch, R., Hanley, W., Levy, H., Matalon, R., Rouse, B., de la Cruz, F., Azen, C., and Gross, F. E. 1990. A preliminary report of the collaborative study of maternal phenylketonuria in the United States and Canada. *J Inherit Metab Dis* 13 (4): 641–50.

National Institutes of Health. 2000. Phenylketonuria (PKU): screening and management. *NIH Consensus Statement* 17 (3): 1–33.

National Institutes of Health, Consensus Conference. 1987. Newborn screening for sickle cell disease and other hemoglobinopathies. *JAMA* 258 (9): 1205–9.

Newborn Screening Task Force. 2000. Serving the family from birth to the medical home: a report from the Newborn Screening Task Force convened in Washington DC, May 10–11, 1999. *Pediatrics* 106 (2 Pt 2): 383–427.

Paul, D. B. 1997. The history of newborn phenylketonuria screening in the US. In *Promoting Safe and Effective Genetic Testing in the United States: Final Report of the Task Force on Genetic Testing*, ed. N. A. Holtzman and M. S. Watson, pp. 137–60. Bethesda, MD: National Institutes of Health.

Pearson, H. A., O'Brien, R. T., McIntosh, S., Aspnes, G. T., and Yang, M. M. 1974. Routine screening of umbilical cord blood for sickle cell diseases. *JAMA* 227 (4): 420–21.

Powars, D., Overturf, G., Weiss, J., Lee, S., and Chan, L. 1981. Pneumococcal septicemia in children with sickle cell anemia: changing trend of survival. *JAMA* 245 (18): 1839–42.

Rappaport, E. 1989. Improving newborn screening with peer review and consultation. In *Proceedings of the Sixth National Neonatal Screening Symposium, May 22–25, 1988, Portland, Oregon*, ed. M. Skeels, N. Buist, and J. M. Tuerck, pp. 15–16. Washington, DC: Association of State and Territorial Public Health Laboratory Directors.

Rouse, B., Azen, C., Koch, R., Matalon, R., Hanley, W., de la Cruz, F., Trefz, F., Friedman, E., and Shifrin, H. 1997. Maternal Phenylketonuria Collaborative Study (MPKUCS) offspring: facial anomalies, malformations, and early neurological sequelae. *Am J Med Genet* 69 (1): 89–95.

Scott, R. B. 1970. Health care priority and sickle cell anemia. *JAMA* 214 (4): 731–34.

Serjeant, B. E., Forbes, M., Williams, L. L., and Serjeant, G. R. 1974. Screening cord bloods for detection of sickle cell disease in Jamaica. *Clin Chem* 20 (6): 666–69.

Sinnette, C., Smith, J., and Smith, C. 1974. Sickle cell disease: legislation, insurability and employability. In *Proceedings of the Addresses to the Legislative and Economic Conferences from New York, New Jersey and Connecticut* (Harlem Hospital Sickle Cell Center, New York, January 12, 1973, and February 23, 1973). New York: Harlem Hospital Sickle Cell Center.

Therrell, B. L., and Hannon, W. H. 2006. National evaluation of US newborn screening system components. *Ment Retard Dev Disabil Res Rev* 12 (4): 236–45.

Therrell, B. L., Johnson, A., and Williams, D. 2006. Status of newborn screening program in the United States. *Pediatrics* 117 (1): 212–52.

Therrell, B. L., Panny, S. R., and Davidson, A. 1992. US Newborn Screening System Guidelines: statement of the Council of Regional Networks for Genetic Services. *Screening* 1 (2): 135–47.

Therrell, B. L. Jr., Simmank, J. L., and Wilborn M. 1989. Experiences with sickle hemoglobin testing in the Texas newborn screening program. *Pediatrics* 83 (5 Pt 2): 864–67.

Therrell, B., Tuerck, J., and McCabe, E. R. B. 1992. Newborn screening systems in the United States: a critical review. In *Neonatal Screening in the Nineties*, ed. B. Wilcken and D. Webster, pp. 18–24. Sydney, Australia: Kelvin Press.

Therrell, B. L., Williams, D., Johnson, K., Lloyd-Puryear, M., Mann, M. Y., and Ramos, L. R. 2007. Financing newborn screening issues and future considerations. *J Public Health Manag Pract* 13 (2): 207–13.

Watson, M. S., Mann, M. Y., Lloyd-Puryear, M. A., Rinaldo, P., and Howell, R. R. 2006. Newborn screening: toward a uniform screening panel and system—executive summary. *Pediatrics* 117 (Suppl): 297–307.

CHAPTER 10

What Is the Role for Evidence-Based Decision Making in Expanded Newborn Screening?

VIRGINIA A. MOYER, M.D., M.P.H.
NED CALONGE, M.D., M.P.H.
STEVEN M. TEUTSCH, M.D., M.P.H.
JEFFREY R. BOTKIN, M.D., M.P.H.
ON BEHALF OF THE UNITED STATES
PREVENTIVE SERVICES TASK FORCE

All U.S. states and territories have state-sponsored public health programs that screen newborns for selected hereditary and congenital conditions. The purpose of screening is to initiate treatment or preventive interventions before the onset of serious health consequences. Phenylketonuria (PKU) is the paradigm condition for newborn screening. This genetic metabolic disorder can cause permanent mental retardation unless infants with the disorder are identified and placed on a special diet very early in life. State-mandated screening for PKU began in the 1960s and 1970s. Over time, individual states added other conditions to their screening panels, based on local perceptions of efficacy, program support, and local advocacy (Newborn Screening Task Force 2000). This process led to major differences among states in the conditions included on test panels and in other program policies and procedures. The differences were not justifiable on the basis of standard screening principles and raised serious equity issues. In 2000, a national task force sponsored by the American Academy of Pediatrics and the Health Resources and Services Administration (HRSA) called for more federal involvement in newborn screening programs and in efforts to develop a standard list of conditions that should be screened for in all states (Newborn Screening Task Force 2000).

In response, HRSA funded the American College of Medical Genetics (ACMG) to convene an expert group to fashion recommendations for a uniform newborn screening panel (American College of Medical Genetics 2006; American College of Medical Genetics Newborn Screening Expert Group 2006). In a report released in 2005 (published in 2006), the ACMG group called for all states to adopt a core screening panel consisting of 29 primary disorders for which evidence of benefit was regarded as compelling and an additional 25 secondary disorders that would be detected incidentally in the process of detecting the core disorders (American College of Medical Genetics 2006). Advocacy and professional organizations as well as the Advisory Committee on Heritable Disorders and Genetic Diseases in Newborns and Children, an official advisory body to the secretary of the Department of Health and Human Services, endorsed the report. The ACMG group's recommendations had begun to circulate even before the report was released and, by the time the full report was available, some states had already begun to expand their newborn screening panels to include the entire list of disorders.

In this chapter, we express serious reservations about the rapid expansion of newborn screening that is currently taking place. We believe that screening recommendations for public health programs should be developed through a process that is transparent, unbiased, evidence-based, and attentive to important societal ethical values. This is especially important for programs that affect every child born in the United States. We discuss the ACMG process and explain why we believe it failed to conform to that standard. We conclude that state and federal policymakers should subject each of the recommended conditions to further objective evaluation before recommending its inclusion in mandated screening panels.

The Technological Imperative: Tandem Mass Spectrometry

A newborn screening program is not just screening tests; it is also parental education, follow-up, diagnosis, treatment and management, and program evaluation. Except for the test for hearing impairment, the tests for conditions in the ACMG's uniform panel are blood analyses. The newborn's heel is stuck, blood is collected on an absorbent card, the card is sent to a laboratory, and the tests are carried out. Babies who test positive for a condition are referred for follow-up testing to confirm the diagnosis, because for every true positive there are false positives—children who do not have the condition. Children found to be true positives must then be linked to appropriate long-term treatment and management. False negatives—children who have the condition but are not identified by the test—can also occur, and usually there is a tradeoff: changing test cutoff levels to reduce the number of false negatives increases the number of false positives. In all, newborn screening is a complex system, and the various parts of the system must be in place and working well if the potential benefits of screening are to be realized.

The invention of the original PKU test and the card (Guthrie card) used to store and transport the blood sample to the laboratory made public newborn screening programs possible. In the past, adding another condition to a program meant adding a new test, and the different tests used a variety of laboratory methods to identify affected children. In contrast, most of the additional conditions recommended by the ACMG group are detected using a single method: tandem mass spectrometry (MS/MS). MS/MS produces results with a high degree of precision and accuracy and permits multiplex testing, in which a single blood analysis screens for many conditions at once (Marsden, Larson, and Levy 2006). It can replace the tests formerly used to screen for PKU and simultaneously screen for a large number of other metabolic abnormalities, some clinically significant and treatable, some clinically significant but not yet treatable, and others of unknown significance.

The availability of this new technology has been important in the creation of political pressure on states to increase their newborn screening efforts. Parents of children with disorders that are candidates for screening, health professionals who treat these disorders, and private firms that sell screening tests and equipment have all advocated for adoption of MS/MS and expansion of state programs (see chapters 2, 4, and 6).

Campaigns inspired by the deaths of children with undiagnosed medium-chain acyl-CoA dehydrogenase deficiency (MCAD), a disorder of fatty acid metabolism, have been particularly influential. People with MCAD cannot go without food for long; fasting may cause them to suddenly experience hypoglycemia, vomiting, lethargy, seizures, encephalopathy, coma, apnea, respiratory arrest, or cardiac arrest, or suffer sudden unexpected death (Centers for Disease Control and Prevention 2000). Treatment includes avoidance of fasting and encouraging the use of nutritional supplements. Advocates have argued that newborn screening programs should invest in MS/MS to prevent mortality and morbidity through identification of children with MCAD and, once the technology is in place, the state might as well test for the whole range of conditions that MS/MS can detect. The ACMG's evaluation methodology was influenced by this perspective; it placed considerable weight on the multiplex capability of MS/MS, giving an advantage to conditions detectable by MS/MS and making it more likely that they would be selected for the uniform panel.

Critics of this perspective have responded that many of these disorders are poorly understood or are not treatable, or both, and screening for such disorders on a population basis departs from standard public health practice. Moreover, they argue that a newborn screening panel should be expanded only if the newborn screening program is fully prepared to make all the components of the complex system available for the added disorders. This would be costly and might not be the best use of scarce health care resources, given the existence of many other unmet child health needs.

A Conceptual Framework for Analysis of Expanded Newborn Screening

Atkins, Seigel, and Slutsky (2005) suggest a framework for use by policymakers in resolving controversy regarding the adoption or implementation of a new technology. The framework asks six major questions:

1 What is the ultimate goal, and how does the intervention achieve those ends?
2 How good is the evidence that the intervention can improve important outcomes?
3 How good is the evidence that the intervention will work in the setting specific to the policymaking under discussion?
4 How do the potential benefits compare with the possible harms or costs of the intervention?
5 What constitutes "good enough" evidence for a policy decision?
6 What other considerations are relevant to policy decisions?

We use this framework to organize our critique of the ACMG group's process, its uniform panel recommendations, and the current expansion of newborn screening.

The Ultimate Goal and the Intervention

The intervention in this case is the *mandatory screening of all newborns* for certain rare hereditary and congenital disorders through a *public health program*, with follow-up to definitive diagnosis and ongoing treatment and management of the condition. The primary goal of the intervention is to improve health outcomes in the screened population of newborns. Given this goal, screening makes sense only if early detection and treatment through screening leads to better health outcomes than would be seen if treatment were initiated when the condition became symptomatic. Achieving this requires the availability of a suitable test and an effective treatment that works better if delivered before the onset of symptoms. Such treatments should have demonstrated benefit with an acceptable degree of confidence.

The mandatory feature of this intervention requires special justification. Medical screening of children for a health condition normally requires parental informed consent, especially when the condition is not a threat to others in the community. Newborn screening has been an exception to this basic ethical standard. When PKU screening was introduced, it was argued that the consequences to a child's health if not identified and treated soon after birth were so dire that they justified creation of a public program that mandated screening and ensured that affected children received treatment. Currently, newborns are screened without parental informed consent in all but a few states; in some states, parents may refuse the mandated screening, but parents often are not aware that they have that option. Not everyone accepts the urgency argument for foregoing informed consent, even for PKU, and this feature has been a source of continuing controversy about the programs (see chapter 6).

In newborn screening, some advocates have advanced secondary goals in addition to the primary goal of improved health outcomes for the infants (see chapter 4). One such goal is the identification of infants with rare abnormalities in order to facilitate the research necessary to develop effective therapeutic interventions. We find this goal to be ethically questionable. Mandated screening to recruit human research subjects does not conform to standard ethical requirements. In response to this criticism, some argue that identification may directly benefit infants by giving their parents the opportunity to enroll them in clinical trials (Alexander and van Dyck 2006). In pediatric cancer care, for example, it is generally accepted that access to clinical trials enhances the overall quality of care, especially for children with poor prognoses. However, in the case of cancer, there is no mandated testing of asymptomatic children before offering access to clinical trials of cancer treatment. At the very least, informed decision making by the parents should be required before screening if there is no direct health benefit to the infant from the screening and the primary goal is to identify potential subjects for research on unproven treatments. Further, there is no research infrastructure in the United States that supports collaborative clinical trials on rare metabolic conditions, as there is for childhood cancer. The generation of useful information from clinical trials requires the development of such an infrastructure. This needs to be a national priority that should be addressed before screening panels are expanded to include a large number of poorly characterized conditions.

Another secondary goal is the provision of information to parents about a child's health status. Advocates make several points in arguing that providing information is an appropriate screening goal, even when a condition has no proven medical treatment.

- The family can avoid the "diagnostic odyssey," a protracted search for an explanation when a child becomes symptomatic.
- The parents can avoid the impact of a second affected child on the family by incorporating information about an inherited condition into their future reproductive decisions (Alexander and van Dyck 2006).
- Parents can use advance knowledge of a child's future health problems to make plans for managing the impact of the condition on the child and the family.
- Simply knowing the information is valuable in itself.

We find these points insufficient to justify mandated public health screening of all newborns. First, a diagnostic odyssey does not begin until a condition manifests clinically. If treatment need not begin until after clinical symptoms appear, why is the solution to odysseys a mandated screening in the newborn period? Screening should not be mandated, and it might be more appropriate to offer testing at the initial onset of symptoms because this strategy would result in fewer false positives. Strategies to enhance early clinical diagnosis in children with symptoms of rare conditions should be more thoroughly considered. Better clinical strategies would reduce the probability of odysseys, and such strategies are important even if universal newborn screening is done. Because screening always produces some false negatives, physicians must be able to recognize the clinical presentation of a condition whether or not it is included in a mandatory screening panel.

On the second point, some parents may welcome information about the risk of an inherited disorder in a future pregnancy, but others may not. In this country, there is a strong ethical presumption that adults should decide what genetic information they wish to have about themselves, and an even stronger presumption that they should make their own reproductive decisions. If the provision of information for reproductive decisions, not health benefit to the child, is to be the goal of screening, parents should give their informed consent to the screening.

Similarly, some parent advocates speak eloquently about their desire to know of a child's condition in advance so they can prepare themselves to provide appropriate care; however, other parents may prefer to remain in ignorance until symptoms appear, if there is no treatment that must be provided before that happens. Given the wide range in clinical presentations and the consequent uncertainty about how an individual child will be affected, the latter preference is reasonable. Obtaining parental informed consent is the ethically appropriate approach because it respects individual values.

Finally, in proposing the provision of information as a secondary goal of newborn screening, some have argued that families have a "right to know" about genetic diseases in their children even if an effective treatment is not available (Alexander and van Dyck 2006). In particular, some argue that if MS/MS is used at all, it should be used to test for all the abnormalities it is capable of detecting and the information should be provided to parents. This goal seems far removed from the goal of improved health outcomes and violates a time-honored tenet of medicine that clinicians should not order a test if the results will not change management. Moreover, receiving this information may have negative consequences for some children and families, such as labeling, anxiety, changes in family relationships and dynamics, and unnecessary treatments.

Obtaining information about a child's health status is a goal that some parents might want to pursue in a clinical care context with informed consent. If mandated public health screening of newborns is justified on other grounds, the information it produces might reasonably be considered an additional benefit to at least some parents, provided any harms and costs to parents and society resulting from the information are also taken into account.

However, the secondary goals of identifying potential research subjects and providing parents with information about a child's future health status do not in themselves justify mandated public health screening of all newborns for a disorder. It is inappropriate for policymakers to consider disorders that have no proven treatment, or have treatments that are relevant only after clinical presentation, as equivalent to PKU in terms of urgency of detection (Grosse et al. 2006; see chapters 4, 5, 6, and 14 for additional perspectives).

In the next section, we focus on the primary goal of improving health outcomes for infants when we discuss the evidence on the effectiveness of interventions.

Evidence of Improvement in Important Health Outcomes and Effectiveness in a Given Setting

To assess whether an intervention can improve health outcomes as expected, policymakers need a great deal of information about the conditions being assessed, the associated screening tests, and the entire newborn screening program structure. For each condition, they need information on the incidence and natural history. How many infants will be identified as having the condition and, of those identified, how many will go on to develop clinically important disease? Even when the natural history of clinically detected cases of a condition is known, the natural history for screen-detected cases is often poorly understood. Many children with screen-detected conditions may never develop clinically important morbidity and mortality, or they may have milder manifestations than those whose conditions are clinically detected.

Policymakers need information on the availability of effective treatments and the extent to which there are advantages to early detection. To justify mandatory public health screening of all newborns, proven effective therapies or preventive strategies should be available, and should be more effective when provided before clinical presentation. Information on the risks of treatment is also important. Unproven treatments that can cause harm are particularly unfortunate for children whose condition would not have progressed to clinically important disease in the first place.

Policymakers also need information on the characteristics of the screening tests, such as false positive and false negative rates. The conditions being tested for are generally rare. When the entire newborn population is tested, even low rates of false positives with an accurate test will lead to follow-up testing of many babies. This may cause parental anxiety and long-term worry. The acceptability of a large number of false positives depends on the extent to which important morbidity and mortality is being prevented or ameliorated.

Finally, to ensure effectiveness in local settings, policymakers must have information about the extent to which a state can put all the relevant pieces in place and create a unified system that works well for each disorder over the entire range of circumstances prevailing throughout the state. Even when there is demonstrated efficacy of a screening intervention under controlled or experimental circumstances, the efficacy of the program in actual practice may be substantially lower (see chapter 11).

How good is the evidence of improvement and effectiveness for the current expansion of newborn screening to many additional disorders? This is difficult to answer because the push for expanded newborn screening has bypassed traditional evidence-based decision-making processes at both the state and federal levels. The ACMG panel's task was to review the evidence on the various conditions and decide which should be included in the uniform panel; however, the expert group developed its own process for carrying out its duties.

The process was neither transparent nor open to independent review. No experts in systematic reviews or development of evidence-based recommendations were invited to participate or comment. At the national level, the U.S. Preventive Services Task Force (USPSTF), the Evidence-Based Practice Centers sponsored by the Agency for Healthcare Research and Quality, the Task Force on Community Preventive Services at the Centers for Disease Control and Prevention, and the Institute of Medicine—none of these groups were invited to participate in or review the process. Other than specific newborn screening specialists, state policymakers were not involved, even though most states have newborn screening advisory committees to advise the executive and legislative branches of state government, and two states (Massachusetts and Washington) have a policy of conducting structured reviews of evidence pertaining to screening tests. The process and the grounds for the ACMG group's recommendations were eventually outlined in a lengthy report (American College of Medical Genetics Newborn Screening Expert Group 2006), and HRSA announced a 60-day public comment period. However, the report's release for review and public comment did not occur until months after the recommendations had become public knowledge and were being endorsed and promoted by advocacy groups.

The detailed report describes a seriously flawed process. In determining the recommended panel of tests, the ACMG group relied on an opinion survey of mostly disease experts, screening specialists, and lay and professional advocates, supplemented by nonsystematic reviews conducted by selected disease experts. The ACMG group developed its own criteria and numerical weighting system to prioritize disorders for inclusion. The system seemed to give as much (or more) weight to the testing technology used as it gave to the health benefits of early detection, with strong preference given to the capability of detecting multiple disorders. Supplemental information related to the estimated prevalence of these disorders demonstrated a lack of robust epidemiological data. Concerns about the quality of the evidence of health effects, the costs of expansion, or potential harms from false positive screening results or potentially unnecessary treatments received little attention.

The ACMG group's recommended core panel consists of 29 disorders that, according to the members of the group, met three "minimum" criteria: a condition identifiable between 24 and 48 hours after birth; availability of a high-throughput screening test with appropriate sensitivity and specificity; and demonstrated benefits of early detection, timely intervention, and efficacious treatment. The first criterion is straightforward, but the second is not, because it requires the interpretation of "appropriate" for each condition. The ACMG group did not provide specific guidance to the survey respondents or selected disease experts on how to do this; moreover, for many of the conditions, there has been little or no recorded experience with large-scale population screening. Thus, it is hard to know what it means to say the criterion is met in all cases.

The third criterion is the most important, and the unequivocal statement that all 29 core disorders satisfy it is also difficult to assess from the information in the report. In the group of metabolic abnormalities identified through MS/MS testing, there are some conditions for which the evidence seems to be fairly strong in support of early detection and screening; for example, good cases can be made for early identification and management of PKU and MCAD. There is substantial experience with population-based screening and treatment of PKU. For MCAD, there is fair information on the prevalence of the disorder, some information about the natural history of the condition, an intervention that seems to reduce at least the risk of fatal metabolic crisis, and little in the way of anticipated harms, although the possible harms are not well characterized in the current literature (Grosse and Dezateux 2006).

For most other abnormalities identified through MS/MS, simple logic and close reading of the report suggest a much greater uncertainty about the incidence of the abnormality and its natural history in individuals identified through screening rather than through clinical presentation. Given this fact, inevitably there is less direct evidence of benefit and more uncertainty about

TABLE 10.1

Evidence Levels in the American College of Medical Genetics Report

Level 1	Derived from well-designed randomized controlled trials or diagnostic studies on relevant populations
Level 2	Derived from well-designed randomized controlled trials or diagnostic studies with minor limitations and/or overwhelming, consistent evidence from observational studies
Level 3	Derived from observational studies (case-control and cohort design)
Level 4	Derived from expert opinion, case reports, and reasoning from first principles

the health consequences of treating children who might never have become symptomatic. Studies of some individual conditions identify variants that do not affect health outcomes, and this variation supports a recommendation against routine screening for such conditions (van Maldegem et al. 2006). Even for MCAD, population-screening studies have suggested that there are less severe genetic variants for which the impact of early detection and treatment is uncertain (Wilcken et al. 2003).

In its report "Conceptualizing and Combining Evidence for Health System Guidance" (Lomas et al. 2005), the Canadian Health Services Research Foundation discusses three types of evidence that are referenced in evidence-based decision making: colloquial evidence, context-free scientific evidence, and contextual scientific evidence. In the foundation's framework, colloquial evidence includes evidence about resources, expert opinion, political judgment, values, habits and traditions, lobbyists, and other elements of the specific issue. Context-free scientific evidence consists of truths that are valid in any context, and is what researchers most often refer to in evidence-based medicine. Contextual scientific evidence consists of truths that depend on the characteristics of the setting in which the intervention takes place.

All of the conditions on the ACMG core list can be considered to be supported by at least colloquial evidence, but it is clear from the report that only a smaller number are well supported by either type of scientific evidence. The opinion survey was (at best) colloquial evidence. In the second tier of the process, the evidence base was assessed and a fact sheet was prepared for each disorder. At least two recognized experts on each disorder validated the fact sheets. In the process, they used a four-level scale (table 10.1) to rank the available evidence related to the condition, the test, the diagnosis, and the treatment; for each disorder, their rankings are shown in Appendix 1 of the report (American College of Medical Genetics 2006). For many conditions, at least one expert categorized the available evidence as level 3 or 4.[1]

To support screening for MS/MS-detectable conditions without good scientific evidence of demonstrated benefit, the ACMG group and other advocates of screening have used extrapolation and supposition to support a conclusion of health benefit. They also argue that the other types of benefits discussed above as secondary goals should be used to justify screening when evidence of direct health benefit is lacking (Howell 2006).

In addition to assessing the evidence related to specific disorders, the ACMG group assessed the ability of states to carry out the activities required to make screening for conditions on the uniform panel effective in local settings. The report identifies significant barriers to the construction of a model newborn screening system, including inadequate state financing, fragmentation of service delivery, limited availability of metabolic disorder specialists, and the absence of universal health coverage. The Newborn Screening Task Force report (2000) and the ACMG report indicate that many states have been struggling to overcome these barriers for the conditions already in their panels; adding many new conditions will be a major undertaking. In our judgment, the ACMG group's assessment provides reason for concern about the extent to which its uniform panel can be effectively implemented nationally.

Comparison of Potential Benefits with Potential Harms or Costs

In addition to the potential risks associated with treatment, all screening tests have more general potential harms, such as parental worry, labeling of children as having serious health problems, and long-term impacts on insurability and employability. In the setting of an intervention with at least fair evidence of effectiveness, benefits may be large enough and certain enough to allow a rough judgment that they outweigh potential harms. When both the benefits and harms are not well characterized, however, a more cautious approach, as advocated by Botkin et al. (2006), is warranted.

Making policy decisions based on an inadequate risk-to-benefit evaluation creates a risk of implementing programs that could potentially do more harm than good or that provide no demonstrable health benefit but expend scarce health care resources. Given tight state budgets for newborn screening programs and for other essential child care services such as Medicaid, resource consumption without benefit must be considered a potential harm.

Sufficiency of Evidence

The evidence evaluations by the U.S. Preventive Services Task Force are produced to inform decisions about whether to introduce services such as screening tests into routine clinical care. Without performing our own full-scale evidence reviews we cannot be sure, but based on the ACMG's fact sheets and the validation reports characterizing the evidence, we believe that if the structured approach of the USPSTF were used to evaluate the list of core conditions, we would come to the following conclusions. A few conditions would be recommended with an A or B grade (having at least fair evidence that benefits outweigh harms); perhaps a few would receive C grades (at least fair evidence, but benefits and harms too closely balanced to support an across-the-board recommendation); and the majority would receive I grades (insufficient evidence to recommend for or against). Therefore, it is troubling that the ACMG group is recommending that these conditions be adopted by all state newborn screening programs. Good public health practice and good ethics require the evidence threshold to be at least as high for a recommendation for mandatory screening of all newborns through a public health program as it is for recommendation of any test for use in clinical care with informed consent.

That the ACMG's expert group was primarily composed of people in the newborn screening field is a matter for concern. Current U.S. practice suggests that interpretations of the sufficiency of evidence relate to how closely an evaluation is linked to advocates of screening versus an independent decision-making body that incorporates health policy experts. In many states, colloquial evidence provided by advocates and medical experts has been the dominant influence. Two states that conducted structured reviews of scientific evidence, Massachusetts and Washington, have implemented MS/MS programs that mandate screening for far fewer conditions than those on the ACMG core panel (Atkinson et al. 2001; Grosse and Gwinn 2001). Massachusetts mandates screening for MCAD but makes other MS/MS testing optional. Washington State currently includes MCAD in its screening panel and is in the process of reconsidering other disorders in the ACMG core panel.

Other Relevant Considerations

The paradigm of evidence-based medicine recently shifted somewhat to be inclusive of nonscientific inputs such as the values of the individual being tested or treated. At the policy level, the inclusion of other considerations is evident in Kohatsu's definition of evidence-based public health as the integration of science-based interventions with community preferences (Kohatsu, Robinson, and Toner 2004). The Canadian Health Services Research Foundation states that colloquial evidence, context-free scientific evidence, and context-sensitive scientific evidence require a deliberative process including consultation with relevant stakeholders in order to be combined and interpreted to reach an evidence-based judgment (Lomas et al. 2005). The same is true of the decisions on newborn screening: those ultimately responsible for setting health policy at the national, state, or even health care system level must balance the scientific evidence, both context-free and contextual, with the evidence that supports a belief in the value of screening for a set of conditions for which the evidence on early detection and treatment is not well developed. Because collective resources, both public and private, support public newborn screening programs, decision makers must also take care to consider the preferences of the entire community concerning the use of those resources, not just the preferences of those directly concerned with newborn screening. Finally, they should ensure that their decisions respect societal ethical values relating to the nature of benefit and harm, and to consent to treatment and research.

It seems clear that the ACMG's approach, which relied mostly on colloquial evidence, failed to be adequately inclusive of the science of demonstration of effectiveness and balance of benefit and harm. It also failed to seek out and incorporate the views of the community at large on the proper place of newborn screening in the allocation of health care resources to child health needs.

Conclusion

At least some of the ACMG's list of 29 core conditions do not meet conventional population-screening criteria at the present time, including the minimum criteria proposed by the ACMG report itself. We do not know how many of these conditions would meet objective criteria for population screening, because the process by which this list was produced excluded the evidence-based approaches accepted by the research community in evaluating medical and public health interventions. The rarity of candidate conditions for screening and the desire to support a politically popular program for the nation's most vulnerable population, newly born infants, may have hindered this process.

The multiplex screening technology was favored in the priority-setting process. The evidence for benefits of early detection for many of these disorders has not been adequately assessed or balanced with potential risks of harm and costs. State policymakers would be well advised to ask probing questions before making decisions about whether to mandate that all newborns be screened for disorders for which evidence of benefit is lacking or incomplete. In particular, we argue that on ethical as well as pragmatic grounds, parents should have a right to choose whether their children are screened for disorders for which the evidence on benefits and harms is equivocal or limited. It is reasonable to expect that a high standard of evidence should be met before a state requires all infants to be screened for any particular disorder. Additional attention is required on how to better involve parents as active participants in newborn screening systems. Research on prenatal education and prenatal permission for unproven newborn screening interventions would be appropriate.

Both states and the federal government should objectively evaluate each condition on the basis of prevention potential and medical rationale, availability of treatment, public health rationale, available technology, and cost-effectiveness, before recommending its inclusion in mandated screening panels. Stakeholders including experts in genetic disorders and advocacy organizations should participate in this process, but not to the exclusion of evidence-based policy experts who are experienced in the objective evaluation of scientific evidence. Because scientific evidence is rapidly evolving, states should regularly revisit their screening lists (e.g., every three to five years).

Finally, we urge that states choosing to expand newborn screening to include disorders for which the evidence of benefits and harms is incomplete commit to collecting longitudinal data on infants who test positive. Although these data will be strongly biased (as all or nearly all children identified by screening are likely to be treated, regardless of whether the treatment will alter health outcomes), this information should help us learn from our experiences and, it is to be hoped, implement truly effective, evidence-based screening programs. Given the imminent arrival of other screening technologies such as DNA microarrays, it is vital that we get the processes in place now to ensure sound, evidence-based decisions that promote the health of our children through the early detection of treatable disorders.

ACKNOWLEDGMENTS AND DISCLAIMER

An earlier version of this chapter was previously published as Virginia A. Moyer, Ned Calonge, Steven M. Teutsch, and Jeffrey R. Botkin, on behalf of the United States Preventive Services Task Force, "Expanding Newborn Screening: Process, Policy, and Priorities," *Hastings Center Report* 38 (3): 32–39 (copyright © 2008 by the Hastings Center; used with permission).

We are grateful to Scott Grosse, Iris Mabry, Barbara Yawn, Alissa Johnson, Mary Ann Baily, and an anonymous reviewer for their thoughtful comments on this chapter. The opinions expressed herein represent the thinking of the U.S. Preventive Services Task Force and the authors alone and do not represent the official position of the Agency for Healthcare Research and Quality or the U.S. Department of Health and Human Services.

NOTE

1. For 12 of the 29 core conditions, the experts' rankings of the evidence levels differed by more than one category (e.g., the evidence for the benefit of treatment might be considered level 1 by one expert and level 3 or 4 by another). This is surprising because the definitions of the levels are clear. One would expect more agreement from experts reviewing a single body of literature.

REFERENCES

Alexander, D., and van Dyck, P. C. 2006. A vision of the future of newborn screening. *Pediatrics* 117 (5): S350–54.

American College of Medical Genetics. 2006. Newborn screening: toward a uniform screening panel and system. *Genet Med* 8 (Suppl 1): 1–252S.

American College of Medical Genetics Newborn Screening Expert Group. 2006. Newborn screening: toward a uniform screening panel and system—executive summary. *Pediatrics* 117 (5 Pt 2): S296–307 (available at www.pediatrics.org/cgi/content/full/117/5/SE1/e296).

Atkins, D., Seigel, J., and Slutsky, J. 2005. Making policy when the evidence is in dispute. *Health Aff (Millwood)* 24 (1): 102–13.

Atkinson, K., Zuckerman, B., Sharfstein, J. M., Levin, D., Blatt, R. J., and Koh, H. K. 2001. A public health response to emerging technology: expansion of the Massachusetts newborn screening program. *Public Health Rep* 116 (2): 122–31.

Botkin, J. R., Clayton, E. W., Fost, N. C., Burke, W., Murray, T. H., Baily, M. A., Wilfond, B., Berg, A., and Ross, L. F. 2006. Newborn screening technology: proceed with caution. *Pediatrics* 117 (5): 1793–99.

Centers for Disease Control and Prevention, National Office of Public Health Genomics. 2000. HuGENet: fact sheets: MCAD deficiency medium-chain acyl-CoA dehydrogenase. www.cdc .gov/genomics/hugenet/factsheets/FS_MCAD.htm.

Grosse, S. D., Boyle, C. A., Kenneson, A., Khoury, M. J., and Wilfond, B. S. 2006. From public health emergency to public health service: the implications of evolving criteria for newborn screening panels. *Pediatrics* 117 (3): 923–29.

Grosse, S. D., and Dezateux, C. 2006. New evidence on the effectiveness of newborn screening for inherited metabolic disease. *Lancet* 369 (9555): 5–6.

Grosse, S. D., and Gwinn, M. 2001. Assisting states in assessing newborn screening options. *Public Health Rep* 116 (2): 169–72.

Howell, R. R. 2006. We need expanded newborn screening. *Pediatrics* 117 (5): 1800–1805.

Kohatsu, N. D., Robinson, J. G., and Toner, J. C. 2004. Evidence-based public health: an evolving concept. *Am J Prev Med* 27 (5): 417–21.

Lomas, J., Culyer, T., McCutcheon, C., McAuley, L., and Law, S., for the Canadian Health Services Research Foundation. 2005. Conceptualizing and combining evidence for health system guidance. www.chsrf.ca/other_documents/evidence_e.php.

Marsden, D., Larson, C., and Levy, H. L. 2006. Newborn screening for metabolic disorders. *J Pediatr* 148 (5):577–84.

Newborn Screening Task Force. 2000. Serving the family from birth to the medical home: a report from the Newborn Screening Task Force convened in Washington DC, May 10–11, 1999. *Pediatrics* 106 (2 Pt 2): 383–427.

van Maldegem, B. T., Duran, M., Wanders, R. J. A., Niezen-Koning, K. E., Hogeveen, M., Ijlst, L., Waterham, H. R., and Wijburg, F. A. 2006. Clinical, biochemical, and genetic heterogeneity in short-chain acyl-coenzyme A dehydrogenase deficiency. *JAMA* 296 (8): 943–95.

Wilcken, B., Wiley, V., Hammond, J., and Carpenter, K. 2003. Screening newborns for inborn errors of metabolism by tandem mass spectrometry. *JAMA* 348 (23): 2304–12.

CHAPTER 11

Research for Newborn Screening

Developing a National Framework

JEFFREY R. BOTKIN, M.D., M.P.H.

Newborn metabolic screening is conducted for approximately four million infants per year in the United States and represents the largest single application of genetic testing in medicine. Newborn screening programs traditionally are run by state public health departments, although there is an emerging commercial sector for the provision of these services. Screening for phenylketonuria (PKU) was initiated in the 1960s, and subsequently the number of conditions on the newborn screening panels increased considerably. However, there is a broad range among states in the number of conditions targeted, from 4 to more than 40. With the advent of new technology such as tandem mass spectrometry (MS/MS) and the recognition of the substantial variability among programs, an active national discussion has emerged to support states in bringing to children high-quality services that are effective and efficient (Newborn Screening Task Force 2000).

Unfortunately, there are significant barriers to conducting research on the efficacy of newborn screening programs. The basic question relevant to efficacy is whether morbidity and/or mortality rates are reduced for affected children identified through a universal screening program, compared with outcomes after clinical diagnosis or selective screening. Assessing the efficacy of universal screening requires a basis on which to make this comparison, with both short-term and long-term outcomes in mind. However, state departments of health often do not have the funds to conduct evaluations of established programs beyond counts of true positive, false positive, and true negative results and laboratory quality assessments. Programs typically do not make systematic attempts to identify affected children who had false negative results or to evaluate formally the longer-term health benefits for affected children. Also, many of the conditions targeted in newborn screening programs are rare, meaning that most states identify only a few affected children with each condition per year. This makes outcome studies with sufficient statistical power through state-based projects virtually impossible in all except the largest states.

A more fundamental barrier to research in newborn screening is an ethical concern regarding the use of randomized controlled trials (RCTs), which are usually considered the standard in research design. The ethical concern arises when an apparently clinically beneficial intervention for affected children is proposed as a component of a population-based screening program. It becomes ethically problematic to propose a control arm for a study in which screening is not provided to a segment of the population, even though the efficacy of the screening approach is unproven. This is a question of scale; can we be confident that interventions that are effective on a smaller, project scale will be effective when implemented on a population basis? To date, the only RCT of newborn screening in the United States is the Wisconsin cystic fibrosis (CF) project. The Wisconsin CF project has been valuable in addressing the efficacy of newborn screening for CF, but the project design, involving randomization, has been the focus of criticism in the lay press and ethical discussion in the professional literature (Begley 2002; Taylor and Wilfond 2004). This project is discussed in more detail below. In the absence of randomized designs, research on newborn screening often is observational, after implementation of screening, with either historical control data or control through comparisons with similar populations that are not screened.

These barriers to research are formidable. Despite the use of this screening technology for four million infants per year in the United States, and many more internationally, in the past three decades, the research basis remains relatively poor. The New York State Task Force on Life and the Law stated, in its 2000 publication on genetic testing: "In fact, only a minority of newborn screening tests that are currently performed have been demonstrated formally to have both clinical validity and utility" (p. 143). Wilcken et al. (2003) concluded more broadly: "Formal evidence of the clinical effectiveness of newborn screening is lacking." Currently, many states are adopting MS/MS for newborn screening programs, despite uncertainties about the sensitivities and specificities of the tests and the natural history and treatability of many conditions identified. Of the 30 or more conditions detectable with MS/MS, medium-chain acyl-CoA dehydrogenase deficiency (MCAD) shows the greatest promise in terms of screening efficacy for children. Nevertheless, as Elliman, Dezateux, and Bedford (2002) observed, "Despite international experience of screening well over a million newborn infants [for MCAD] . . . there has been no report of a systematic follow-up of longer term outcome in affected infants detected by screening" (p. 6). Therefore, although we know that MS/MS can detect affected children and that early intervention can be lifesaving, we remain uncertain about the nature and magnitude of the longer-term benefits of population screening programs.

The implication of these concerns is not only that some modalities of newborn screening may prove to be ineffective when evaluated formally. Experience over several decades and a body of observational research lend support to many of these programs. In this era of evidence-based medicine, however, a less than rigorous approach to research on these large, expensive, and important public health programs is no longer appropriate (A. B. Miller 1988; Wilfond 1995; Grimes and Schulz 2002). The recent history of medicine illustrates how research on popular screening programs can reveal limited efficacy; hospital-admission chest films (U.S. Preventive Services Task Force 2004) and breast self-examinations (Kosters and Gotzsche 2003) are prominent examples. Furthermore, not only does research identify screening programs that are ineffective and/or harmful (Feldman 1990), but formal evaluation can identify aspects of valuable programs that reduce their efficacy in critical ways. Thus the goals of research are not just to make policy decisions to adopt or forgo population screening but also to design programs to maximize benefits and minimize harm. This chapter reviews several examples of newborn screening that illustrate the strengths and weaknesses of the empirical foundation for screening. A proposal to develop a national framework for research on newborn screening is then outlined.

Examples of Challenges in Newborn Screening
Hemoglobinopathies

Screening for hemoglobinopathies is a component of newborn screening programs in 49 states and the District of Columbia. Sickle cell disease (SCD) is the primary condition of interest, although other hemoglobinopathies are also detected (American Academy of Pediatrics 1996). In the United States, SCD occurs most commonly among African Americans, with an incidence at birth of 1 in 375 infants. Other population groups are affected with incidences of 1 in 3000 Native American infants, 1 in 20,000 Hispanic infants, and 1 in 60,000 white infants. Young children with SCD are susceptible to systemic infections with *Streptococcus pneumoniae* at a rate of 8 episodes per 100 person-years, with a case fatality rate of about 35 percent (U.S. Preventive Services Task Force 1996). Early detection of SCD for an infant permits the prophylactic administration of penicillin to prevent pneumococcal infections, in addition to vaccination with *Haemophilus influenzae* type b and pneumococcal vaccines.

The seminal study demonstrating the efficacy of preventive therapy for SCD was published in 1986 by Gaston et al. This multicenter clinical trial randomized children under three years of age with SCD to either penicillin or placebo. The study was terminated after 15 months of follow-up monitoring when results indicated substantial reductions in infection and mortality rates in the treatment group. These impressive results led to a federally sponsored consensus conference in 1987. The conference concluded: "The benefits of screening are so compelling that universal screening should be provided. State law should mandate the availability of these services while permitting parental refusal." Furthermore, "To be effective, neonatal screening must be part of a comprehensive program for the care of sickle cell patients and their families" (National Institutes of Health, Consensus Conference 1987, p. 1207).

The study by Gaston et al. (1986) clearly demonstrated the efficacy of penicillin prophylaxis in reducing morbidity and mortality rates for young children with SCD who were monitored in a longitudinal research environment. However, a key question is whether the efficacy of a preventive treatment can be maintained when expanded to a population level as part of a routine public health program. The impressive benefits of penicillin prophylaxis demonstrated by Gaston and colleagues were for children diagnosed clinically, not through newborn screening. Therefore, the benefits added by newborn screening are for the subsets of affected children who die or become seriously ill before a clinical diagnosis.

Newborn screening is more than a test and an intervention; it must be viewed as a system involving a chain of decisions and actions from the heel stick of the infant through the laboratory, the health department, the primary care provider, and the parents to the effective delivery and maintenance of long-term treatment for the child. Any system is only as good as its weakest link, and the efficacy of all newborn screening programs is contingent on the integrity of this chain.

Gaston et al. (1986) recognized that compliance with the penicillin regimen was critical to the success of prophylaxis, and one of the valuable aspects of their study was the administration of penicillin by mouth rather than injection. Prophylaxis with penicillin administered through injection is painful and requires frequent visits to the clinic, leading to poor compliance. However, compliance can also be poor for many orally administered medicines or diets among both adults and children (Ramgoolam and Steele 2002). A parallel problem involves physicians who are not compliant with standard-of-care measures.

A report by the Centers for Disease Control and Prevention (2000) presented data from 1998 on compliance in newborn screening programs for SCD in California, Illinois, and New York. Parents reported that 93 percent of the children received regular penicillin therapy and 75 percent had received the pneumococcal vaccine. However, 76 percent of physicians reported providing penicillin prophylaxis to their patients and estimated that only 44 percent of parents were compliant. Only 25 percent of patients had received the pneumococcal vaccine. A recent study of children with SCD in Washington State and Tennessee who received their health care through Medicaid found that enough prophylactic antibiotic was dispensed to cover only 40 percent of the year-long study period (Sox et al. 2003). Teach, Lillis, and Grossi (1998) found a penicillin compliance rate of 43 percent among children with SCD, as measured with urine assays. Other reports also illustrated compliance problems with the SCD prophylactic regimen (Wurst and Sleath 2004).

The implication of these data is that it is difficult to know the magnitude of the benefit for newborn screening for SCD. The general consensus in the literature is that mortality and morbidity rates for young children are decreased with newborn screening (Quinn, Rogers, and Buchanan 2004), but acquiring definitive data to draw this conclusion is challenging, for several reasons. First, there has been no formal controlled trial of newborn screening for SCD.

Comparison with historical mortality rates can provide useful information, but historical control data may be biased because of changes in health care with time. Second, the adverse outcomes preventable with screening for SCD occur for a minority of affected children, whether or not prophylactic interventions are used; therefore, it is difficult to identify the benefits of screening without carefully tracking large populations of affected children over time. The ability to track the health outcomes of a large cohort of children is not a feature of our health care system. Third, the almost universal use of newborn screening for SCD makes it impossible to compare otherwise comparable states that use and do not use newborn screening for this condition.

A recent Cochrane review did not identify any RCTs of newborn screening for SCD. The reviewers concluded: "There is however evidence of benefit from early commencement of treatment in SCD, which is made possible by screening in the neonatal period . . . Information from a well designed prospective RCT of neonatal screening is desirable to make recommendations for practice. However such trials may now be considered unethical in view of the proven benefit of early prophylactic treatment with penicillin" (Lees, Davies, and Dezateux 2000).

The conclusion here is that newborn screening for SCD probably is effective in saving many lives per year, but we do not have solid data to demonstrate this efficacy or to define the magnitude of the benefits. It is too late to conduct an efficacy trial of population screening, but additional work on enhancing compliance is warranted. This is a frustrating state of affairs for an intervention that has been adopted for virtually all infants born in the United States and its territories.

Galactosemia

Newborn screening for galactosemia is performed in every state and the District of Columbia. This condition is attributable to a genetic defect in an enzyme responsible for breaking down sugars present in milk, and occurs at a rate of approximately 1 in 60,000 neonates. Affected infants appear normal at birth but within two weeks can develop vomiting, irritability, hepatomegaly, jaundice, and sepsis. Evidence suggests that in the absence of early detection, death in the neonatal period occurs for about 20 to 30 percent of patients. Galactosemia among surviving children is associated with developmental delays. Treatment consists of a diet low in lactose/galactose.

Enthusiasm for newborn screening for galactosemia developed in the 1960s and 1970s, with the identification of a valid test that uses dried bloodspots. Clinical observations demonstrated that affected children experienced prompt resolution of symptoms with initiation of the appropriate diet. However, an important feature of galactosemia is that symptoms develop rapidly in the first two weeks of life, which means that the newborn screening system must be efficient to identify affected children before death or serious illness occurs. Evidence indicates that approximately two-thirds of infants are symptomatic at the time of the report of a positive newborn screening result (American Academy of Pediatrics 1996).

As the technology developed to screen for this devastating condition, there was a strong push to initiate universal screening. Levy, an effective early advocate of newborn screening, wrote an article with Hammersen, in which they stated: "Galactosemia screening should be routine for all newborn infants. It is a disorder with definite and severe complications, but one in which the complications can be prevented with simple and inexpensive treatment" (Levy and Hammersen 1978, p. 875). Subsequently, outcome studies showed that the situation is more complicated. In a study of 350 affected children (mean age nine years) published in 1990, Waggoner, Buist, and Donnell (1990) compared the outcomes of children diagnosed (before the advent of newborn screening) on the basis of clinical symptoms alone and children diagnosed shortly after birth by virtue of having an affected sibling. In this context, early detection on the basis of family history is a surrogate for early detection through population screening. The children diagnosed following the appearance of clinical symptoms had a mean age of diagnosis of 63 days, whereas those diagnosed on the basis of family history had a mean age of diagnosis of 1 day. If early detection and treatment are effective in reducing morbidity rates, then we would expect children diagnosed at birth to have better outcomes than children diagnosed late, after clinical symptoms appear. Unfortunately, the results reported by Waggoner and colleagues showed no statistical differences in intellectual function between these groups. The authors concluded: "It is clear that current methods of treatment, even if carefully followed, do little to ameliorate the long-term complications which occur in the majority of cases regardless of when treatment was begun or how successfully galactose intake was restricted" (Waggoner, Buist, and Donnell 1990, p. 815). Other authors also raised concerns about our current understanding and treatment of galactosemia (Gitzelmann and Steinmann 1984; Matalon 1997; Widhalm, Miranda da Cruz, and Koch 1997).

The study by Waggoner, Buist and Donnell (1990) did not address the efficacy of newborn screening for galactosemia in terms of reduced infant mortality rates. It may be that the goals of newborn screening for galactosemia should be stated only in terms of saving lives and not in terms of protecting intellectual function. However, because of the lack of relevant research trials, it is difficult to determine the reduction in mortality rates resulting from newborn screening. In an Irish study published in 1996, the authors reported 9 deaths among 62 affected children (15%) identified previously through screening, over a 20-year period (Badawi et al. 1996). Eight of the deaths occurred in the first 10 years of life. This mortality rate compares with 7 unexplained infant deaths among 84 siblings of affected children before the era of screening. With the assumption that 25 percent of siblings would be affected with galactosemia (an autosomal recessive condition), approximately 21 of the 84 siblings would have had galactosemia. Therefore, a mortality rate of 7 (33%) of 21 affected siblings can be estimated. This evidence suggests a reduction in mortality rate from 33 to 15 percent with screening, although there is potential for historical bias as well as uncertainty about the affected status of the siblings. In addition, advances in neonatal care over the past 30 years might have produced a lower contemporary mortality rate among affected infants in the absence of screening. Comparable data from the United States are not available, but a reduction in mortality rate of this magnitude would result in about 12 fewer infant deaths resulting from galactosemia per year nationwide with screening, or about 3 lives saved per 1 million children screened. By comparison, the sixth leading cause of infant death in the United States in 2002 was injuries, with a rate of 235 deaths per 1 million children (National Center for Health Statistics 2005).

This brief analysis suggests several conclusions. The early enthusiasm for the efficacy of newborn screening for galactosemia has not been supported by the subsequent data, with respect to the preservation of cognitive function among affected children. These data on the relative efficacy of newborn screening were acquired two decades after some states initiated screening. Early intervention seems to reduce infant mortality rates for galactosemia, but the magnitude of this benefit remains uncertain. Some children still die as a result of galactosemia, despite newborn screening, and clinical diagnosis can be achieved in the absence of screening. Approaches other than universal newborn screening have been evaluated, with promising results (Shah et al. 2001). Again, the purpose of this discussion is not to suggest that newborn screening for galactosemia does not have value but to highlight the limited knowledge on which this enormous public health effort is based.

Neuroblastoma

Neuroblastoma is the most common extracranial tumor among young children, with an incidence of approximately 1 in 7000 children (Castleberry 1997). Better prognoses are associated with younger age and earlier stages of the disease at diagnosis. These features of the condition suggested that pre-symptomatic diagnosis and early treatment might improve the mortality rate. In addition, the tumor secretes a characteristic pattern of catecholamines, which enables detection through blood testing before the emergence of clinical symptoms. Enthusiasm for a screening approach to neuroblastoma led to the development of programs in Japan in the early 1970s. However, there was sufficient uncertainty about the efficacy of screening that two large screening trials were conducted, one in Germany by Schilling et al. (2002) and the other in Canada by Woods et al. (2002).

In the German study, almost 2.6 million children were screened for neuroblastoma in 6 of 16 German states from 1995 to 2000; 2.1 million children served as control subjects in the other German states. The incidence and outcomes of neuroblastoma cases were compared between the screened and control populations over the same time period. In the Canadian study, 476,654 children were screened in Quebec Province between 1989 and 1994, and the results were compared with those for children in separate control populations in Ontario, Minnesota, Florida, and the Greater Delaware Valley. The results of both studies did not demonstrate any benefit from population screening, in terms of mortality rates. Of particular interest was the finding that screening identified many more children than would have been predicted on the basis of the clinical incidence of the disease. This confirmed other observations that neuroblastomas can arise and then resolve spontaneously without producing symptoms. These children might be accurately labeled as having the condition, but they represent false positive results in the sense that they are not destined to be ill with their neuroblastomas. However, all children identified as having neuroblastomas are considered for treatment because physicians may not be able to discriminate between children who will become ill and those who have tumors that will resolve spontaneously. In this situation, screening may seem to lead to improved survival rates for children with neuroblastomas, compared with historical control subjects, but this is only because screening identifies a subset of asymptomatic children who would have fared well anyway.

To illustrate this point, imagine that 20 children in a population have neuroblastomas identified clinically and all are treated. Assume that treatment cures 10 children, and 10 children die as a result of their disease. Therefore, the cure rate is 50 percent. After the introduction of screening, 40 children with neuroblastomas are identified but, unbeknownst to the screeners, in 20 cases the tumor would have resolved spontaneously. All 40 children are treated for their cancer and 10 die, as observed previously (before screening). The apparent cure rate is now 75 percent, an improvement of 25 percentage points that might be falsely attributed to the benefits of the screening program.

This problem is directly relevant to screening for metabolic diseases, because metabolic conditions usually entail a spectrum of severity and the spectrum may include a proportion of individuals with "abnormal" biochemical test results who will never become sick with the disease (Wilcken et al. 2003; Refsum et al. 2004). These neuroblastoma studies are excellent illustrations of the value of population-based research for assessing the efficacy of screening approaches.

Another notable aspect of these studies is the use of separate but relevantly similar populations as control groups. Rather than randomize children within a region to screening versus clinical diagnosis, these studies screened an entire population and compared the outcomes with those for a comparable unscreened population during the same time period. This approach eliminates the problems with historical control data and avoids the complexities of randomizing children to two different groups within a population.

The final aspect of the neuroblastoma studies worth emphasizing is the ability to conduct large-scale, population-wide studies within a reasonable time frame. The German study required the collaboration of 6 of 16 states for the screening intervention and that of the remaining states for clinical data only, as control populations. With uncommon conditions, no individual state could generate a sufficient number of cases to conduct such a study. Obviously this situation pertains to the United States, in which collaboration among multiple states would be essential to obtain a sufficient number of cases in a reasonable time with a population that is representative of the national population. The complexity of this interstate collaboration should not be underestimated, but the obstacles should be confronted in an effort to generate high-quality data on population-based screening programs.

These examples—hemoglobinopathies, galactosemia, and neuroblastoma—illustrate the need for a more consistent and comprehensive approach to evaluating screening tests and programs before their population-wide implementation.

Collaborative Research Agenda

A number of commentators, professional bodies, and state programs have developed criteria for deciding when a condition should be added to newborn screening programs (Wilson and Junger 1968; Committee for the Study of Inborn Errors of Metabolism 1975; Andrews et al. 1994; National Institutes of Health 1997). These criteria typically address the nature of the disease, the availability of a valid test, evidence for the benefits of screening, and the presence of all necessary service elements for a complete screening program. Here we are concerned primarily about the evidence for the benefits of screening. The criteria for what constitutes adequate evidence of benefit have not been established at the national level, leaving this determination up to individual state programs. The lack of established criteria and sufficient data on benefits is a central reason for the substantial variation among states and countries in the conditions targeted in newborn screening programs.

We can imagine the confusion in the United States if drugs and devices were regulated and funded at the state level. Fortunately, we have a national system of drug evaluation and approval through the Food and Drug Administration, by which drugs and devices proposed for human medical use are evaluated through a standard series of research protocols (U.S. Food and Drug Administration 2006). Generally, human studies are pursued only after collection of data on safety in animals, when feasible. In phase I human studies, a small number of participants are involved, primarily for evaluation of safety and pharmacokinetic features. If the drug seems safe, then phase II studies involving up to several hundred participants are pursued to evaluate effectiveness. If these results are promising, then phase III studies are conducted with several hundred to thousands of individuals to assess safety, effectiveness, and dosage. Phase II studies may be performed with or without a control group, and phase III studies often use a randomized, double-blind, controlled protocol to maximize the quality of the data. With the results of these studies, the Food and Drug Administration is in a position to determine whether a drug should be licensed nationally for specific indications for specific population groups (such as adults or children). After approval, phase IV studies may be conducted for postmarketing evaluations of safety and efficacy in new or larger patient populations. The method is long, expensive, and by no means foolproof in terms of safety or efficacy, but it is a remarkably robust approach to the scientific assessment of drugs for medical applications.

A similar framework for the methodical evaluation of screening tests is necessary. The Institute of Medicine Committee on Assessing Genetic Risks concluded, in 1994: "The committee recommends the systematic develop-ment of basic data on the full range of genetic testing and screening services that is needed to provide a sound basis for policy development in the future" (Andrews et al. 1994, p. 306). Other authors also support a standardized approach to genetic test evaluation (Burke et al. 2002). The following is a preliminary proposal for a framework to study newborn screening tests and programs.

There are three basic questions for research to address. First, does early detection and treatment of affected infants or children reduce morbidity and/or mortality rates? Second, if early detection seems beneficial, does a population-based screening approach result in net benefits to affected chil-dren, compared with alternative methods of detection? Third, if there are net benefits from population screening, are these benefits sufficient to warrant the use of public health resources for this purpose? The proposed research framework is designed to answer these questions in sequence.

Does early detection produce better outcomes? There is strong public con-fidence in the ability of medical science to identify signs of future disease and to act decisively to save lives (Russell and Milbank 1994). Screening tests have become prevalent in medicine, including mammograms, Pap tests, digital rectal examinations, sigmoidoscopies, amniocentesis, and measurements of blood pressure and of blood glucose, cholesterol, and prostate-specific antigen levels, to name only a few. Commercial providers are now prominently ad-vertising full-body computed tomography to the public as a method for early detection of a host of potential problems (U.S. Preventive Services Task Force 2005).

However, early detection is not beneficial if medicine does not have the abil-ity to affect the course of the disease. This is more common than popularly thought. The U.S. Preventive Services Task Force (2005) conducts exhaustive analyses of preventive measures. The task force supports screening for breast cancer, colon cancer, and cervical cancer, but it does not advocate popula-tion screening for cancers of the prostate, bladder, pancreas, ovaries, or lung. These decisions are based in large measure on the absence of data indicating that early detection improves outcomes.

An inability to improve outcomes may mean that there is no ability to treat the condition at all or no net benefit to early detection, as measured in a population of individuals. For some conditions, certain individuals may benefit from early detection whereas others are harmed. This can occur particularly when diagnostic or treatment procedures carry substantial risk. As noted above, this is also a concern when there is a broad spectrum of disease severity. In these situations, it may be that the individuals who are most severely affected do not benefit from early detection, those with mild or subclinical disease may be harmed by unnecessary interventions, and those with intermediate severity can obtain benefit from early detection. If clinicians cannot discriminate between these degrees of severity at the time of diagnosis, then affected individuals may experience burdensome or harmful interventions as often as an improved outcome resulting from a screening program.

Stage I Research

For the purposes of this discussion, stage I research refers to projects that seek to determine whether early detection and intervention can improve clinical outcomes. This kind of research can be performed in a variety of ways that do not require population screening. For genetic conditions (the majority of newborn screening conditions), significant information can be obtained by comparing the outcomes of second affected siblings versus first affected siblings when there are discrepancies in the time of diagnosis. A first affected sibling is often diagnosed only after clinical symptoms emerge, and frequently much later, after parents have pursued a "diagnostic odyssey." Once parents have been alerted to the risk for subsequent siblings, the second affected child can be diagnosed prenatally or in early infancy. If a proposed early treatment or preventive strategy is available, then a comparison of the outcomes for the first versus second (and subsequent) affected siblings provides evidence for the efficacy of the intervention. This approach can be used retrospectively, if an intervention is in use for the condition, or prospectively, through enrollment of sibling pairs at the time of diagnosis of the second affected child. The galactosemia study by Waggoner, Buist, and Donnell (1990) noted above is an example of this method.

A second option for stage I research is a RCT of the intervention among children diagnosed clinically. This approach is useful when the initial presentation of the condition is not devastating for the majority of children. Stated differently, it is more useful when only a subset of affected children experience the serious adverse outcome to be prevented. This is because investigators need to know which children are affected before they can be randomized, and the children cannot have already experienced the adverse outcome at the time of randomization. A good example here is penicillin prophylaxis for children with SCD. As discussed above, the study by Gaston et al. (1986) demonstrated that children with SCD fared much better with penicillin prophylaxis, and it is an excellent example of stage I research.

A third approach to stage I research is a small-scale screening project. If a high-risk group can be targeted for screening to detect a sufficient number of affected children, then a RCT of screening for the proposed intervention can be conducted. However, most conditions considered appropriate for population-wide newborn screening are rare enough in the general population, and not sufficiently strongly associated with a particular racial or ethnic group, that targeted screening is not feasible.

An approach that is not as useful for stage I research is the use of historical data comparing children identified at a younger versus older age. Particularly when there is an association between an earlier medical/technological era and the later age of diagnosis, many factors may bias the comparison. More specifically, an earlier age of diagnosis in more recent eras may occur in conjunction with many other improvements in care.

The purpose of stage I research is to provide definitive data on the efficacy of early intervention. The move to population-wide screening should be made only when there is solid evidence that early detection and intervention can lead to improved morbidity and/or mortality rates.

Stage II Research

Stage II research addresses the second question: does a population-based screening approach result in net benefits to affected children, compared with alternative methods of detection? The central point here is that improvements in clinical outcomes that are demonstrable through stage I research may not be achievable in population-wide programs. Rather, the benefits of early detection may be brought to affected children through clinical detection schemes in the absence of population screening. After stage I research, the question is how best to bring the benefits of early detection to affected children.

As noted above, newborn screening programs entail a series of activities from the heel stick through the laboratory to the physician, the family, and ultimately a sustained intervention. Systematic weaknesses in any of these components can seriously hamper the efficacy of the program. The benefits of the SCD program, for example, may be significantly reduced by poor compliance of physicians and parents with prophylaxis and vaccination. In galactosemia and congenital adrenal hyperplasia (CAH) screening programs, the primary value of screening is largely contingent on the ability of the program to provide a rapid test result before the decline and death of some infants at about two weeks of age. Even for PKU, which represents the paradigm program for newborn screening, the efficacy of the program may be impaired substantially by the inability of families to obtain the special foods or to comply with the diet over time (National Institutes of Health, Consensus Development Panel 2001).

An ideal design, from a scientific perspective, is the RCT. Newborns can be randomized to receive either screening for the target condition or no screening. The morbidity and/or mortality rates for the condition can be compared between affected children identified through screening and those identified clinically. To date, the only RCTs of newborn screening are the Wisconsin CF project initiated in 1984 (Farrell et al. 2001) and a CF screening project in the United Kingdom (Chatfield et al. 1991). All newborns in Wisconsin were screened after parental permission was obtained. Tests were run on all samples, but results were reviewed and disclosed for only one-half of the newborns. For infants in the "unscreened" control group, results were disclosed at four years of age. Outcomes have been compared for the screened and unscreened groups over the past 20 years. Although the magnitude and nature of the benefits of newborn screening for CF remain controversial, the Wisconsin trial has been critical in providing data for policy development (Grosse et al. 2004).

A number of potential problems arise with a randomized, controlled design, from methodological and ethical perspectives. First, if screening itself is randomized, then it may be difficult or impossible to identify all cases in the unscreened group. This creates a significant potential for bias. In the unscreened group, those who come to medical attention by virtue of clinical symptoms, or who do so at a younger age (within the window of a research project), tend to be those who are more severely affected with the condition. In contrast, a screened population would include children across the full spectrum of severity, including those who are mildly affected and those who may never become ill with the condition. Given this difference in sensitivity for detection, a comparison of outcomes for the screened and unscreened populations would show improved outcomes for the screened group even if the intervention conferred no benefit. This problem is similar to "length bias" (National Center for Biotechnology Information 1996) and is primarily a concern for studies that calculate outcome data in terms of number of deaths per affected population. This occurs because the denominator is expanded through screening to include mildly affected individuals, thereby decreasing the apparent death rate compared with a group composed of only severely affected individuals.

There are at least two ways to address this problem. The neuroblastoma studies measured their outcomes in terms of deaths per 100,000 population in the screened and unscreened populations. This eliminated the bias created by calculating death rates for the affected population. Another approach to eliminating this source of bias is to follow the approach used in the Wisconsin CF screening trial, in which blood samples were obtained for all infants but screening test results were disclosed on a randomized basis. As noted, for the "unscreened" group the results were reviewed and disclosed when the children were four years of age. This allowed the research team to obtain outcome data for all affected members of the unscreened group as if they had been screened at the outset. Through this approach, subclinical cases could be identified in the unscreened group that were never identified clinically.

A second practical problem with RCTs arises from the low incidence of most conditions targeted by newborn screening. Because RCTs require at least two approximately equivalent groups for comparison and the groups must be of a size to allow determination with sufficient power that a significant difference exists in the outcome measure, trials for most newborn screening conditions must be large. This issue is discussed in greater detail below.

The more fundamental challenges to the performance of RCTs in stage II research are ethical concerns. If early intervention has been shown to be effective in stage I research, is it ethical to randomize infants to an unscreened group (Wilcken 2003)? In addressing this question, a standard approach in research ethics is to ask whether there is equipoise between the two study groups (Freedman 1987; Miller and Weijer 2003). That is, is there genuine uncertainty in the professional community about whether an intervention under study is preferable to an alternative? If there is general consensus that one option is preferable to another on the basis of solid scientific evidence, then randomization is not ethically acceptable. Conversely, if there is legitimate uncertainty about the best approach, then randomization is acceptable.

The newborn screening context and the proposed stage I and stage II approach offer a greater level of complexity than most questions about equipoise. If stage I research demonstrates benefit, then there is no longer equipoise with respect to earlier intervention versus later intervention. However, equipoise may still exist with respect to whether the benefits of earlier intervention can be achieved through the complex mechanism of a newborn screening program. Therefore, the "test article" is the program (i.e., the method of delivering the key intervention, rather than the intervention itself).

Let us look at the issue as if the research were to address the efficacy of a delivery method for an intervention that we know to be effective. Would it be ethical to compare a particular delivery method with no delivery at all? This is analogous to comparing a placebo in a trial with an intervention of known efficacy. This is generally considered unethical, unless the risks to the placebo group are minor or there are other compelling scientific reasons to consider a placebo group (World Medical Association 2004). In the context of newborn screening, however, population-wide screening may not be the only approach to early detection. For example, neonatal deaths resulting from CAH or galactosemia usually occur after symptoms have been present for several days. This symptomatic period offers the opportunity for clinical diagnosis. The more effective parents and the health care system are in recognizing and responding to characteristic symptoms in individual cases, the less marginally effective a population screening approach would be. Therefore, for these conditions, screening is an alternative not to nothing (as with a placebo) but to the health care system that is designed to respond to sick infants. When there is no ability to detect an affected child before permanent damage has been done, as with PKU and congenital hypothyroidism, then an unscreened group in a RCT would be analogous to a placebo group; this study design would not be appropriate. Therefore, randomization need not be framed in terms of screening versus nothing, depending on the condition, but can be regarded as diagnosis through screening versus diagnosis through clinical care or selective screening.

Attempts can be made to promote efficient diagnosis through clinical care, with education programs for clinicians and perhaps parents, or through selective screening. A recent study in Toronto evaluated the possibility of screening for galactosemia by testing every infant under two weeks of age who presented to the hospital for any reason and infants over two weeks of age with clinical suspicion of galactosemia (Shah et al. 2001). The authors suggested that this selective approach to screening identifies severely affected infants with galactosemia as rapidly as does population screening.

The conclusion is that RCTs for phase II screening are ethical in the context of newborn screening when population screening is compared with a potentially effective method of delivering a timely clinical diagnosis or with a more selective screening approach. RCTs of screening for conditions similar in their presentation to CAH, CF, or SCD can be justified, particularly in conjunction with efforts to enhance the education of care providers about early clinical detection. In contrast, for conditions with no prospect of early clinical detection before significant morbidity or death, a stage II RCT would not be justified.

If a RCT is not deemed ethical or feasible, an alternative is a cohort design. A prospective cohort design compares the outcomes of two groups that differ by virtue of the intervention in question. In this context, a screened cohort of children is compared with an unscreened cohort with respect to morbidity and mortality rates over time. For newborn screening, a cohort could consist of a state's entire newborn population or the population of a group of states. There are several significant advantages to a cohort design for stage II screening research. Logistically, it is easier to implement a screening program in a population in a uniform manner. From an ethical perspective, the cohort design avoids explicitly assigning children to an unscreened group when screening could have been made available. Of course, infants in the unscreened cohort do not receive screening, but this is already the situation in the absence of the research project. After a new screening modality is introduced, some states take years to consider or to implement the program, whereas others are more rapid adopters; this provides the opportunity for a comparison of cohorts according to state.

There are two principal drawbacks to the cohort design. The first is the potential bias created by comparing populations that may differ in a number of variables in addition to the variable in question (screening). State populations may differ with respect to factors such as socioeconomic status, racial/ethnic composition, disease prevalence, health care services, insurance coverage, and efficacy of the newborn screening programs. If differences in morbidity or mortality rates are found between cohorts, there may be residual concern that the explanation does not depend on screening. The second problem inherent in the cohort design in this context involves the ability to identify and monitor affected individuals in the unscreened cohort. A screening program establishes the population prevalence at an individual level and creates the infrastructure for tracking. Without a screening program, there is unlikely to be a comprehensive registry of affected children. Furthermore, children who might have died at a young age as a result of the condition under study might not have been identified as affected, or their condition might not have been recorded in such a manner that the information was retrievable. Many affected children may be known to subspecialty physicians in regional referral centers, but these are likely to be more severely affected children.

This latter problem of defining the affected group in the unscreened population is a fundamental challenge. If a cohort design is used for stage II research, then the unscreened cohort must be evaluated as thoroughly as possible to identify affected children. One way to address this problem adds a retrospective component to the project. In many states, residual newborn screening samples are stored for variable lengths of time, from months to decades (Therrell et al. 1996; Mandl et al. 2002). If the analyte is stable with time, then stored newborn screening samples can be screened for the condition in question at a time when differences in morbidity or mortality rates between the screened and unscreened groups would be expected. Children identified as affected through retrospective screening of residual samples could be traced and their health status measured and compared with that of children identified prospectively through screening. Children who died before a diagnosis was made also could be identified through this approach. Furthermore, children who were mildly affected and never came to clinical recognition would also be identified. Identification and tracking would not be 100 percent complete with this method, but this approach is likely to be much more comprehensive than other forms of identification. This method would require the retention and availability of residual newborn screening samples. A discussion of the extent and content of parental information or permission for this kind of research would be important (Taylor and Wilfond 2004).

For stage II research, the best approach from a scientific perspective is a RCT. This approach is likely to be expensive, however, and ethical concerns may be prominent. Nevertheless, a randomized design is justifiable in some circumstances. In other circumstances, a cohort design with retrospective screening of the initially unscreened cohort is most appropriate from both scientific and ethical perspectives.

Stage III and Stage IV Research

Stage III research addresses the relative costs of a population-wide screening program. Stage II research may demonstrate benefits of screening, but decisions about implementation will depend on estimates of the costs necessary to achieve the benefits. Cost-benefit and cost-effectiveness analyses may be feasible with data obtained in stage II projects. An economic analysis may reveal that the benefits do not justify the costs of the program.

To date, cost-benefit and cost-effectiveness analyses of newborn metabolic screening have been limited by the lack of solid data on some variables. Economic analyses are often contingent on a variety of assumptions under the best of circumstances, including program costs, health care costs, test parameters, effectiveness of interventions, and the economic value of intangible factors such as anxiety associated with false positive results and knowledge for future reproductive decision making. Overall, the track record for cost-benefit analyses for newborn screening has been described as "unimpressive" (Pollitt 2001). Nevertheless, economic analyses are important for policy decisions. Several recent reports addressed MS/MS as an emerging technology. Schoen et al. (2002) found that MS/MS compares favorably with other mass screening programs on a cost-benefit basis. In contrast, Pandor et al. (2004), in a systematic analysis in the United Kingdom, concluded that the evidence supports the use of MS/MS for PKU and MCAD but sufficient evidence for screening for other conditions is lacking. Both studies revealed the need for additional data to estimate actual costs and benefits. Despite the volume of literature on newborn screening for CF, Grosse et al. (2004) noted, a full cost-effectiveness analysis has not been performed. Under the proposed research scheme, stage II projects could be designed to collect data on costs and benefits in a manner conducive to stage III economic analysis.

Stage IV research involves projects designed for the ongoing evaluation of established programs. As yet, state newborn screening programs have a limited ability to conduct formal program evaluations and quality assurance activities. The American Academy of Pediatrics and Health Resources and Services Administration's Newborn Screening Task Force (Newborn Screening Task Force 2000) and the Council of Regional Networks for Genetic Services (Pass et al. 2000) place a strong emphasis on the funding and development of these activities. Effective programs require periodic evaluation because of changes in test technology, program organization, population demographic features, and health care resources.

Collaboration

Central to the ability to conduct stage II and stage III research is a population of sufficient size. Because of the low incidence of many conditions detectable by newborn screening, multiple states must collaborate with a single protocol to achieve adequate statistical power that will allow timely conclusions about the efficacy of a screening strategy. Traditionally, development of multistate research collaborations has been a significant challenge, and such collaborations have not been common in the newborn screening literature beyond survey projects. New federal initiatives may help foster larger-scale, multistate projects.

Title XXVI of the Children's Health Act of 2000, Screening for Heritable Disorders, establishes a program to improve the ability of states to provide newborn and child screening. The act authorizes the secretary of the Department of Health and Human Services "to award grants to States, or a political subdivision of a State, or a consortium of two or more States, or political subdivisions of States to enhance, improve or expand the ability of States and local public health agencies to provide screening, counseling or health care services to newborns and children having or at risk for heritable disorders" and "to award grants to eligible entities to provide for the conduct of demonstration programs to evaluate the effectiveness of screening, counseling or health care services in reducing the morbidity and mortality caused by heritable disorders in newborns and children" (Health Resources and Services Administration 2005, §1109). To assist in this process, the secretary recently established the Advisory Committee on Heritable Disorders in Newborns and Children. The tasks of the committee are to provide advice and recommendations to the secretary concerning the grants and projects authorized under the act.

In addition, Title V of the Social Security Act provided funding for two new initiatives. A national coordinating center for newborn screening is being established, and regional genetic services and collaborative newborn screening systems are now in place. Seven national regions have been created to "enhance and support the genetics and newborn screening capacity of States across the nation by undertaking a regional approach toward addressing the maldistribution of genetic resources. These grants are expected to improve the health of children and their families by promoting the translation of genetic medicine into public health and health care services" (Title V of the Social Security Act, §501 [a][2]).

These national priorities and funding opportunities represent an exciting development in the care of children. The state-level organization of newborn screening services is an accident of history, but should not be a barrier to evidence-based analyses of the benefits and risks of these complex programs. The adoption of an accepted sequence of research protocols through multistate collaborations should greatly facilitate the translation of research into effective public health programs. Ultimately, there are no serious methodological or ethical barriers to conducting stage I, stage II, and stage III research to demonstrate the efficacy of newborn screening modalities before the implementation of population-based programs.

ACKNOWLEDGMENTS

An earlier version of this chapter was previously published in *Pediatrics* 116: 862–71, copyright © 2005 by AAP, and is used with permission.

My thanks go to Mary Ann Baily and colleagues at the Hastings Center for supporting this work under grant 1 R01 HG02579.

REFERENCES

American Academy of Pediatrics, Committee on Genetics. 1996. Newborn screening fact sheets. *Pediatrics* 98 (3): 473–501.

Andrews, L. B., Fullarton, J. E., Holtzman, N. A., and Motulsky, A. G. 1994. *Assessing Genetic Risks: Implications for Health and Social Policy.* Washington, DC: National Academy of Sciences.

Badawi, N., Cahalane, S. F., McDonald, M., Mulhair, P., Begi, B., O'Donohue, A., and Naughten, E. 1996. Galactosaemia: a controversial disorder: screening and outcome, Ireland, 1972–1992. *Ir Med J* 89 (1): 16–17.

Begley, S. 2002. Research involving tests on newborn highlights need for stricter ethics. *Wall Street Journal,* May 3.

Burke, W., Atkins, D., Gwinn, M., Guttmacher, A., Haddow, J., Lau, J., Palomaki, G., Press, N., Richards, C. S., Wideroff, L., and Wiesner, G. L. 2002. Genetic test evaluation: information needs of clinicians, policy makers, and the public. *Am J Epidemiol* 156 (4): 311–18.

Castleberry, R. P. 1997. Biology and treatment of neuroblastoma. *Pediatr Clin North Am* 44 (4): 919–37.

Centers for Disease Control and Prevention. 2000. Update: newborn screening for sickle cell disease: California, Illinois, and New York, 1998. *JAMA* 284 (11): 1373–74.

Chatfield, S., Owen, G., Ryley, H. C., Williams, J., Alfaham, M., Goodchild, M. C., and Weller, P. 1991. Neonatal screening for cystic fibrosis in Wales and the West Midlands: clinical assessment after five years of screening. *Arch Dis Child* 66 (1 Spec No): 29–33.

Committee for the Study of Inborn Errors of Metabolism, Division of Medical Sciences, Assembly of Life Sciences, National Research Council. 1975. *Genetic Screening: Programs, Principles, and Research*. Washington, DC: National Academy of Sciences.

Elliman, D. A., Dezateux, C., and Bedford, H. E. 2002. Newborn and childhood screening programmes: criteria, evidence, and current policy. *Arch Dis Child* 87 (1): 6–9.

Farrell, P. M., Kosorok, M. R., Rock, M. J., Laxova, A., Zeng, L., Lai, H. C., Hoffman, G., Laessig, R. H., and Splaingard, M. L. 2001. Early diagnosis of cystic fibrosis through neonatal screening prevents severe malnutrition and improves long-term growth. Wisconsin Cystic Fibrosis Neonatal Screening Study Group. *Pediatrics* 107 (1): 1–13.

Feldman, W. 1990. How serious are the adverse effects of screening? *J Gen Intern Med* 5 (5 Suppl): S50–53.

Freedman, B. 1987. Equipoise and the ethics of clinical research. *N Engl J Med* 317 (3): 141–45.

Gaston, M. H., Verter, J. I., Woods, G., Pegelow, C., Kelleher, J., Presbury, G., Zarkowsky, H., Vichinsky, E., Iyer, R., and Lobel, J. S. 1986. Prophylaxis with oral penicillin in children with sickle cell anemia: a randomized trial. *N Engl J Med* 314 (25): 1593–99.

Gitzelmann, R., and Steinmann, B. 1984. Galactosemia: how does long-term treatment change the outcome? *Enzyme* 32 (1): 37–46.

Grimes, D. A., and Schulz, K. F. 2002. Uses and abuses of screening tests. *Lancet* 359 (9309): 881–84.

Grosse, S. D., Boyle, C. A., Botkin, J. R., Comeau, A. M., Kharrazi, M., Rosenfeld, M., and Wilfond, B. S. 2004. Newborn screening for cystic fibrosis: evaluation of benefits and risks and recommendations for state newborn screening programs. *MMWR Recomm Rep* 53 (RR-13): 1–36.

Health Resources and Services Administration, Maternal and Child Health Bureau. 2005. Advisory Committee on Heritable Disorders and Genetic Diseases in Newborns and Children Charter. www.mchb.hrsa.gov/programs/genetics/committee/charter.htm.

Kosters, J. P., and Gotzsche, P. C. 2003. Regular self-examination or clinical examination for early detection of breast cancer. *Cochrane Database Syst Rev*, no. 2:CD003373.

Lees, C. M., Davies, S., and Dezateux, C. 2000. Neonatal screening for sickle cell disease. *Cochrane Database Syst Rev*, no. 2:CD001913.

Levy, H. L., and Hammersen, G. 1978. Newborn screening for galactosemia and other galactose metabolic defects. *J Pediatr* 92 (6): 871–77.

Mandl, K. D., Feit, S., Larson, C., and Kohane, I. S. 2002. Newborn screening program practices in the United States: notification, research, and consent. *Pediatrics* 109 (2): 269–73.

Matalon, R. 1997. Galactosemia: promise, frustration and challenge. *J Am Coll Nutr* 16 (3): 190–91.

Miller, A. B. 1988. The ethics, the risks and the benefits of screening. *Biomed Pharmacother* 42 (7): 439–42.

Miller, P. B., and Weijer, C. 2003. Rehabilitating equipoise. *Kennedy Inst Ethics J* 13 (2): 93–118.

National Center for Biotechnology Information. 1996. *Guide to Clinical Preventive Services*. 2nd ed.

Health Services/Technology Assessment Text. Washington, DC: National Library of Medicine (available at: www.ncbi.nlm.nih.gov/books/bv.fcgi?rid=hstat3.chapter.10062).

National Center for Health Statistics. 2005. Infant deaths/mortality. www.cdc.gov/nchs/data/dvs/LCWK7_2002.pdf.

National Institutes of Health. 1997. *Promoting Safe and Effective Genetic Testing in the United States: Final Report of the Task Force on Genetic Testing.* Bethesda, MD: National Institutes of Health.

National Institutes of Health, Consensus Conference. 1987. Newborn screening for sickle cell disease and other hemoglobinopathies. *JAMA* 258 (9): 1205–9.

National Institutes of Health, Consensus Development Panel. 2001. Conference statement: phenylketonuria: screening and management, October 16–18, 2000. *Pediatrics* 108 (4): 972–82.

New York State Task Force on Life and the Law. 2000. *Genetic Testing and Screening in the Age of Genomic Medicine.* New York: New York State Task Force on Life and the Law.

Newborn Screening Task Force. 2000. Serving the family from birth to the medical home: a report from the Newborn Screening Task Force convened in Washington DC, May 10–11, 1999. *Pediatrics* 106 (2 Pt 2): 383–427.

Pandor, A., Eastham, J., Beverley, C., Chilcott, J., and Paisley, S. 2004. Clinical effectiveness and cost-effectiveness of neonatal screening for inborn errors of metabolism using tandem mass spectrometry: a systematic review. *Health Technol Assess* 8 (12): iii, 1–121.

Pass, K. A., Lane, P. A., Fernhoff, P. M., Hinton, C. F., and Panny, S. R. 2000. US newborn screening system guidelines II: follow-up of children, diagnosis, management and evaluation. Statement of the Council of Regional Networks for Genetic Services (CORN). *J Pediatr* 137 (4 Suppl): 1–46.

Pollitt, R. J. 2001. Newborn mass screening versus selective investigation: benefits and costs. *J Inherit Metab Dis* 24 (2): 299–302.

Quinn, C. T., Rogers, Z. R., and Buchanan, G. R. 2004. Survival of children with sickle cell disease. *Blood* 103 (11): 4023–27.

Ramgoolam, A., and Steele, R. 2002. Formulations of antibiotics for children in primary care: effects on compliance and efficacy. *Paediatr Drugs* 4 (5): 323–33.

Refsum, H., Fredriksen, A., Meyer, K., Ueland, P. M., and Kase, B. F. 2004. Birth prevalence of homocystinuria. *J Pediatr* 144 (6): 830–32.

Russell, L. B., and Milbank, M. F. 1994. *Educated Guesses: Making Policy about Medical Screening Tests.* Berkeley: University of California Press.

Schilling, F. H., Spix, C., Berthold, F., Erttmann, R., Fehse, N., Hero, B., Klein, G., Sander, J., Schwarz, K., Treuner, J., Zorn, U., and Michaelis, J. 2002. Neuroblastoma screening at one year of age. *N Engl J Med* 346 (14): 1047–53.

Schoen, E. J., Baker, J. C., Colby, C. J., and To, T. T. 2002. Cost-benefit analysis of universal tandem mass spectrometry for newborn screening. *Pediatrics* 110 (4): 781–86.

Shah, V., Friedman, S., Moore, A. M., Platt, B. A., and Feigenbaum, A. S. 2001. Selective screening for neonatal galactosemia: an alternative approach. *Acta Paediatr* 90 (8): 948–49.

Sox, C. M., Cooper, W. O., Koepsell, T. D., DiGiuseppe, D. L., and Christakis, D. A. 2003. Provision of pneumococcal prophylaxis for publicly insured children with sickle cell disease. *JAMA* 290 (8): 1057–61.

Taylor, H. A., and Wilfond, B. S. 2004. Ethical issues in newborn screening research: lessons from the Wisconsin cystic fibrosis trial. *J Pediatr* 145 (3): 292–96.

Teach, S. J., Lillis, K. A., and Grossi, M. 1998. Compliance with penicillin prophylaxis in patients with sickle cell disease. *Arch Pediatr Adolesc Med* 152 (3): 274–78.

Therrell, B. L., Hannon, W. H., Pass, K. A., Lorey, F., Brokopp, C., and Eckman, J. 1996. Guidelines for the retention, storage and use of residual dried blood spot samples after newborn screening analysis: statement of the Council of Regional Networks for Genetic Services. *Biochem Mol Med* 57 (2): 116–24.

U.S. Food and Drug Administration. 2006. From test tube to patient: protecting America's health through human drugs. www.fda.gov/fdac/special/testtubetopatient/default.htm.

U.S. Preventive Services Task Force. 1996. Screening for hemoglobinopathies. In *Guide to Clinical Preventive Services*, 2nd ed., pp. 485–494. Washington, DC: U.S. Preventive Services Task Force (available at www.ahrq.gov/clinic/2ndcps/hemoglob.pdf).

———. 2004. Lung cancer screening. www.ahrq.gov/clinic/uspstf/uspslung.htm#summary.

———. 2005. Guide to clinical preventive services. www.ahcpr.gov/clinic/cps3dix.htm#cancer.

Waggoner, D. D., Buist, N. R., and Donnell, G. N. 1990. Long-term prognosis in galactosaemia: results of a survey of 350 cases. *J Inherit Metab Dis* 13 (6): 802–18.

Widhalm, K., Miranda da Cruz, B. D., and Koch, M. 1997. Diet does not ensure normal development in galactosemia. *J Am Coll Nutr* 16 (3): 204–8.

Wilcken, B. 2003. Ethical issues in newborn screening and the impact of new technologies. *Eur J Pediatr* 162 (Suppl 1): S62–66.

Wilcken, B., Wiley, V., Hammond, J., and Carpenter, K. 2003. Screening newborns for inborn errors of metabolism by tandem mass spectrometry. *N Engl J Med* 348 (23): 2304–12.

Wilfond, B. S. 1995. Screening policy for cystic fibrosis: the role of evidence. *Hastings Cent Rep* 25 (3): S21–23.

Wilson, J. M. G., and Jungner, G. 1968. *Principles and Practice of Screening for Disease*. Geneva: World Health Organization.

Woods, W. G., Gao, R. N., Shuster, J. J., Robison, L. L., Bernstein, M., Weitzman, S., Bunin, G., Levy, I., Brossard, J., Dougherty, G., Tuchman, M., and Lemieux, B. 2002. Screening of infants and mortality due to neuroblastoma. *N Engl J Med* 346 (14): 1041–46.

World Medical Association. 2004. Declaration of Helsinki. www.wma.net/e/policy/b3.htm.

Wurst, K. E., and Sleath, B. L. 2004. Physician knowledge and adherence to prescribing antibiotic prophylaxis for sickle cell disease. *Int J Qual Health Care* 16 (3): 245–51.

CHAPTER 12

Ethical and Policy Issues Involving Research with Newborn Screening Blood Samples

KAREN J. MASCHKE, PH.D.

As of November 2007, all 50 states and the District of Columbia mandated the collection of blood samples from newborns to screen for six conditions: classical galactosemia, congenital hypothyroidism, sickle cell anemia, sickle-C disease (sickle-hemoglobin C disease), S-β-thalassemia (sickle-β-thalassemia), and phenylketonuria/hyperphenylalaninemia. Some states also mandate screening for other conditions, and several states offer parents the opportunity to have their newborn screened for conditions not on the state's mandated screening panel (see table 1.1).

Newborn screening programs generally retain newborn blood samples after using them for disease screening, with retention ranging from two weeks in Louisiana to indefinitely in at least four states (National Newborn Screening and Genetics Resource Center 2000). Varying retention policies reflect the needs, goals, and priorities of each newborn screening program. For example, newborn screening programs have used stored samples to confirm disease screening results and to assess the quality of new screening tests (Olshan 2007). The purpose of such activities is to make newborn screening programs more evidence-based and more efficiently managed.

Newborn screening samples have also been used in a wide range of population- and disease-based studies. Researchers have investigated the "prevalence of *in utero* exposure to drugs and environmental agents; the allele frequency of genes associated with significant morbidity, mortality, or disability in infancy or childhood; and the prevalence of serious maternal or intrauterine infections" in various populations (Newborn Screening Task Force 2000, p. 415). Samples have also been used to assess "the feasibility of screening for various diseases of the newborn and infant, and to determine risk factors for birth defects and developmental disabilities" (p. 415), to assess the prevalence of HIV antibodies in childbearing women (Hoff et al. 1988), and for a host of environmental epidemiological studies (Olshan 2007).

Research with newborn screening samples is potentially beneficial to newborn screening programs as well as to children and families. Nevertheless, several ethical, regulatory, and policy issues are implicated when human biospecimens are collected, stored, and used for research. This chapter describes these issues and identifies the unresolved ethical challenges involving research with human biospecimens; examines existing policy recommendations for research with newborn screening samples and the current policy landscape across state newborn screening programs; and identifies the unresolved ethical and policy challenges faced by newborn screening programs as they continue to collect and store newborn screening samples. (See chapters 13 and 14 for additional perspectives on these issues and challenges.)

Research with Human Biospecimens

Research with human biospecimens is on the rise in the United States and other countries, particularly for genetic research. Numerous government advisory bodies (Nuffield Council on Bioethics 1995; Tri-council Policy Statement 1998; National Bioethics Advisory Commission 1999; German National Ethics Council 2004), professional organizations (American Society of Human Genetics 1988, 1996; American College of Medical Genetics 1995), and international bodies[1] have identified and examined several ethical issues that arise when human biospecimens are collected, stored, and used in research. These issues include matters related to informed consent, privacy and confidentiality, ethics review of research proposals, access to research results, and commercial and other benefits derived from the research.

Informed Consent, Privacy and Confidentiality, and Ethics Review

The issue of informed consent when research involves human biospecimens has generated considerable attention. Requiring researchers to obtain informed consent from individuals who participate in research satisfies the ethical principle of respect for persons, which reflects the right to self-determination (i.e., the right to make autonomous decisions about what is done to and with one's body) (National Commission for the Protection of Human Subjects of Biomedical and Behavioral Research 1979). In addition to fulfilling the function of honoring the individual, informed consent fulfills the functions of disclosing risk and addressing lack of trust in the research enterprise (Clayton et al. 1995). Providing individuals with information about a study's purpose, its potential risks, and other elements related to the study reflects a commitment to transparency, which is an important factor in fostering trust in research (Kass et al. 1996).

However, many commentators have questioned whether informed consent is always required for research with human biospecimens and whether consent must be for specified research purposes. Rothstein and others have pointed out that the nature and degree of risk of harm arising from research with biospecimens "depends on (1) the identifiability of the sample and any linked health information, and (2) whether the samples are extant or to be collected prospectively" (Rothstein 2005, p. 90). Potential risks of harm include the nonconsensual disclosure of sensitive information about the biospecimen contributor, the use of the biospecimen in research to which the contributor objects (e.g., genetic research on behavior or cloning research), and stigma and discrimination resulting from research findings on genetic traits of the contributor and family members. Although there is no evidence that genetic discrimination in insurance or employment is common, many people fear they will have trouble getting or keeping health insurance (or a job) because of their genetic profile. To allay these fears, President Bush signed the Genetic Information Nondiscrimination Act (GINA) in May 2008. GINA prohibits health insurer or employer discrimination against individuals based on their genetic information (Genetics and Public Policy Center 2008).

For prospective collection of identifiable biospecimens for research, there is consensus that researchers must obtain informed consent from the individuals who provide the biospecimens. Consensus has been elusive, however, regarding the scope of informed consent at the time of collection. Can individuals give true informed consent for unspecified future research with their biospecimens? Should individuals be given the opportunity to prohibit use of their biospecimens for research that does not conform to their values? Several commentators suggest using a tiered, rather than a blanket, consent approach in response to these concerns (Weir, Olick, and Murray 2004). With tiered consent, individuals are given options for how their biospecimens can be used in current and subsequent studies. For example, individuals might agree to allow use of their biospecimens for arthritis research but not for behavioral genetics research. On the other hand, a blanket consent approach would only give individuals the choice of opting in or out of unspecified current or future research. The U.K. Biobank (www.ukbiobank.ac.uk), which will collect biospecimens from adults throughout the United Kingdom for population-based genetic research, uses the blanket consent approach, as does the Estonian Genome Project (www.geenivaramu.ee/3829), another national population-based biobank.

Others ask whether broad authorization rather than blanket consent for future unspecified uses of biospecimens is an acceptable alternative consent framework. According to Greely (1999), blanket consent is "far short of true informed consent" because what individuals consent to is too general for meeting the requirement of being "informed" about research purposes. Thus, Caulfield, Upshur, and Daar (2003) proposed an authorization model that resembles a health care directive. Under this model, individuals would give informed consent when the biospecimen is collected and would authorize subsequent unspecified uses of the biospecimen subject to review and approval by an ethics review board (known in the U.S. as an institutional review board, or IRB). In the view of these authors, the authorization model "preserves aspects of autonomy, but is neither restrictive of future uses as a full consent model, nor is as permissive as proposed blanket consent models." Hannson et al. (2006) endorse a similar approach—broad and future consent—when researchers collect biospecimens for a research biobank. Individuals would give consent for broad and future use of their biospecimens under the condition that the research-related information is handled safely, that the donors can withdraw their consent at any time, and that changes to the legal or ethical authority of the biobank or proposals for new studies are approved by an ethics review board.

In the United States, whether informed consent is required for research with human biospecimens depends on whether the research constitutes human subjects research as defined by the Department of Health and Human Services' human research regulations (Protection of Human Subjects, Subparts A–D, Code of Federal Regulations, 45 CFR 46).[2] The Office for Human Research Protections (OHRP), which oversees compliance with the regulations, issued guidance on the matter in 2004. According to OHRP, research with only coded biospecimens is not considered human subjects research: (1) when the biospecimens were not collected specifically for a currently proposed research project through interaction or intervention with living individuals; and (2) when the researchers cannot readily ascertain the identity of the biospecimen contributors to whom the coded private information pertains. Examples of situations in which the researchers cannot readily ascertain a biospecimen contributor's identity include: (1) when the key to decipher the code is destroyed before the research begins; (2) when the researchers and the holder of the key enter into an agreement that prohibits the release of the key to the researchers under any circumstances, until the biospecimen contributors are deceased; (3) when IRB-approved written policies and procedures for a repository or data management center prohibit releasing the key to researchers under any circumstances, until the biospecimen contributors are deceased; and (4) when other legal requirements are in place prohibiting release of the key to researchers, until the biospecimen contributors are deceased (Office for Human Research Protections 2004).

For research with coded biospecimens that does not meet OHRP's guidance criteria and for research with prospectively collected identifiable biospecimens, researchers must obtain informed consent from the biospecimen donors. Yet even in these scenarios, the regulatory requirement for informed consent and IRB review and approval of research protocols is not absolute. The regulations permit IRBs to waive or alter the requirement for informed consent when four conditions are met: (1) research risks are no more than minimal; (2) the rights and welfare of individuals are not adversely affected by the waiver or alteration; (3) the research could not practicably be carried out without the waiver or alteration; and (4) when appropriate, participants will be provided with pertinent information about the research in which they participated (Protection of Human Subjects, Subparts A–D, 45 CFR 46.117).

OHRP has also said that an IRB should oversee the operation of a biospecimen repository, including its data management center. The IRB is expected to "review and approve a protocol specifying the conditions under which data and specimens may be accepted and shared" and should ensure that adequate provisions are in place "to protect the privacy of subjects and maintain the confidentiality of data" (Office for Protection from Research Risks 1997). Yet, when research does not meet the definition of human subject research—as is the case for research with anonymized and some coded biospecimens (i.e., biospecimens that can be linked to individual contributors)—IRB review and approval of research protocols is not required.

Research Results and Benefits

Recent commentary on research results reveals differing opinions about whether researchers should provide research subjects with information on a study's findings, including clinically relevant information (Fernandez, Kodish, and Weijer 2003; Quaid, Jessup, and Meslin 2004; Partridge et al. 2005; Pelias 2005; Shalowitz and Miller 2005; Ravitsky and Wilfond 2006). Of particular concern is whether research results that identify genetic risk should be conveyed to biospecimen contributors. Obtaining genetic information about newborns and children may be problematic, especially if an adult-onset disorder is identified and/or no treatments for the condition are available. Moreover, genetic information about an individual may be relevant for other family members, which raises issues about risks faced by living relatives, including breaches of privacy and confidentiality.

Because most population-based research will not generate information that could lead directly to an evidence-based intervention, some commentators contend that researchers are not obligated to provide biospecimen contributors with information on findings derived from such studies. Even if studies produce results that can be linked to specific individuals, some argue that there still is no obligation to notify individuals of the results, especially if potentially clinically relevant results were not obtained from a laboratory that performed tests in compliance with the Clinical Laboratory and Improvement Act (CLIA) of 1988 (CLIA 42 CFR 493.2).[3] Other commentators contend that the principle of respect for persons requires researchers to provide study participants with research results if they want such information (Quaid, Jessup, and Meslin 2004; Shalowitz and Miller 2005). Although consensus has not been reached on this issue, there is general agreement that if researchers are willing to share information, biospecimen contributors should be asked whether they want to know about research results. Forms of information sharing include contacting specific individuals or publishing results through newsletters, websites, and other forms of mass communication.

In the area of possible commercial benefits from research, at least two courts in the United States have ruled that biospecimen contributors do not have property rights in their biological material and therefore researchers are not obligated to share financial benefits with biospecimen contributors (*Moore v. Regents of the University of California*, 793 P.2d 479 [Cal. 1990]; *Greenberg v. Miami Children's Hosp. Research Inst., Inc.*, 254 F. Supp. 2d 1064 [S. D. Fla. 2003]). Nevertheless, many IRBs require researchers to at least inform tissue contributors that while researchers and sponsors may derive commercial benefits from research with their biospecimen, those benefits will not be shared with them.[4]

Newborn Screening Samples: Existing Policy Recommendations

Although several professional and government bodies have issued recommendations for research with newborn screening blood samples, the recommendations do not address all of the issues described above (table 12.1). In 1994, the Institute of Medicine (IOM) Committee on Assessing Genetic Risks issued a report that addressed the social, legal, and ethical implications of

.

TABLE 12.1

Recommendations for Research with Newborn Screening Samples

	IOM	CORN	AAP	NY State Task Force
Informed consent				
No consent required for use of unidentifiable samples.	✓	✓*	✓	✓
Consent required for use of identifiable samples.	✓	✓	✓†	✓
Type of research				
When more than minimal risk, research should benefit child or improve knowledge of childhood diseases.				
Review and oversight				
IRB review and approval of research required.		✓	✓‡	✓
IRB oversight of repository required.				
Parental information				
Inform parents about policies on retention/storage/ access/research/privacy.	✓			✓§
Provide research results to parents.		✓#		
Inform parents about commercial benefits and/or researchers' financial interests.				

Note: IOM, Institute of Medicine; CORN, Council of Regional Networks for Genetic Services; AAP, American Academy of Pediatrics; IRB, institutional review board.

  * Give parents written opt-out option for research on birth defects, newborn disorders, and public health protection.

  † Five conditions must be met: (1) IRB approval of proposed research; (2) parental/guardian consent; (3) newborn samples the optimal source of available tissue; (4) unlinked samples not sufficient; (5) acceptable samples from consenting adults not available. The task force also recommends reconsent when research is not covered by original consent.

  ‡ Not required when unidentifiable samples are used for hospital and laboratory quality assurance activities.

  § Inform parents about anonymization and research uses.

  # Release results to a laboratory or physician with parental permission.

genetic testing. The federal government created the IOM as a nonprofit organization to provide information on biomedical science, medicine, and health
to policymakers, professionals, and others. The IOM committee investigated a
wide range of issues, including issues associated with genetic screening and
testing of children.

Two years after the IOM report was issued, the Council of Regional Networks for Genetic Services (CORN) issued guidelines for policy development
on the collection, storage, and use of newborn screening samples (Therrell
et al. 1996). CORN was a federally funded consortium of representatives from
10 regional genetic networks. It was developed in 1985 to respond to a perceived need to coordinate the activities of the genetic services networks in
operation at that time. CORN developed guidelines on the use of newborn
screening samples for the purpose of helping "newborn screening programs
make decisions about developing protocols and justifications for length of
retention" of samples (Therrell et al. 1996, p. 117), providing information
about sample release and use, and addressing concerns with potential banking of DNA obtained from samples.

The American Academy of Pediatrics (AAP) is a membership organization of 60,000 physicians. It convened the Newborn Screening Task Force
to "review issues and challenges for state newborn screening systems" at the
request of the Maternal and Child Health Bureau of the U.S. Department of
Health and Human Services. Cosponsors included the National Institutes of
Health (NIH), the Agency for Healthcare Research and Quality, the Genetic
Alliance (a coalition of advocacy groups for various genetic conditions; www
.geneticalliance.org), and the Association of State and Territorial Health Officials. The New York State Task Force on Life and the Law was created in 1985
by executive order. It was charged with recommending legislative and regulatory policy as well as public education for New York State on a wide range of
issues raised by medical advances, including the determination of death, the
use and withdrawal of life-sustaining treatments, organ transplantation, and
assisted reproductive technologies. Its report on the ethical, legal, and social
implications of genetic testing and screening (New York State Task Force on
Life and the Law 2001) was issued in response to developments of the Human
Genome Project, which opened the door to the era of genomic medicine.

On the matter of informed consent, all of the recommendations state that
parental consent should be required for research use of identifiable samples,
but not for use of samples that cannot be traced to their source.[5]

As table 12.1 shows, the AAP's Newborn Screening Task Force also recommended that five conditions be met for research with identifiable newborn screening samples: (1) an IRB approves the proposed research; (2) the child's parents or guardians give consent; (3) the samples are the sole optimal source of tissue available for the specific research; (4) the use of samples unlinked to individuals is not sufficient; and (5) acceptable samples from consenting adults are unavailable. The Newborn Screening Task Force (2000) also recommended that "any research on identifiable samples that is not covered by the original consent should require recontacting parents" (p. 417) and that before doing so an oversight body should approve such a plan. The Newborn Screening Task Force was the only organization that took into account the federal regulations governing research with children (Protection of Human Subjects, Subpart D: Additional Protections for Children Involved as Subjects in Research, 45 CFR 46.401). The task force recommended that "in accordance with current federal regulations regarding research involving children, use of [identifiable] samples for research, that poses more than minimal risk, should be limited to activities that benefit the child or that are of importance to understanding a condition affecting children" (Newborn Screening Task Force 2000, pp. 416–17). The task force's recommendation reflects concern about conducting research with children's samples when treatments are not available for the condition under study or when the research involves adult diseases (Knoppers et al. 2002).

None of the recommendations mention the issue of informed consent for anonymizing samples or address whether the scope of consent should be narrow or broad. Although several of the recommendations mention access to samples and priority use of samples, only the AAP offered specific guidance for how samples should be used. In addition, none of the recommendations mention whether research results should be provided to parents and/or children or whether parents should be informed about researchers' and commercial entities' financial interests in particular research studies.

Newborn Screening Program Policies

Recent surveys of newborn screening programs reveal a patchwork of policies on collection, retention, storage, and research. The surveys provide little detailed information about whether and how newborn screening programs have addressed the ethical and policy issues surrounding research with newborn screening samples. In addition, no explanation is offered for the policy variations. State policies vary for many reasons. Government officials may be uninformed about specific issues or may believe certain issues deserve greater priority than others. Even when issues are deemed a priority, a state may lack the resources to address them. Policy variation may also reflect normative and political disagreements about the need for and nature of policy initiatives.

Mandl et al. reported in 2002 that at least 31 programs stored newborn screening samples with personal identifiers attached. Survey respondents for 3 programs said they used a coding system to protect the identity of the biospecimen sources but allowed decoding if needed. Soon thereafter Olney et al. (2006) reported that 9 programs stored identifiable samples, 12 stored samples without identifying links, 9 stored both identifiable and unlinked samples, and 12 were unsure about their storage practices. Respondents for 37 programs said that samples should be stored with identifiers, whereas 8 said samples should be unlinked.[6]

Lloyd-Puryear (2003) reported that by the end of 2003, at least seven states addressed the retention and use of newborn screening samples in their statutes or regulations. In another survey, Lewis, McCabe, and McCabe (2002) found that at least one newborn screening program had statutory authority to release samples for confidential, anonymous research, whereas in two states statutory authority to authorize research use of samples lay with the department of health. Two additional states require their state departments of health to develop a schedule for the retention and disposal of samples and to permit use of the samples for medical research during the retention period. According to Seo (2004), in 6 states an IRB at the institution with jurisdiction over the newborn screening program is required to approve access to blood samples, whereas in 16 states the IRB at the state laboratory or at the newborn screening program has authority over access. Mississippi, by contrast, prohibits all research with newborn screening samples.

There are few data on newborn screening programs' consent policies for use of samples in research or on whether parents are told that their child's sample may be used in research. In 2002, Lewis, McCabe, and McCabe reported that at least two states informed parents about potential research, though only one state required written informed consent from parents for research use. Doyle reported in 2002 that the Washington State Department of Health released identified samples only if a parent or legal guardian signed a release or the state attorney general issued a subpoena for their release. The department also permitted the release of anonymized samples when all newborn screening testing was completed, when a significant health benefit could be derived from the intended use of the samples, when there were adequate safeguards in place to protect the anonymity of the sample source, and when the agency had sufficient resources to compile the samples.

Lawmakers in three states—South Carolina, Nebraska, and Minnesota—recently passed legislation to regulate the collection, storage, and research use of newborn screening samples. In 2002, the South Carolina legislature passed a law in response to public outcry over release by the Department of Health and Environmental Control (DHEC) of 500 newborn screening samples to a private research company and another 500 to the state's law enforcement division. According to media reports, the private company wanted to use the samples for research on a new genetic test, and the law enforcement division wanted to conduct baseline studies of DNA markers (Hawkins 2002). Although the released samples did not contain personal identifiers, they were linked to the sex and race of the newborns and to the geographic area of the state in which the babies were born (Barnes 2002).

At the time the South Carolina legislation was introduced, the DHEC stored newborn screening samples indefinitely, because the state had no formal retention policy. Moreover, there was no policy for telling parents about the indefinite retention, for obtaining parental consent for research with the samples, or for ensuring the privacy of tissue contributors and the confidentiality of information derived from research with the samples. Under the new law, the newborn screening program must inform parents about the program's storage policy and give parents the opportunity to opt out of having their newborn's sample stored after it is used for disease screening (Barnes 2002). The statute is less restrictive than the original version, which would have prohibited research with newborn screening blood samples without explicit parental consent; let parents decide whether the samples would be stored; required DHEC to inform parents through a website and toll-free number about how they could have the samples destroyed; and made it a felony to obtain or release data from the samples (Lamb 2002).

In 2003, Nebraska lawmakers passed legislation requiring the Department of Health and Human Services Regulation and Licensure to adopt and promulgate rules and regulations for the retention, storage, and use of samples, to satisfy the mandate that samples be used only for public health purposes in compliance "with all applicable provisions of federal law" (Nebraska Slip Bill, Legislative Bill 119, approved by the governor March 20, 2003). That same year, the Minnesota legislature passed a bill giving parents the option to decide whether their newborn's blood samples and records of disease-screening test results should be destroyed within 24 months of the testing (Minnesota Statutes §144.125 Subd. 3 and §144.966 Subd. 3) (Minnesota Department of Health 2007).[7]

Ethical and Policy Challenges

Research with human biospecimens is moving forward at a rapid pace, and it is likely that researchers will want greater access to newborn screening samples, especially for genetic research. Thus, newborn screening programs should set policies on whether samples will be released, to whom, and for what purposes. In addition, there should be policies for ethics oversight, informed consent, and release of research results. These policies should be shared with parents, health care professionals, researchers, and other stakeholders. Because nearly all newborn screening programs provide educational materials to parents that explain newborn disease screening, information about collection, storage, retention, research, and consent policies could easily be incorporated into these materials. The policies could also be posted on newborn screening program websites, in addition to the information currently posted about newborn disease screening. Providing information on program websites would be especially useful to researchers who want access to stored samples. However, the AAP recently reported that only 11 percent of the 47 programs that provide educational materials include information about storage and use of newborn screening samples (Fant, Clark, and Kemper 2005). In addition, as of November 2007, only three of the active newborn screening program websites provided information about storage, access, and other policies, though the scope of information varies across programs.[8]

Although there are still normative disagreements about when and what kind of informed consent should be obtained to satisfy the principle of respect for persons, the four sets of recommendations for research with newborn screening samples examined here are generally consistent with various national guidelines, and with the international guidelines, on consensus regarding informed consent for research with human biospecimens. Thus, newborn screening programs should obtain parental consent for research use of identifiable newborn screening samples. Indeed, the Newborn Screening Task Force

(2000) recommended that "an up-front mechanism of informed consent, at the point of the heelstick, is one logical way of initiating the process of informed consent" (p. 417).

Developing policies in areas where no consensus has been reached raises concerns about policy variation across newborn screening programs. From a policy perspective, it would be less burdensome for researchers requesting samples from multiple newborn screening programs if policies on sample access, informed consent, ethics oversight, and research results were harmonized. Uniformity may also be desirable from an ethical perspective. If harmonizing policies across programs is a desirable goal—and perhaps ethically required—what options are available to achieve this goal, especially where consensus on some issues remains elusive?

One option would be for newborn screening programs to convene a national consensus conference to harmonize policies. The NIH Consensus Development Program is one of many models for consensus building (http://consensus.nih.gov). Another option would be for federal officials to require newborn screening programs to develop policies consistent with those of the NIH's Office of Human Subjects Research as a condition of receiving federal funding (National Institutes of Health 2006a, 2006b, 2006c). Although 65 percent of financing for newborn screening programs comes from fees paid by hospitals or third-party payers, up to 17 percent of funding comes from federal dollars, including the Medicaid program (Association of State and Territorial Health Officials 2005).

An additional policy option would be to create a national biobank of newborn screening blood samples. This could be accomplished by newborn screening programs voluntarily providing samples to the national biobank. In 2002, the U.S. Centers for Disease Control and Prevention held a conference that addressed the desirability and feasibility of developing a biobank in partnership with state newborn screening programs, though no proposal has emerged from that discussion. Another option would be to create a biobank independent of newborn screening programs that invites parents to contribute a blood sample from their infants to the repository. This type of biobank could be funded and managed by federal and or state dollars, by private industry, or by a public-private partnership. A first effort of this sort is the recently created DNA bank at the Children's Hospital of Philadelphia. The hospital is hoping to collect blood samples from up to 100,000 of its child patients to create a DNA database that researchers can use to study the children's genetic profiles (Regalado 2006). A national biobank modeled after the Estonian Genome Project or the U.K. Biobank is another possibility. The Estonian Genome Project will collect biospecimens from adults and children, and the U.K. Biobank will collect biospecimens from adults between the ages of 40 and 69. However, it is unclear whether parents would be willing to have their child's DNA included in a national biospecimen repository. The most extensive public dialogue on biobanking is taking place in the United Kingdom; nothing on that scale has occurred in the United States.[9]

A national biobank of newborn screening samples would probably be attractive to researchers, although creating one would not eliminate policy variation across state newborn screening programs, which would continue to collect samples for disease screening and retain them for research and other purposes. Moreover, it is not clear whether the current state-based "banking" of newborn screening samples should be replaced or supplemented with a different approach. However, as newborn screening programs move forward in developing policies for expanded screening and educational materials for parents and health professionals, they should not lose sight of the fact that good stewardship of newborn screening samples includes having ethically sound and transparent policies for the collection, storage, and research use of such samples.

ACKNOWLEDGMENTS

Thanks to Mary Ann Baily, Andrea Bonnicksen, Jeff Botkin, Anne Comeau, George Cunningham, Scott Grosse, and Thomas Murray for their helpful comments during preparation of this chapter.

NOTES

1. See, for example, Human Genome Organization Ethics Committee, "Statement on DNA Sampling: Control and Access" (www.gene.ucl.ac.uk/hugo/sampling.html).

2. The regulations cover federally funded and sponsored research and also cover industry-funded studies conducted at sites that have a Federal Wide Assurance on file with the Office for Human Research Protections, specifying that all research conducted by their investigators or at their site will abide by the Federal Policy for the Protection of Human Subjects.

3. CLIA establishes quality standards for all laboratory testing to ensure the accuracy, reliability, and timeliness of patient test results, regardless of where the test was performed.

4. See, for example, New York School of Medicine Institutional Review Board, "Genetic Studies" (www.med.nyu.edu/irb/information_sheets/gen_std.html).

5. Subpart D of the Federal Policy for the Protection of Human Subjects specifies that parents give "permission" rather than consent for their children to participate in research, but consistent with the human research literature, the term parental "consent" is used here.

6. The discrepancy in results from these two reports may be due to the populations sampled. In the Mandl et al. study, data were obtained from newborn screening program supervisors; Olney et al. reported data obtained from state laboratory directors or their designees.

7. In March 2007, a state administrative law judge ruled that the statute does not expressly authorize the Minnesota Department of Health to store genetic information from newborn bloodspots indefinitely or disseminate that information to researchers without written informed consent by parents. In August 2007, the Department of Health withdrew a proposed rule that would have addressed this issue. See Citizens' Council on Health Care website (www.cchconline.org).

8. Minnesota (www.health.state.mn.us/divs/fh/mcshn/nbsparents.htm); Nebraska (www .hhs.state.ne.us/hew/fah/nsp/NewDocs/ParentsPage/ParentsGuideEnglish.pdf); and Washington State (www.doh.wa.gov/ehsphl/phl/newborn/privacy.htm).

9. See "Consultations" on the U.K. Biobank website for materials on the consultative process used in the United Kingdom (www.ukbiobank.ac.uk/ethics/consultations.php).

REFERENCES

American College of Medical Genetics. 1995. Storage of Genetics Materials Committee: statement on storage and use of genetic materials. *Am J Hum Genet* 57 (6): 1499–1500.

American Society of Human Genetics. 1988. DNA banking and DNA analysis: points to consider. Ad Hoc Committee on DNA Technology, American Society of Human Genetics. *Am J Hum Genet* 42 (5): 781–83.

———. 1996. Statement on informed consent for genetic research. *Am J Hum Genet* 59 (2): 471–74.

Association of State and Territorial Health Officials. 2005. *Financing State Newborn Screening Systems in an Era of Change*. Washington DC: Association of State and Territorial Health Officials.

Barnes, P. 2002. Baby steps to a genetic dossier. ABCNews.com. http://abcnews.go.com/sections/ scitech/TechTV/techtv_babyDNA020615.html.

Caulfield, T., Upshur, R. E., and Daar, A. 2003. DNA databanks and consent: a suggested policy option involving an authorization model. *BMC Med Ethics* 4 (1): 1–4.

Clayton, E. W., Steinberg, K. K., Khoury, M. J., Thomson, E., Andrews, L., Kahn, M. J., Kopelman, L. M., and Weiss, J. O. 1995. Informed consent for genetic research on stored tissue samples. *JAMA* 274 (22): 1786–92.

Doyle, D. L. 2002. Washington newborn screening program laws and privacy policies. PowerPoint presentation, Olympia, WA, January 3. www.sboh.wa.gov/Goals/Past/Genetics/ GTF2002_01-03/documents/Tab06-DebDoylePowerpoint.ppt#1.

Fant, K. E., Clark, S. J., and Kemper, A. R. 2005. Completeness and complexity of information available to parents from newborn-screening programs. *Pediatrics* 115 (5): 1268–72.

Fernandez, C. V., Kodish, E., and Weijer, C. 2003. Informing study participants of research results: an ethical imperative. *IRB* 25 (3): 12–19.

Genetics and Public Policy Center. 2008. Issue briefs: the Genetic Information Nondiscrimination Act. June 18. www.dnapolicy.org/policy.issue.php?action=detail&issuebrief_id=37 &print=1.

German National Ethics Council. 2004. *Biobanks for Research*. Berlin: German National Ethics Council.

Greely, H. T. 1999. Breaking the stalemate: a prospective regulatory framework for unforeseen research uses of human tissue samples and health information. *Wake Forest Law Rev* 34 (3): 737–66.

Hansson, M. G., Dillner, J., Bartram, C. R., Carlson, J. A., and Helgesson, G. 2006. Should donors be allowed to give broad consent to future biobank research? *Lancet Oncol* 7 (3): 266–69.

Hawkins, D. 2002. As DNA banks quietly multiply, who is guarding the safe? *US News & World Report*, December 2.

Hoff, R., Berardi, V. P., Weiblen, B. J., Mahoney-Trout, L., Mitchell, M. L., and Grady, G. F. 1988. Seroprevalence of human immunodeficiency virus among childbearing women: estimation by testing samples of blood from newborns. *N Engl J Med* 318 (9): 525–30.

Institute of Medicine, Committee on Assessing Genetic Risks. 1994. *Assessing Genetic Risks: Implications for Health and Social Policy*, ed. L. B. Andrews, J. E. Fullarton, N. A. Holtzman, and A. G. Motulsky. Washington, DC: National Academy Press.

Kass, N. E., Sugarman, J., Faden, R., and Schoch-Spana, M. 1996. Trust, the fragile foundation of contemporary biomedical research. *Hastings Cent Rep* 26 (5): 25–29.

Knoppers, B. M., Avard, D., Cardinal, G., and Glass, K. C. 2002. Science and society: children and incompetent adults in genetic research: consent and safeguards. *Nat Rev Genet* 3 (3): 221–25.

Lamb, L. H., 2002. Frozen blood samples raise hopes, worries. *The State* (South Carolina), February 14.

Lewis, M. H., McCabe, L. L., and McCabe, E. R. B. 2002. State laws regarding the retention and use of newborn screening blood specimens [abstract]. Presentation at Newborn Screening: State Policies for Educating Parents about Newborn Screening and the Storage of Newborn Residual Blood Spots, UCLA, Los Angeles, November 21–22.

Lloyd-Puryear, M. A. 2003. State of newborn screening privacy. PowerPoint presentation at the National Conference of State Legislatures, November 17.

Mandl, K. D., Feit, S., Larson, C., and Kohane, I. S. 2002. Newborn screening program practices in the United States: notification, research, and consent. *Pediatrics* 109 (2): 269–73.

Minnesota Department of Health. 2007. Instructions for birth facilities regarding parental newborn screening options. www.health.state.mn.us/divs/fh/mcshn/Docs/nbsrefuseinst .doc.

National Bioethics Advisory Commission. 1999. *Research Involving Human Biological Materials: Ethical Issues and Policy Guidance*. Rockville, MD: Government Printing Office.

National Commission for the Protection of Human Subjects of Biomedical and Behavioral Research. 1979. *The Belmont Report: Ethical Principles and Guidelines for the Protection of Human Subjects of Research*. Washington, DC: Department of Health, Education and Welfare.

National Institutes of Health. 2006a. *Guidance on the Research Use of Stored Samples or Data*. Sheet 14. Office of Human Subjects Research. Bethesda, MD: National Institutes of Health.

————. 2006b. *Points to Consider in Development of Informed Consent Documents that Include the Collection and Research Use of Human Biological Materials*. Sheet 15. Office of Human Subjects Research. Bethesda, MD: National Institutes of Health.

————. 2006c. *Procurement and Use of Human Biological Materials*. Sheet 17. Office of Human Subjects Research. Bethesda, MD: National Institutes of Health.

National Newborn Screening and Genetics Resource Center. 2000. National newborn screening report—2000 (final report February 2003), p. 31. http://genes-r-us.uthscsa.edu/re sources/newborn/00/2000report.pdf.

New York State Task Force on Life and the Law. 2001. *Genetic Testing and Screening in the Age of Genomic Medicine*. New York: New York State Department of Health.

Newborn Screening Task Force. 2000. Serving the family from birth to the medical home: a report from the Newborn Screening Task Force convened in Washington DC, May 10–11, 1999. *Pediatrics* 106 (2 Pt 2): 383–427.

Nuffield Council on Bioethics. 1995. Human tissue: ethical and legal issues. www.nuffieldbio ethics.org/go/ourwork/humantissue/introduction.

Office for Human Research Protections. 2004. *Guidance on Research Involving Coded Private Information or Biological Specimens*. Rockville, MD: Office for Human Research Protections.

Office for Protection from Research Risks. 1997. Issues to consider in the research use of stored data or tissues. www.hhs.gov/ohrp/humansubjects/guidance/reposit.htm.

Olney, R. S., Moore, C. A., Ojodu, J. A., Lindegren, M. L., and Hannon, W. H. 2006. Storage and use of residual dried blood spots from state newborn screening programs. *J Pediatr* 148 (5): 618–22.

Olshan, A. F. 2007. The use of newborn bloodspots in environmental research: opportunities and challenges [meeting report]. *Environ Health Perspect* 115 (12): 1767–69.

Partridge, A. H., Wong, J. S., Knudsen, K., Gelman, R., Sampson, E., Gadd, M., Bishop, K. L., Harris, J. R., and Winer, E. P. 2005. Offering participants results of a clinical trial: sharing results of a negative study. *Lancet* 365 (9463): 963–64.

Pelias, M. K. 2005. Research in human genetics: the tension between doing no harm and personal autonomy. *Clin Genet* 67 (1): 1–5.

Quaid, K. A., Jessup, N. M., and Meslin, E. M. 2004. Disclosure of genetic information obtained through research. *Genet Test* 8 (3): 347–55.

Ravitsky, V., and Wilfond, B. S. 2006. Disclosing individual genetic results to research participants. *Am J Bioeth* 6 (6): 8–17.

Regalado, A. 2006. Plan to build children's DNA database raises concerns. *Wall Street Journal*, January 7.

Rothstein, M. A. 2005. Expanding the ethical analysis of biobanks. *J Law Med Ethics* 33 (1): 89–101.

Seo, K. 2004. *Newborn Disease Screening in the United States: A Policy and Administrative Overview*. Cambridge, MA: Council for Responsible Genetics.

Shalowitz, D. I., and Miller, F. G. 2005. Disclosing individual results of clinical research: implications of respect for participants. *JAMA* 294 (6): 737–40.

Therrell, B. L., Hannon, W. H., Pass, K. A., Lorey, F., Brokopp, C., and Eckman, J. 1996. Guidelines for the retention, storage and use of residual dried blood spot samples after newborn screening analysis. Statement of the Council of Regional Networks for Genetic Services. *Biochem Mol Med* 57:116–24.

Tri-council Policy Statement. 1998. *Ethical Conduct for Research Involving Humans.* Report by a working group of the three federal funding councils: Medical Research Council of Canada, Natural Sciences and Engineering Research Council of Canada, and Social Sciences and Humanities Research Council of Canada. Gatineau, Québec: Public Works and Government Services.

Weir, R. F., Olick, R. S., and Murray, J. C. 2004. *The Stored Tissue Issue: Biomedical Research, Ethics, and Law in the Era of Genomic Medicine.* New York: Oxford University Press.

CHAPTER 13

Parental Permission for Research in Newborn Screening

JEFFREY R. BOTKIN, M.D., M.P.H.

Expanding the evidence base for newborn screening programs is a national priority requiring collaborative research projects at the state, regional, and national levels. Newborn screening programs in most states are conducted without parental permission, and the lack of an informed permission process in clinical application means there is no established foundation for an informed permission process for research. This chapter argues that a waiver of parental permission is justified for population-based newborn screening research in some circumstances, including the use of identifiable residual bloodspot samples. Several measures are recommended to mitigate risks, including parental notification, public awareness, a careful protocol for results disclosure, and approval by a genetics advisory committee.

Newborn screening using dried bloodspots is an important component of child health services that is implemented through public health departments in all 50 U.S states and territories and the District of Columbia. The number of tests used in each state program varies widely, due to different criteria, local opinions about efficacy, local advocacy, and different decision-making processes (Newborn Screening Task Force 2000). The advent of new technology, tandem mass spectrometry (MS/MS) in particular, has led to a rapid expansion in the number of tests in many states. Yet the evidence base for many tests remains limited, and there is uncertainty about the clinical validity, clinical utility, and cost-to-benefit ratio for some of the tests on newborn screening panels (see chapter 11). More specifically, there is uncertainty about the ability to treat some rare conditions, the need to intervene clinically for some atypical findings on metabolic profiles, and the ability of complex newborn screening systems to bring effective interventions to children through population-based programs.

Strengthening the evidence base for newborn screening programs is a national priority (Newborn Screening Taskforce 2000; Natowicz 2005). Much of our information on the management of many of the conditions identified through MS/MS comes from small, uncontrolled observational studies (Steiner 2005). To date, the only newborn screening condition for which population screening has been evaluated through a randomized controlled trial is cystic fibrosis (CF) (Farrell et al. 2001). Therefore, as newborn screening programs expand and as new screening technologies become available, state, regional, and national collaborative research programs are essential to evaluate the efficacy and cost of each component of screening programs.

There are a number of barriers to the conduct of newborn screening research. Challenges include the low incidence of many conditions in the general population, the state-based organization of programs, the limited ability of programs to track affected children and identify false negatives, and ethical concerns over the use of randomized controlled trials. An additional barrier is the lack of informed permission by parents for current newborn screening programs in almost all states. By "informed permission," in this context, I mean a process by which a health professional informs the parent(s) of key elements of the screening program and receives formal permission, usually documented with a signature, before screening interventions. Of course, in the research context, informed consent or parental permission is usually much more thorough than for most clinical interventions. Newborn screening is a mandated component of newborn care in all programs except those in Maryland, Wyoming, and the District of Columbia, and therefore may be conducted without parental permission (U.S. General Accounting Office 2003). Parents have the ability to refuse newborn screening in all but five states for religious or philosophical reasons, but parents are often not informed of this option (Farrell et al. 2001).

The original justification for mandating newborn screening services was based on the substantial benefits and limited burdens and risks of screening for conditions such as phenylketonuria (PKU) and congenital hypothyroidism. The belief in most state programs is that the benefits to newborn are sufficiently great that parental permission need not be sought (Newborn Screening Task Force 2000). There also is a common concern among program and nursery personnel over the effort and time that would be required for a permission process during the hectic postnatal period (Faden et al. 1982; Newborn Screening Task Force 2000). Newborn screening simply is not a high-priority item given the many other demands on the attention of care providers and parents with a new baby. Nursery stays are often less than 24 hours, so time devoted to discussing newborn screening is time away from other priorities such as rest and immediate infant care and feeding responsibilities.

In contrast to the traditional *parens patriae* and the practical justifications for mandated screening, a number of national and state professional bodies have advocated a permission process for newborn screening, including the Institute of Medicine and a president's commission (National Research Council 1975; President's Commission for the Study of Ethical Problems in Medicine and Biomedical and Behavioral Research 1983; Andrews et al. 1994). The arguments in support of permission focus on respect for parental authority, the value of parental education in fostering effective participation, potential reductions in parental distress following false positive results, and challenges to the presumed impracticality of a permission process (Annas 1982; Press and Clayton 2000; Clayton 2005). Research in Maryland suggested that the permission process was relatively brief and did not lead to a substantial rate of refusal (Faden et al. 1982). However, legitimate questions remain on whether a sufficiently streamlined process of permission for busy nursery personnel and postpartum parents could entail a meaningful exchange of information and considered choices by parents (Ballard et al. 2004). Further, surveys of parents on this issue reveal that a majority do not want a permission process (Faden et al. 1982; Campbell and Ross 2003). The American Association of Pediatricians (AAP) Committee on Bioethics called for additional research on permission processes for newborn screening to evaluate feasibility and impact (Nelson et al. 2001). The AAP and the American College of Obstetricians and Gynecologists also called for education about newborn screening in the prenatal period (Newborn Screening Task Force 2000; American College of Obstetricians and Gynecologists 2003), although permission during pregnancy may not be feasible for an intervention that occurs in the newborn nursery. Additional attention to this possibility is warranted. In general, there is no significant pressure within programs to change the current approach to mandated screening.

These considerations suggest that a permission requirement is unlikely to be a component of routine newborn screening programs in the foreseeable future. Whether or not parental signatures are obtained for screening, the challenges posed by the postnatal environment are too great to expect a thoughtful, informed decision-making process between care providers and parents. This has two implications for this discussion. First, new newborn screening tests are being added to panels that, arguably, do not meet traditional criteria for efficacy (Botkin et al. 2006). To the extent that mandatory screening is justified by clear and substantial benefits to children, mandating tests of uncertain benefit is ethically problematic. Second, no established clinical permission process is in place on which to build a permission process for research. This latter issue is a potentially serious obstacle to research in a population-based screening program. I argue that waivers of consent/permission should be considered to overcome this problem and thereby foster quality research on newborn screening programs, while maintaining compliance with contemporary ethical and regulatory standards.

Research on Newborn Screening

Research relevant to newborn screening programs takes a number of forms. As I have argued elsewhere, several stages of research might be conceptualized (Botkin 2005; see also chapter 11). Stage I does not involve population screening but rather is focused on a demonstration of whether early detection improves the outcomes of affected children. Once benefits of early detection are demonstrated with reasonable assurance, stage II involves an assessment of whether population screening brings net benefits to children. At this stage, a "test article" in the research is the population-based screening program itself. The primary purpose of this stage is to assess whether and how an apparently effective intervention can be delivered and maintained through a population-based program. An additional focus of stage II research is to assess the impact of programs on children whose test results are of uncertain clinical significance and on those with false positive results.

Newborn screening involves a complex system that includes parental education (often minimal), bloodspot acquisition, laboratory analysis, results disclosure, confirmation of the diagnosis, initial interventions, and long-term management. Weaknesses in any of these elements of the system may lead to limited efficacy or a failed program. For example, screening for sickle cell disease will have a substantially reduced efficacy if a significant proportion of physicians and/or parents fail to administer the prophylactic antibiotics and vaccinations (Teach, Lillis, and Grossi 1998; Centers for Disease Control and Prevention 2000; Sox et al. 2003). Similarly, dietary management of a metabolic condition may be beneficial in a shorter-term, tightly monitored study, but fail to bring benefits in the "real world" where parents may be unable to sustain the diet due to cost, availability, poor understanding, unavailable professional expertise, multiple caretakers, poor palatability, and/or a child's resistance. Research in this stage must accommodate these kinds of variables and thus involve early detection of affected children followed by short- and long-term surveillance under a uniform management plan, and a comparison group.

A different mode of research in newborn screening uses residual dried bloodspots. Residual bloodspots usually remain after screening, and state programs store these resources for variable lengths of time, from 3 months to 21 years (Therrell et al. 1996; Newborn Screening Task Force 2000; Mandl et al. 2002; see also chapter 12). These specimens represent blood and DNA samples for the entire U.S. newborn population and, if stored over decades, could represent a large portion of the entire population. The specimens can be used to ascertain population prevalence of genetic conditions and prenatal infections (Gwinn et al. 1991; Fitzgerald et al. 2004). Such epidemiological studies may or may not be directly relevant to newborn screening.

Investigators also could employ these specimens in the direct evaluation of additional conditions for newborn screening panels. If residual specimens collected over, say, a five-year period are analyzed retrospectively for the condition, the affected children can be found and evaluated. These children represent a "prescreening" cohort. Their clinical outcomes can be compared with the outcomes of affected children identified through newborn screening once the program is implemented on a pilot or experimental basis. This "retrospective screening" approach provides a comparison group within the same population, while avoiding the ethical complexities of creating a control group by prospectively randomizing newborns to screened and unscreened groups. This approach also avoids the potential detection bias created by comparing outcomes in a screened population, including both mildly and severely affected children, with a group of affected children identified clinically that may be enriched with more severely affected individuals (see chapter 11).

Therefore, if residual specimens are useful for newborn screening research, the question arises of whether the analysis of these specimens requires the informed permission of parents.

Consent and Waivers of Consent

Let us assume a new test is proposed for inclusion in a newborn screening panel, but there is insufficient evidence to mandate the new test as part of the routine panel. Initial implementation under a research protocol is proposed. The obvious initial option is to consider seeking informed permission from all parents. This approach honors parental decision making and may reduce risks posed by screening programs. However, there are a number of obstacles to consider. Given the low incidence of many conditions, a research project may need to involve tens or hundreds of thousands of infants and their parents. The permission process would need to be implemented across numerous delivery centers involving a large number of care providers, research coordinators, and institutional review boards (IRBs). Logistically and financially this would be an enormous challenge. But an even more significant concern is that the permission process would alter the object of study—that is, the program itself.

If the program is a test article, then the research protocol must model the clinical program to draw valid conclusions. Assuming a permission process will not become a feature of clinical newborn screening in the foreseeable future, then including a permission process in a research implementation alters the object of study. This creates problems in several respects. Recruitment levels are likely to fall far below coverage levels achieved by routine newborn screening. Low recruitment might be due to parental refusal of permission, but more often will be due to nursery staff's forgoing the research protocol during busy clinical schedules. Recruitment levels approaching the entire newborn population may be critical for the research, because infants with true positive and false positive results are the subjects of interest. Recruitment also may be biased against inclusion of minority and non-English-speaking populations, given the additional communication challenges. Because many conditions considered for newborn screening panels have differences in incidence among racial and ethnic groups, recruitment that is unrepresentative of the entire population impairs the assessment of a population-based program.

Several newborn screening research protocols have used variants of the

traditional informed permission process. A Massachusetts study was organized to pilot the introduction of MS/MS in 1999 (Zytkovicz et al. 2001).
This study used a "population-based" consent approach that used oral permission (see chapter 14). Parents received a written brochure describing the
mandatory and optional screening measures, were informed of their ability
to obtain the optional tests, and were given a copy of the written documentation of their permission or dissent. The proportion of parents who refused
the optional testing was never more than 2 percent. A French program of
newborn screening for CF used a permission process during a 2002–2003
pilot study (Dhondt 2005). French law requires informed consent for all genetic testing. Permission was documented with a parental signature on the
bloodspot sampling paper itself. The information provided to parents is described as follows: "New educational materials were designed for parents that
approach screening in a general manner with equal emphasis on the diseases
covered. These materials present the screening as a routine matter to minimize anxiety" (Dhondt 2005, p. S107). The refusal rates in this study were
consistently less than 1 percent. In Wisconsin, the pilot study of CF screening
organized in 1984 was more complex (Mischler et al. 1998). The protocol
involved running an analysis for CF on all children born in the state, but ran-
domly disclosing results to parents of only half the children. After four years,
all the undisclosed results were reviewed, and the CF-positive children were
located and evaluated for health status. The health status of children with
CF identified shortly after birth by screening was then compared with that
of children whose results were not disclosed. With respect to permission, "all
parents were informed about the voluntary nature of the CF screening with
a pamphlet given to mothers in the hospital at the time of delivery" (Mischler
et al. 1998, p. 45).

The limited experience from these studies illustrates that a permission process is feasible in newborn screening research, but that models fall far short
of the informed permission process that is typically required for research.
Signatures per se may be relatively easy to obtain, but it is the full discussion of relevant information that is difficult to achieve if enrollment of large
numbers of newborns is necessary. Ultimately, a standard research permission process might sufficiently limit and bias recruitment to the extent that a
population-based study would not be feasible or valid.

A second option is to consider a waiver of consent. The federal regulations
governing human subjects research (Protection of Human Subjects, Subparts A–D, Code of Federal Regulations, 45 CFR 46.116d) permit a waiver of

consent if four criteria are met: "(1) the research involves no more than minimal risk to the subjects; (2) the waiver or alteration will not adversely affect the rights and welfare of the subjects; (3) the research could not practicably be carried out without the waiver or alteration; and (4) whenever appropriate, the subjects will be provided with additional pertinent information after participation." It is up to the IRB with oversight responsibilities to determine whether these criteria are met for a particular protocol.

Can the criteria for waiver be met in this context? The first criterion is that of minimal risk. This criterion is key and is discussed in detail below. The second criterion poses the question of whether any other parental or child rights would be infringed through a waiver. Currently, parents typically get only a limited amount of information about newborn screening, so a waiver would not decrease this information (Fant, Clark, and Kemper 2005). As outlined more fully below, a research project might well entail an effort to educate the population and/or pregnant women about the study. Therefore, a waiver would not involve a withholding of information or services that would be otherwise available. No other apparent legal or ethical rights would be infringed by a waiver, although any relevant state laws and regulations should be considered. On the third criterion, as argued above, permission from virtually all parents is not practicable if one hopes to model and study a population-based program. The fourth criterion, notification after the research intervention, is not required, unless it is relevant to the specific project. In this context, research results are likely to be available to all health care providers and potentially to parents. A postresearch notification for those with negative screening results is expected. However, a formal debriefing process by investigators for all parents of children with negative results would not be feasible. Parents of children with positive results would receive detailed information, as described more fully below.

The most significant question with respect to a waiver in this context is whether the experimental introduction of a newborn screening test confers only minimal risk. The definition of minimal risk in the federal regulations is tied to the risks of everyday life and to routine clinical and psychological examinations. This will be a subjective call by the IRB, but an argument can be made for minimal risk in this case, given several considerations and stipulations. A new test does not involve any additional direct interventions, because the experimental tests would be run on the same bloodspots originally collected. So parents (and infants) will not experience any deviations from the expected routine by virtue of their participation in research. Of course, the primary risks from genetic tests arise from the potential psychosocial impact of the information, including true positive, false positive, and false negative results. The assessment of risk must hinge primarily on these psychosocial effects.

The large majority of parents will learn of negative results on the experimental screening test, if they learn of specific results at all. Children with these normal results (and their parents) will experience no adverse effects from their participation. The rare child who has a false negative result will not experience harm, because the child would not have been otherwise identified in the absence of the experimental screening. While there is some risk that a false negative result would delay a diagnosis later, if care providers believed a negative screening test definitively excluded the condition, this risk is remote.

Therefore, the relevant risks primarily are those conferred by true positive and false positive results. True positive results confer a risk because the early detection and treatment of the condition after screening may be more harmful than no screening. This can be true if early detection and treatment are generally worse than the disease. However, this is unlikely if stage I research has demonstrated the clinical utility of early detection and intervention. Thus the risk of this outcome is low for most affected children if stage I research precedes stage II protocols.

A more likely scenario is that a particular subset of affected children would be harmed by early detection and intervention. These are children with subclinical forms of the condition or benign metabolic variants that need no treatment. These children may be subjected to burdensome or harmful treatments because it may not be possible to distinguish "affected" children who require treatment from those who do not. The early history of PKU screening illustrates this phenomenon. Children with benign hyperpheylalaninemia could not be distinguished from children with classical PKU, and some were harmed from unnecessarily restricted diets (Fost 1992). The magnitude of this phenomenon with conditions amenable to MS/MS screening remains to be determined. In a study of population screening in New Zealand, Wilcken et al. (2003) found substantially more children with medium-chain acyl-CoA dehydrogenase deficiency than had been predicted based on the incidence of children who presented clinically with the disease. Waddell et al. (2006) identified a mutation in the medium-chain acyl-CoA dehydrogenase gene that may be associated with a milder form of the condition, a situation that is likely to be common with genetic metabolic conditions. Conditions that prove to be normal variants also occur. Histidinemia, a condition previously targeted by some newborn screening programs, proved to be benign (Lam et al. 1996). In these circumstances, harm to children may come from unnecessary labeling or stigma but more tangibly from the use of restricted diets, dietary alterations, or medications that are harmful. A central purpose of stage II research is to identify and evaluate these phenomena.

False positive results also confer a risk of harm. False positive results are common in newborn screening, as they are in all screening programs for low-prevalence conditions (Kwon and Farrell 2000). The positive predictive value (PPV) for many newborn screening tests is less than 2 percent, meaning that more than 98 percent of the initial positive results are false positives. MS/MS has a relatively good PPV, estimated to be about 8 to 10 percent (Fost 1992; Zytkovicz et al. 2001). Newborn screening programs are designed to conduct confirmatory testing after an initial positive result, to establish or exclude the diagnosis. Many parents experience substantial anxiety between the time of initial results and the confirmatory testing (Dillard and Tluczek 2005). Unfortunately, research consistently shows that a subset of parents whose children have false positive results continue to have anxiety and uncertainty over the health of their children months or even years later (Bodegard, Fyro, and Larsson 1983; Sorenson et al. 1984; Fyro and Bodegard 1987; Waisbren et al. 2003).

It is possible that the prevalence of significant adverse effects from false positive results can be reduced through improved education of parents before screening and during the disclosure of initial positive test results, but this also remains to be determined through research. False positive results with the attendant distress and potential for longer-term anxiety is a risk for any experimental screening intervention.

Are the risks of true positive and false positive results to parents and children greater than minimal risk? The incidence of adverse outcomes will be low across the whole population of newborns and parents, but the impact of those outcomes on the people who experience them can be significant. We can illustrate the prevalence of adverse events from false positive results using a hypothetical example. Let us assume a condition occurs in 1 in 20,000 infants, so a state with 100,000 births per year will have 5 affected children per year. If the PPV is 10 percent, approximately 50 infants per year will have false positive results. If 10 percent of the parents experience longer-term anxiety about the health of their child, this will affect 5 parent-child dyads per year, or 1 dyad per 20,000 births. Arguably, the magnitude and frequency of this outcome, and the adverse effects of unnecessary treatments, are comparable to the risks of everyday life in the United States.

That is, life normally involves a low incidence of significantly adverse events. By way of comparison, infant deaths from injuries occurred at a rate of 23.1 per 100,000 infants in 2003 (National Center for Health Statistics 2003). Similarly, the risks of routine physical and psychological examinations (to which the federal regulations tie the definition of minimal risk) include the risks of identifying abnormalities, and thus also carry the risk of false positive results with the associated distress. For true positive newborn screening results, of course, infants may benefit from the research if early intervention proves to be helpful.

Risks or adverse events in the context of newborn screening research can be reduced through several efforts. First, a statewide or regional research project can use public education and notification of parents. Newspaper articles, radio announcements, and television segments describing the study can reach a portion of the population and thereby promote a basic level of awareness. Pregnant women and/or parents of newborns can be informed of the study with brochures, videos, or brief presentations. Parents also might be informed of the opportunity to opt out of the study. These mechanisms cannot replace information provided in an informed permission process and they will not reach every new parent, but they might mitigate a "surprise factor" for many of the parents who later receive positive screening results.

A second way to reduce risk is to develop a sensitive, fully informative method to disclose initial positive results to parents. Primary care providers typically have the responsibility to disclose these results to parents and to encourage and arrange confirmatory testing. This will become an increasingly complex challenge as newborn screening panels expand to cover rare and unfamiliar conditions. A potential advantage of a stage II research protocol is an enhanced support for pediatricians in managing the disclosure process. A carefully designed approach to results disclosure and confirmatory testing may reduce the risk of adverse psychological effects resulting from false positive results, and from true positive results as well.

A research project that adequately evaluates the benefits and risks of a new newborn screening test requires longitudinal evaluation of the children. Once an initial result is provided to the parents, there is the opportunity to obtain informed permission for the follow-up component of the study. That is, a waiver of consent would cover only the period from the research analysis of the sample through disclosure of the results. Children with positive results are a small subgroup of the population, and it is not necessary or appropriate to claim that informed permission from parents of these children is not practicable. Obviously, the participation of affected children and their parents in ongoing evaluations is critical to the success of this research. Permission must be obtained at this point for the collection of surveillance data and, of course, for any experimental interventions with the child.

In summary, I suggest that a waiver of consent is justifiable if several criteria are met:

- Stage I research demonstrates with reasonable assurance that early detection and intervention benefit affected children.
- Population education about the research protocol is offered through the mass media.
- A reasonable effort is made to educate and notify pregnant women and parents of newborns about the project. Opt-out opportunities should be offered.
- The waiver covers only the period between testing and results notification and confirmatory testing.
- Protocols are developed to manage results disclosure to minimize the negative psychological effects on parents of children with positive test results.

Permission for Research with Residual Specimens

A modest volume of research has been done with residual dried bloodspots following removal of all individual identifiers (Newborn Screening Task Force 2000). Although IRBs may want oversight over the process of de-identifying tissue samples, the use of anonymous tissue samples in research does not constitute human subjects research. Therefore, research with de-identified samples is exempt from IRB oversight and from the regulatory requirements for consent. Residual specimens also are commonly used for quality control efforts in the laboratory. This use for quality assessment does not create concerns over consent.

The question of parental permission arises when investigators wish to use identifiable samples or samples that are coded but linked to individual identifiers. If only a small subset of samples were needed, parental permission would not pose a significant challenge from a practical perspective. But if samples from a large segment of the population, or the entire infant population, were necessary for the research, then a prospective consent process in the newborn nursery would face the same challenges noted above. A consent process initiated after the specimens were stored would be even more difficult, given the need to contact parents anew, mail and request the return of signed documents, and so forth. Thus individual parental consent for the use of large numbers of residual samples poses an enormous challenge.

Despite these potential difficulties, several professional organizations advocate informed permission for use of identifiable residual samples from newborn screening. These include the Institute of Medicine Committee on Assessing Genetic Risk (Andrews et al. 1994), the Council of Regional Networks for Genetic Services (Therrell et al. 1996), the Newborn Screening Task Force (2000) of the AAP, and the New York State Task Force on Life and the Law (2000). The Newborn Screening Task Force (2000) specifically states: "Parental permission should be sought for the use of identifiable samples in research to validate tests for additional diseases, or for epidemiologic research" (p. 416). These committees do not speak to the possibility of a waiver of permission, so it is uncertain whether they assume that research on identifiable samples never involves minimal risk.

Genetic tests have raised concerns in recent decades, due to the ethical, legal, and social implications of the results. Yet a number of authors argue that genetic information is not inherently more problematic than other forms of medical information (Murray 1997; Green and Botkin 2003). The impacts and risks of genetic information depend heavily on the nature of the specific information being generated and the context of the testing. Research on the effects of various forms of genetic testing illustrates that the large majority of people deal well with adverse diagnostic information (Lerman and Shields 2004) and that the risks of social discrimination, including insurance and employment discrimination, are low (Hall and Rich 2000). Therefore, it is not accurate to claim that genetic testing inherently involves a greater than minimal risk. Waivers of consent are applicable to genetic research as long as the required criteria are met.

Is a waiver of permission justified in some circumstances for use of residual samples in newborn screening research? The criterion that a consent process is not practicable is met in this case, assuming investigators need to use thousands of samples. The central question is whether such research poses more than a minimal risk. This assessment depends on the nature of the research being proposed. Let us look at the "retrospective screening" protocol outlined above. This use would involve retention of samples over a period of time and analysis for a condition being experimentally evaluated for population screening. Parents of children who test positive would be contacted, given information about the condition and the research project, and asked to permit a health assessment of their child. There would be potential benefits to affected children and their parents if the children were symptomatic or at risk for health consequences from the condition, but had not been diagnosed clinically.

The adverse consequences of the research would be much the same as for a prospective research protocol. That is, there is risk from identification of true positives when such identification is, on the whole, not beneficial, and risk from notifying parents of results that prove to be false positives. That screening is conducted retrospectively does not clearly increase these risks. In fact, the risk of parental distress due to false positive results might be decreased, because parents of older children might be less sensitive than parents of newborns to potentially bad news about their child's health, particularly if they believe the older child is healthy.

A retrospective screening use of stored specimens is likely to be conducted in conjunction with a prospective screening trial. Therefore, several of the methods to reduce risk outlined above would be applicable, including the use of public education to publicize the study and the use of parental notification about the research in the perinatal period. Again, the waiver of permission would apply only to the storage, sample analysis, and notification of parents. Parental permission would be obtained for retention of research data, follow-up, and any experimental interventions for the condition.

Institutional Review Board Oversight

Research conducted on newborn screening programs needs approval from an institutional review board. State departments of health have an affiliated IRB for this purpose, staffed with individuals who are familiar with public health research. If a waiver of consent is sought by the investigator, the IRB would have the responsibility of determining whether a waiver is justified under the regulations in the context of the proposed project. Given the wide variability among IRBs that review pediatric research in their assessments of risk (Shah et al. 2004), it would not be surprising if different IRBs came to different determinations about the justification for waivers of consent.

The central ethical challenge of this proposal for waiving consent for newborn screening research is, of course, the potential enrollment of tens of thousands of individuals and their parents in research without their permission. The sheer magnitude of this enterprise, the use of genetic testing, and the fact that research is being conducted by, or through, a government agency may raise the level of concern about a waiver of consent. For this reason, any research in this domain should be conducted in the full light of public scrutiny. IRB review and approval is a form of independent scrutiny that involves non-scientists, but IRB approval does not suffice for public awareness and support. I also argued above for public and parental education about such projects as they are conducted. But these measures, too, are not sufficient. It would be advisable to plan all prospective and retrospective newborn screening research with the active involvement of community representatives. Here "community" means the lay public, health care providers, public health professionals, hospitals, and relevant advocacy groups. Many state health departments have genetic advisory groups that are increasingly active in providing advice on policies and procedures related to newborn screening. Support from these groups for specific newborn screening research protocols, and for the waivers of consent as proposed here, would be essential. Thus, the research would be conducted as a highly visible enterprise with broad public awareness and support, but without individual parental permission.

Conclusion

The primary recommendation in this analysis is to pursue a waiver of consent for research on newborn screening for the types of projects described. This approach has the obvious advantage of remaining within the existing regulations. Yet, as noted, there is and should be considerable public anxiety about the conduct of any research without the explicit knowledge and permission of participants or their surrogates. This anxiety arises in part from the poor fit between standard research ethics, designed largely for projects with a limited number of participants, and the need to address some health problems through broad public health measures.

Biomedical knowledge increasingly may provide opportunities to address health problems through public health measures rather than through individual interactions and decisions. Fluoridation and chlorine-treatment of our water supplies are examples of valuable public health measures whose efficacy is due to uniform implementation for the entire population. Folate supplementation of foods to reduce neural tube defects is another example of a public health approach to disease prevention. This approach functions without the individual consent of all those receiving the risks and benefits of the intervention. These types of public health intervention are justified when risks are low, benefits are substantial, public dialogue has occurred, and individual choice is not conducive to an effective program.

How, then, to make the transition from small-scale research projects to uniform or mandated population-based programs? Population-based pilot programs are the answer. Unfortunately, in the context of newborn screening, the more typical answer has been to simply implement promising new tests in mandated programs on the assumption that they will be effective. The translational research between small clinical trials and mandated population programs often is skipped. Years or decades later, we may find that measures are worthless or even harmful. Thus, there is a need to reevaluate the normal expectations for individual consent that serves as a barrier to research when dealing with public health interventions. Consent can be a barrier both because of the prohibitive practicalities involved and because the consent process itself alters the programs under study—specifically, when individual decisions will not be a feature of the program once implemented.

The recommendations outlined in this chapter are an attempt to bridge this gap between small research projects where consent is essential and fully implemented public health programs that preclude individual choice. While it might be desirable for the federal regulations to be more explicitly sensitive to public health research, changes in the regulations would be a serious bureaucratic challenge, particularly if the current regulations are sufficiently flexible. Changes in state regulations or in public health department policies and procedures may be more feasible.

To foster education and reduce risks, investigators and programs conducting population-based newborn screening research without individual consent should consider using the following measures:

- Public education about the research through mass media outlets
- Notification of parents about the project, with an opt-out provision
- Dialogue with the lay and professional communities about the research during planning and implementation
- Approval and periodic review by a genetics advisory board or similar body external to the health department that can give force to community concerns and expectations
- Approval by an IRB

Of course, these measures would not replace all the ethical and educational functions of individual informed consent. Yet they may be sufficiently protective of individuals' rights and welfare in low-risk research while permitting new public health interventions to be implemented on a solid evidence base.

REFERENCES

American College of Obstetricians and Gynecologists. 2003. Committee on Genetics opinion: newborn screening. *Obstet Gynecol* 102 (4): 887–89.

Andrews, L. B., Fullarton, J. E., Holtzman, N. A., and Motulsky, A.G. 1994. *Assessing Genetic Risks: Implications for Health and Social Policy.* Washington DC: National Academy of Sciences.

Annas, G. J. 1982. Mandatory PKU screening: the other side of the looking glass. *Am J Public Health* 72 (12): 1401–3.

Ballard, H. O., Shook, L. A., Desai, N. S., and Anand, K. J. 2004. Neonatal research and the validity of informed consent obtained in the perinatal period. *J Perinatol* 24 (7): 409–15.

Bodegard, G., Fyro, K., and Larsson, A. 1983. Psychological reactions in 102 families with a newborn who has a falsely positive screening test for congenital hypothyroidism. *Acta Paediatr Scand Suppl* 304:1–21.

Botkin, J. R. 2005. Research for newborn screening: developing a national framework. *Pediatrics* 116 (4): 862–71.

Botkin, J. R., Clayton, E. W., Fost, N. C., Burke, W., Murray, T. H., Baily, M. A., Wilfond, B., Berg, A., and Ross, L. F. 2006. Newborn screening technology: proceed with caution. *Pediatrics* 117 (5): 1793–99.

Campbell, E., and Ross, L. F. 2003. Parental attitudes regarding newborn screening of PKU and DMD. *Am J Med Genet A* 120 (2): 209–14.

Centers for Disease Control and Prevention. 2000. Update: newborn screening for sickle cell disease—California, Illinois, and New York, 1998. *JAMA* 284 (11): 1373–74.

Clayton, E. W. 2005. Talking with parents before newborn screening. *J Pediatr* 147 (3 Suppl): S26–29.

Dhondt, J. L. 2005. Implementation of informed consent for a cystic fibrosis newborn screening program in France: low refusal rates for optional testing. *J Pediatr* 147 (3 Suppl): S106–8.

Dillard, J. P., and Tluczek, A. 2005. Information flow after a positive newborn screening for cystic fibrosis. *J Pediatr* 147 (3 Suppl): S94–97.

Faden, R., Chwalow, A. J., Holtzman, N. A., and Horn, S. D. 1982. A survey to evaluate parental consent as public policy for neonatal screening. *Am J Public Health* 72 (12): 1347–52.

Fant, K. E., Clark, S. J., and Kemper, A. R. 2005. Completeness and complexity of information available to parents from newborn-screening programs. *Pediatrics* 115 (5): 1268–72.

Farrell, P. M., Kosorok, M. R., Rock, M. J., Laxova, A., Zeng, L., Lai, H. C., Hoffman, G., Laessig, R. H., and Splaingard, M. L. 2001. Early diagnosis of cystic fibrosis through neonatal screening prevents severe malnutrition and improves long-term growth. Wisconsin Cystic Fibrosis Neonatal Screening Study Group. *Pediatrics* 107 (1): 1–13.

Fitzgerald, T., Duva, S., Ostrer, H., Pass, K., Oddoux, C., Ruben, R., and Caggana, M. 2004. The frequency of GJB2 and GJB6 mutations in the New York State newborn population: feasibility of genetic screening for hearing defects. *Clin Genet* 65 (4): 338–42.

Fost, N. 1992. Ethical implications of screening asymptomatic individuals. *FASEB J* 6 (10): 2813–17.

Fyro, K., and Bodegard, G. 1987. Four-year follow-up of psychological reactions to false positive screening tests for congenital hypothyroidism. *Acta Paediatr Scand* 76 (1): 107–14.

Green, M. J., and Botkin, J. R. 2003. "Genetic exceptionalism" in medicine: clarifying the differences between genetic and nongenetic tests. *Ann Intern Med* 138 (7): 571–75.

Gwinn, M., Pappaioanou, M., George, J. R., Hannon, W. H., Wasser, S. C., Redus, M. A., Hoff, R., Grady, G. F., Willoughby, A., and Novello, A. C. 1991. Prevalence of HIV infection in childbearing women in the United States: surveillance using newborn blood samples. *JAMA* 265 (13): 1704–8.

Hall, M. A., and Rich, S. S. 2000. Laws restricting health insurers' use of genetic information: impact on genetic discrimination. *Am J Hum Genet* 66 (1): 293–307.

Kwon, C., and Farrell, P. M. 2000. The magnitude and challenge of false-positive newborn screening test results. *Arch Pediatr Adolesc Med* 154 (7): 714–18.

Lam, W. K., Cleary, M. A., Wraith, J. E., and Walter, J. H. 1996. Histidinaemia: a benign metabolic disorder. *Arch Dis Child* 74 (4): 343–46.

Lerman, C., and Shields, A. E. 2004. Genetic testing for cancer susceptibility: the promise and the pitfalls. *Nat Rev Cancer* 4 (3): 235–41.

Mandl, K. D., Feit, S., Larson, C., and Kohane, I. S. 2002. Newborn screening program practices in the United States: notification, research, and consent. *Pediatrics* 109 (2): 269–73.

Mischler, E. H., Wilfond, B. S., Fost, N., Laxova, A., Reiser, C., Sauer, C. M., Makholm, L. M., Shen, G., Feenan, L., McCarthy, C., and Farrell, P. M. 1998. Cystic fibrosis newborn screening: impact on reproductive behavior and implications for genetic counseling. *Pediatrics* 102 (1 Pt 1): 44–52.

Murray, T. H. 1997. Genetic exceptionalism and "future diaries": is genetic information different from other medical information? In *Genetic Secrets: Protecting Privacy and Confidentiality in the Genetic Era*, ed. M. A. Rothstein, pp. 60–73. New Haven, CT: Yale University Press.

National Center for Health Statistics. 2003. Infant deaths/mortality. www.cdc.gov/nchs/data/hestat/finaldeaths03_tables.pdf#4.

National Research Council, Committee for the Study of Inborn Errors of Metabolism. 1975. *Genetic Screening Programs, Principles, and Research.* Washington, DC: National Academy of Sciences.

Natowicz, M. 2005. Newborn screening—setting evidence-based policy for protection. *N Engl J Med* 353 (9): 867–70.

Nelson, R. M., Botkin, J. R., Kodish, E. D., Levetown, M., Truman, J. T., Wilfond, B. S., Harrison, C. E., Kazura, A., Krug, E. III, Schwartz, P. A., Donovan, G. K., Fallat, M., Porter, I. H., and Steinberg, D. 2001. Ethical issues with genetic testing in pediatrics. *Pediatrics* 107 (6): 1451–55.

New York State Task Force on Life and the Law. 2000. *Genetic Testing and Screening in the Age of Genomic Medicine.* New York: New York State Task Force on Life and the Law.

Newborn Screening Task Force. 2000. Serving the family from birth to the medical home: a report from the Newborn Screening Task Force convened in Washington DC, May 10–11, 1999. *Pediatrics* 106 (2 Pt 2): 383–427.

President's Commission for the Study of Ethical Problems in Medicine and Biomedical and Behavioral Research. 1983. *Screening and Counseling for Genetic Conditions: A Report on the Ethical, Social, and Legal implications of Genetic Screening, Counseling, and Education Programs.* Washington, DC: Government Printing Office.

Press, N., and Clayton, E. W. 2000. Genetics and public health: informed consent beyond the clinical encounter. In *Genetics and Public Health in the 21st Century*, ed. M. J. Khoury, W. Burke, and E. J. Thomson, pp. 505–26. New York: Oxford University Press.

Shah, S., Whittle, A., Wilfond, B., Gensler, G., and Wendler, D. 2004. How do institutional review boards apply the federal risk and benefit standards for pediatric research? *JAMA* 291 (4): 476–82.

Sorenson, J. R., Levy, H. L., Mangione, T. W., and Sepe, S. J. 1984. Parental response to repeat testing of infants with "false-positive" results in a newborn screening program. *Pediatrics* 73 (2): 183–87.

Sox, C. M., Cooper, W. O., Koepsell, T. D., DiGiuseppe, D. L., and Christakis, D. A. 2003. Provision of pneumococcal prophylaxis for publicly insured children with sickle cell disease. *JAMA* 290 (8): 1057–61.

Steiner, R. D. 2005. Evidence based medicine in inborn errors of metabolism: is there any and how to find it. *Am J Med Genet A* 134 (2): 192–97.

Teach, S. J., Lillis, K. A., and Grossi, M. 1998. Compliance with penicillin prophylaxis in patients with sickle cell disease. *Arch Pediatr Adolesc Med* 152 (3): 274–78.

Therrell, B. L., Hannon, W. H., Pass, K. A., Lorey, F., Brokopp, C., and Eckman, J. 1996. Guidelines for the retention, storage and use of residual dried blood spot samples after newborn screening analysis. Statement of the Council of Regional Networks for Genetic Services. *Biochem Mol Med* 57 (2): 116–24.

U.S. General Accounting Office. 2003. Newborn screening characteristics of state programs. www.gao.gov/new.items/d03449.pdf.

Waddell, L., Wiley, V., Carpenter, K., Bennetts, B., Angel, L., Andresen, B. S., and Wilcken, B. 2006. Medium-chain acyl-CoA dehydrogenase deficiency: genotype-biochemical phenotype correlations. *Mol Genet Metab* 87 (1): 32–39.

Waisbren, S. E., Albers, S., Amato, S., Ampola, M., Brewster, T. G., Demmer, L., Eaton, R. B., Greenstein, R., Korson, M., Larson, C., Marsden, D., Msall, M., Naylor, E. W., Pueschel, S., Seashore, M., Shih, V. E., and Levy, H. L. 2003. Effect of expanded newborn screening for biochemical genetic disorders on child outcomes and parental stress. *JAMA* 290 (19): 2564–72.

Wilcken, B., Wiley, V., Hammond, J., and Carpenter, K. 2003. Screening newborns for inborn errors of metabolism by tandem mass spectrometry. *N Engl J Med* 348 (23): 2304–12.

Zytkovicz, T. H., Fitzgerald, E. F., Marsden, D., Larson, C. A., Shih, V. E., Johnson, D. M., Strauss, A. W., Comeau, A. M., Eaton, R. B., and Grady, G. F. 2001. Tandem mass spectrometric analysis for amino, organic, and fatty acid disorders in newborn dried blood spots: a two-year summary from the New England Newborn Screening Program. *Clin Chem* 47 (11): 1945–55.

CHAPTER 14

Population-Based Research within a Public Health Service

Two Models for Compliance with the Common Rule in the Massachusetts Newborn Screening Program

ANNE MARIE COMEAU, PH.D.

DONNA E. LEVIN, J.D.

Routine and universal newborn screening for state-specified lists of disorders is performed on every neonate born in the United States—approximately four million live births per year (Martin, Brady, et al. 2003; National Newborn Screening and Genetics Resource Center 2003; Martin, Hamilton, et al. 2004)—and in most developed countries. Nationally, this public health measure is widely acclaimed for its early disease detection and intervention in clinical outcomes for more than 5000 infants a year who would otherwise suffer severe mental retardation, life-threatening morbidity, and, in many cases, death (data derived from National Newborn Screening and Genetics Resource Center 2003). In general, the following criteria must be met for a disorder to be included in the newborn screening panel: the disorder is treatable, with direct benefit to the infant screened; there is an accurate screening test; and the timing of appropriate clinical intervention is such that it warrants screening in the neonatal period (Wilson and Jungner 1968; Committee for the Study of Inborn Errors of Metabolism 1975; Andrews et al. 1994; Holtzman and Watson 1997; Newborn Screening Task Force 2000). In the United States, each state independently determines the panel of disorders to be screened, in accordance with state law and regulation. In each state, consideration is given to the regional prevalence of the disorder and to the availability of coordinated services, which include timely laboratory testing and specialized clinical follow-up. Every state screens for at least three disorders—congenital hypothyroidism, galactosemia, and phenylketonuria—and most states screen for several more. Some states have been screening for all disorders (see table 1.1) recommended by the Secretary's Advisory Committee on Heritable Disorders and Genetic Diseases in Newborns and Children (a committee of the Department of Health and Human Services), based on a proposal for a national uniform panel of newborn screening disorders (American College of Medical Genetics 2006), and most of these states do so outside a research protocol.

Newborn screening as a public health service is authorized by the state and operates under state privacy laws and regulations. Research that uses specimens and data collected with the authorization of the state is conducted pursuant to the Federal Common Rule 45 CFR 46 governing research on human subjects. Adherence to the Common Rule is mandatory for institutions (such as states) receiving federal funding, and compliance is monitored through mandatory reporting to federally regulated human subjects institutional review boards (IRBs). In contrast, research performed at institutions that operate newborn screening services independent of the state and without federal funds is not necessarily subject to the same monitoring. This chapter discusses two successful models for population-based research run in concert with state-authorized newborn screening services.

Between 1999 and 2004, parents of 482,904 Massachusetts live-born infants were offered optional newborn testing for cystic fibrosis (CF) and for 19 metabolic disorders, as part of a Massachusetts-wide newborn screening research protocol; 98.6 percent, or 476,056 and 476,098 parents, consented to each option, respectively. Results of any individual's optional testing were available from the newborn screening program to each participant through his or her birth or health care provider.

Under another Massachusetts-wide research protocol conducted between 1988 and 1994, newborn specimens were tested for maternal HIV antibody; all live births were enrolled. For this research, parents were not offered an option of enrollment, because all specimens were de-identified before any testing. Because the results of any specific individual's HIV testing in the newborn screening program were not generated, they were not available for review and reporting. However, any individual could be tested at one of many free, anonymous test sites throughout the state to determine confidentially his or her own HIV status.

Both research protocols used population-based residual samples from the routine newborn screening required by Massachusetts law (M.G.L. c.111, §§4E and 110A; 105 CMR 270.000). Each research protocol was implemented by researchers cognizant of Massachusetts legislation or intended legislation for protection of individuals' rights to keep HIV or genetic testing information private and for such testing to be free of coercion (M.G.L. c.111, §70F and §70G, respectively). One protocol required parental consent and the other did not, because de-identified samples were used.

For future studies, how should rules that are conventionally applied to the use of residual samples and data be applied when the samples and data are collected under the authority of the state for a public health service? Under what circumstances would one protocol be appropriate and not the other? That is, do the two protocols provide equal privacy protections for the individuals tested? Do they provide equal opportunity to participating individuals to gain medically relevant information? Do they provide equal protection to individuals in preventing test results from prompting therapeutic applications prematurely? As we move forward with technology that allows for more population-based evaluations, how can we ensure that protections and access to good-quality services are available when public health services such as newborn screening overlap with research? This chapter takes a closer look at these questions, outlining the advantages and disadvantages of each protocol in the light of our experience in Massachusetts and relative to alternative protocols.

The Massachusetts Studies
Expansion of the Number of Disorders Included in Newborn Screening

In 1998, the Massachusetts Department of Public Health issued regulations based on recommendations from its Newborn Screening Advisory Committee (NBSAC) mandating statewide routine newborn screening for 10 disorders (more than any other state at the time). The regulations went into effect on February 1, 1999 (105 CMR 270.000). The 10 disorders included 9 previously required plus medium-chain acyl-CoA dehydrogenase deficiency (MCAD).[1] Given the documented and significant risk of morbidity or mortality if these 10 disorders were untreated in newborns and given that the window of opportunity for timely clinical intervention could be so narrow in the neonatal period, routine and universal newborn screening is mandatory, pursuant to statutory authority, without obtaining parental permission. Massachusetts law, however, does provide for an exemption from mandatory screening when such screening conflicts with the religious tenets and practices of the newborn's parents (M.G.L. c.111, §110A).

Concurrent with its deliberations resulting in the addition of MCAD to the mandatory panel, the NBSAC was faced with the challenge and opportunity to screen for an additional set of disorders, some of which would be detectable by the same multiplex technology (technology capable of identifying multiple disorders in a single run) necessary to detect MCAD. Recognizing a presumed benefit in screening for 20 other disorders that did not meet all the criteria for mandatory newborn screening,[2] the NBSAC recommended that newborn screening services be offered statewide as a pilot study for an expanded list of disorders (Atkinson et al. 2001).

The NBSAC proposed one pilot program for CF and one pilot program for an additional 19 rare metabolic disorders, to gain a better understanding of the following factors. Some of the assays to detect the disorders would, of necessity, include analyses of some newborns' DNA and would be likely to identify some carriers of a disorder (CF in particular). There was an interest in determining the predictive values of a CF screening algorithm that used testing for multiple mutations, as well as the effectiveness of a multitiered program that included genetic counseling for families of identified carriers. Although the program was to collect data on the clinical utility of CF newborn screening, it was expected that analyses of clinical utility would include larger and longer-standing datasets than would be available in Massachusetts alone. In particular, the continuing data accrual from the Wisconsin and U.K. clinical trials (Chatfield et al. 1991; Farrell et al. 1997) and from the Australian cohort study (Wilken and Chalmers 1985) promised the availability of good-quality data on clinical outcomes linked to screening that otherwise would require years, even decades, to obtain. Massachusetts's implementation of a statewide study was in accordance with then-standing recommendations from the Centers for Disease Control and Prevention (1997). In the pilot program for 19 metabolic disorders, the tandem mass spectrometry (MS/MS) technology necessary to detect the mandated disorder, MCAD, would be applicable to the detection of the 19 rare metabolic disorders in the pilot program (not CF). However, little was known at the time about the specificity of MS/MS and whether it would enhance the detection of carriers or the detection of relatively asymptomatic or untreatable cases. Furthermore, because so little was known about the incidence, natural history, spectrum of disease, and/or treatability of many of these 19 disorders, there was an interest in collecting such data. It was predicted, however, that a larger dataset than would be available from the Massachusetts birth cohort would be necessary to understand the clinical utility of screening. Clearly, without any screening, the knowledge base would be static. Also, a larger dataset of cases identified by newborn screening would not, alone, be sufficient; without the clinical trials such as those available for CF, the importance of the quality of the outcomes data to be collected weighed heavily.

The state's Department of Public Health accepted the NBSAC's recommendation and established two pilot programs built on the existing infrastructure of the newborn screening program. The two pilot programs were designed to contribute to the general knowledge about screening for these disorders that would be available to the department and to its NBSAC. The two pilot programs were implemented on February 1, 1999.

In keeping with the NBSAC's recommendations, the Department of Public Health authorized and directed the state's Newborn Screening Program to develop and conduct the two population-based studies in which specimen identifiers would be maintained, allowing study results to be linked to and reported for specific individuals. Two human subjects IRBs, one at the department and one at the University of Massachusetts Medical School, determined that parental permission for these studies was required (noting that the mechanism for unconsented enrollment was mandatory screening). However, both IRBs recognized the NBSAC's assessment of presumed benefit to enrolled infants and did not want to restrict access to the pilot screening. The two IRBs also determined that there would be little if any physical risk (no additional specimens for an infant to be enrolled) and that clinical protocols for follow-up of infants with positive screening results were in place. Furthermore, the IRBs recognized that, operationally, implementation of these evaluations would have to accommodate the need to educate and ask permission from approximately 80,000 parents each year whenever a newborn screening specimen was obtained.

The two IRBs approved an oral permission/consent protocol, with particular requirements for implementation (http://umassmed.edu/nbs/). Briefly, personnel attending the births were instructed to ensure that parents had access to brochures describing the pilot programs (available in nine languages and, ideally, distributed prenatally); to remind parents that in the absence of a religious objection, all Massachusetts newborns would be screened for 10 disorders; to let parents know that optional screening was available at no additional cost for another 20 disorders, if the parents so desired; to ask parents about their wishes for optional screening; and to give parents a copy of the written documentation of the oral permission/consent or dissent.

At the outset, there was little evidence on which to base predictions of the percentage of parents that would decline optional genetic screening through the newborn screening program. The chance that an affected infant would not be identified by the optional screen because a parent declined enrollment would depend on the prevalence of the disorder in the population and the frequency with which parents declined a particular option (table 14.1). Given what was known about the frequencies of disease in the Massachusetts population, the possibility that parents might decline optional testing for an (unknowingly) affected infant seemed to be highest for CF-affected infants, most of whom would be identified at approximately 18 months of age by conventional means (Cystic Fibrosis Foundation, Patient Registry 2006 [1990–1994 data]; note that the then current estimate was for detection by 14.5 months [Grosse et al. 2004; Accurso, Sontag, and Wagener 2005]). That parents might decline optional testing for an infant unknowingly affected with a rapidly progressing metabolic disorder was predicted to become likely only when the frequency of parents' declining optional screening approached 20 percent (table 14.1). After more than six years of optional screening in the Massachusetts program, only one affected infant was identified who was not tested by the optional screen, and this was a CF-affected infant who had a prenatal diagnosis.

The proportion of parents who declined CF testing or metabolic testing thus far is small; in the general population, it has never exceeded 2 percent. The Massachusetts subpopulations with highest rates of parents who decline optional screening are those who give birth at home and at hospitals serving more affluent communities (table 14.2). Most parents who declined CF testing

TABLE 14.1
Projected Annual Incidence of Missed Cases Relative to the Percentage of Parents Declining Optional Genetic Screens in Massachusetts

Percentage of Parents Declining Screens	Projected Number of Cystic Fibrosis Cases Missed	Projected Number of Pilot Metabolic Disorders (combined) Cases Missed
20	5 (1/15,000)	~1 (1/67,000)
3	<1 (1/105,000)	<<<1 (1/440,000)

TABLE 14.2

Relationship between Percentage of Total Births and Percentage of Parents Declining Optional Screens in Particular Birth Hospitals in Massachusetts

Percentage of Parents Declining Optional Screen	Number of Hospitals	Percentage of Total Births
0	7 ⎫	
0.0–0.9	17 ⎬	25
1–1.9	18	50
2.0–7.2	10* ⎫	
10	Home births ⎬	25

* Hospitals serving affluent communities.

also declined metabolic testing, and vice versa. Over time, the percentage of parents who declined optional testing seems to have decreased (table 14.3).

The knowledge base gained from data obtained through the pilot programs has grown considerably. Incidence data for CF-affected infants in the Massachusetts birth cohort were consistent with projections at about 30 in 100,000 births through 2003, and a significantly decreased incidence since then has been documented (Hale, Parad, and Comeau 2008); for CF screening, the feasibility of a multiple mutation–screening algorithm with reasonable predictive value has been demonstrated (Comeau et al. 2004); and multiple parameters on the effectiveness of a multitiered program that includes diagnostic follow-up and genetic counseling are now better understood (Comeau et al. 2005; Parad and Comeau 2005; Parad et al. 2005). Increasing evidence for the clinical utility of CF newborn screening resulted in the CDC's 2004 statement that CF newborn screening is justified (Grosse et al. 2004) and prompted the Cystic Fibrosis Foundation's recommendation (2005) for careful implementation.

The additional 19 metabolic disorders have a combined incidence of approximately 10 in 100,000 infants screened (Roger B. Eaton, personal communication), but such statistics continue to be confounded by the absence of clear case definitions for many of these disorders when detected by screening. Unlike CF, for which the natural history is well understood and diagnostic standards exist (Rosenstein and Cutting 1998), the spectrum of "disease" that is being uncovered by population screening for rare metabolic disorders presents challenges. Case definitions have traditionally relied on clinical presentation; diagnostic and treatment practices for presymptomatic infants need to be reconsidered. A multiplex-technology strategy that selectively tests for markers of disorders for which a parent or a state has authorized screening is known to be technically feasible (Zytkovicz et al. 2001). Observed clinical

TABLE 14.3

Number and Percentage of Parents Declining Optional Screens in Massachusetts

Year	Number of Births*	Total Number of Parents Declining an Optional Screen	Parents Declining Optional CF Screen (%)	Parents Declining Optional Metabolic Screen (%)	Parents Declining Either Optional Screen (%)
1999†	75,485	1,418	1.75	1.77	1.88
2000	83,019	986	1.09	1.12	1.19
2001	82,605	748	0.82	0.85	0.91
2002	82,102	727	0.84	0.81	0.89
2003	81,682	670	0.77	0.75	0.82
2004	79,490	512	0.60	0.59	0.64

* Number of initial specimen requisitions on Massachusetts specimen card.
† Eleven-month period.

outcomes in the affected infants identified from the cohort include a spectrum from "well" (relatively asymptomatic) through "death in later childhood" (preventable?) and "acute presentation with early death" (relatively untreatable); for many of these disorders, the clinical utility of the expanded metabolic screen is still under study.

Initiative to Address an Epidemiological Question of National Importance about the Prevalence of HIV

During the height of the U.S. HIV/AIDS epidemic in the 1980s, there was an urgent need to monitor the epidemic so that public health agencies could plan and evaluate preventive strategies and determine future needs for health resources for those who would become infected. Conventional means, by clinical surveillance, provided data that lagged behind infection incidence by several years. Laboratory sampling of subpopulations yielded results that could not be extrapolated to the general population, because the samplings were obtained from one of two groups with unusual risk profiles: high-risk groups (intravenous drug users or males self-identifying as gay) or low-risk groups (blood donors and military recruits). As described in the seminal publication by Hoff et al. (1988), the development of methods to study the epidemic in an important "bridge group" (i.e., childbearing women) provided a timely and "sensitive measure of the course of the epidemic." The key component that would provide an unbiased sampling of childbearing women was access to residual dried bloodspots from public health newborn screening programs.

The research institute affiliated with the Massachusetts Newborn Screening Program and working with the National Institute for Child Health and Human Development (NICHD) convened a National Advisory Committee to address the legal and ethical issues and survey design of the 1987 proposal for the study of HIV seroprevalence in childbearing women.[3] The technical component of the study called for measuring maternal HIV antibody in the infants' bloodspots; a positive antibody test would indicate that the mother was infected and that the infant was at risk of infection. As in the later study of expanded newborn screening described above, concerns about any additional discomfort to the infant resulting from an additional heel prick were moot because the residual bloodspots would be used. Concern that a consent-based mechanism of enrollment would not give a complete epidemiological picture was confronted with arguments that infants and their mothers should benefit from testing of their samples. Unlike in the consent-based study discussed above, two determining points (both of which were true at the time) justified using de-identified infant samples rather than identified samples after consent, as noted by the committee:

1 "Knowledge of the HIV status of the infant was not beneficial to the infant because there is no specific treatment available . . . at present there are no efficient HIV antibody screening methods that distinguish HIV infection in newborns."

2 "Women who desire anonymous or confidential testing for HIV can obtain these services from a variety of clinics operated by public health departments and the medical care system" (HIV Seroprevalence in Childbearing Women Advisory Committee 1987).

A methodology for de-identification while retaining epidemiological integrity was developed. Residual specimens from newborn screening in the state of Massachusetts were divided according to nine geographic health service areas; for multiple births, all but one birth was removed from the study; and samples were de-identified before testing for HIV antibody status. Results of the testing were reported as raw numbers of specimens tested and as the rate of HIV seropositive specimens per thousand births (number of positive HIV specimens per number of total specimens tested × 1000). Results were interpreted to indicate the number of HIV-infected mothers giving birth in a cohort of all mothers giving birth in a particular geographic area. Approximately 2.3 in 1000 women giving birth in Massachusetts were infected with HIV in each of years from 1988 to 1994 (table 14.4).

With advances in antiretroviral therapy and the possibility that infected infants could be treated, there were calls to halt the anonymous survey and to implement mandatory newborn screening for HIV risk (Dao 1994). When

TABLE 14.4
HIV Seropositivity Rates, Massachusetts, 1988–1994

Year	Number of Initial Residual Bloodspot Specimens	HIV Seropositivity Rate (per 1000 births)
1988	88,924	2.5
1989	92,238	2.2
1990	92,816	2.4
1991	88,292	2.5
1992	87,256	2.5
1993	84,120	2.2
1994	80,551	2.0

results from a clinical trial showed that prenatal use of AZT (azidothymidine) reduced the rate of mother-to-infant transmission from 30 to 10 percent (Connor et al. 1994; Mofenson 2002), several groups, such as the Institute of Medicine, that had been considering addition of HIV risk to newborn screening panels determined that it was more appropriate to offer prenatal HIV testing to pregnant women (McCormick, Davidson, and Stoto 1999; Mofenson 2000). The CDC and the NICHD withdrew funding for the national survey (CDC suspends testing of newborns 1995); as a result, most statewide surveys were halted. However, Connecticut and New York added HIV testing to their newborn screening panel and continued to screen newborns for HIV exposure, in addition to offering women's prenatal HIV testing and treatments (National Newborn Screening and Genetics Resource Center 2006).

Discussion

The circumstances that led to the two very different research protocols described above could be said to apply to many of the disorders already considered for the uniform screening panel recommended by the Secretary's Advisory Committee, based on a report by the American College of Medical Genetics (2006), and certainly to additional disorders and syndromes that will be presented for consideration in the future. Currently, we have either a total lack of or incomplete information about the incidence and natural history for many of the disorders proposed for the national panel. Likewise, we have either a total lack of or incomplete information about the predictive values and clinical utility associated with population-based newborn screening programs for many of the disorders proposed for the national uniform panel (American College of Medical Genetics 2006; Grosse et al. 2006; see also chapters 2 and

10). Standards of care are in development and vary among specialty centers. Genetic discrimination laws in many states prohibit genetic testing without informed consent, some states allow exceptions for newborn screening, and many states have no specific genetic testing laws.[4]

When so much is unknown about the disorders under consideration for screening, including whether screening in the neonatal period is of any benefit for the newborn, the first question that must be answered is whether we are screening to seek generalizable knowledge, which under the Common Rule constitutes human subjects research. There seems to be little question that much of the currently proposed expansion of newborn screening (American College of Medical Genetics 2006) constitutes human subjects research. For the future, new epidemiological questions of national importance undoubtedly will arise for which de-identified samples from a national cohort would be of use (e.g., frequency of a genotype projected to be unresponsive to a new drug or vaccine), and this would constitute human subjects research. Thus, a critical question is, why is there no national research protocol model to address our lack of knowledge as we move toward national standardization for newborn screening, and which we may need to address new epidemiological questions of national importance?

The Common Rule (45 CFR 46) requires IRBs to determine that protocols ensure that research subjects understand the risks and benefits of the research and (absent an IRB waiver of need for consent) give their informed consent before participating. There may be a reluctance to conclude that some newborn screening constitutes research, because conducting research can be time-consuming and expensive, and certain forms of informed consent before enrollment for testing may be impractical in universal population-based datasets (Feuchtbaum et al. 2006). However, there is flexibility in applying the Common Rule and in implementing human subjects protection. The Massachusetts protocols approved for de-identification and for oral consent, such as those described above, provided a balance between the practicalities of the study protocol and the protection of the interests of newborns and their families. This is not to say that the protocols did not involve significant, added expense. For example, implementation of "anonymous HIV test sites" as a "free" parallel testing system available on request to any enrollee in the state's prevalence surveys ensured individual access to potentially useful information. The parallel HIV testing system could have resulted in a doubling of the laboratory costs alone, but because most enrollees did not use the anonymous test site, the two systems were complementary: one performing laboratory tests on 100 percent of individuals in a cohort without any counseling (Hoff et al. 1988), and the other performing laboratory tests on a maximum of 10 percent of individuals in the cohort,[5] who wanted testing and obtained testing consistent with Massachusetts laws requiring that full counseling accompany HIV testing. Additional expenses were also incurred in implementing the Massachusetts consent model, which required ensuring that parents were notified of the research protocol and had the opportunity to decline participation. Expenses were also incurred for the preparation, translation, and distribution of educational materials, training of hospital and non-hospital-based personnel on the consent protocol, and monitoring of the protocol.

For both protocols, there are significant first-time capital expenditures and ongoing expenditures. However, once in place, the existence of a modifiable research protocol provides a mechanism for continuing review and evaluation of otherwise unobtainable data that will contribute to well-informed quality improvements in newborn screening. Policy for newborn screening research should place the highest priority on research that contributes to improvements in newborn screening and lowest priority on studies for general knowledge, for which data can be obtained from other sources. Most newborn screening programs have developed in the context of public funding for the provision of the mandated screening service and must protect allotted funds for this service. It is time for the establishment of national and state policies to identify quality improvement research as part of the fundamental services provided by newborn screening programs and to fund such projects within these programs. Only then will a comprehensive system be in place for finding and tracking affected infants with outcomes research and links to independently run clinical trials for rare disorders.

Informing the entire populace about a nationwide research protocol involving the testing of all individuals for a variety of disorders carries the risk that the protocol will not be acceptable or will be acceptable only under certain circumstances, as was the case in Iceland (Fortun 2001; Gertz 2004). Is the alternative of not informing those who are involved in the research ethical? If there is a presumed but unproven benefit to more screening, does the marketing of expanded newborn screening to a national population to ensure that most individuals embrace the expansion as a benefit violate the principles of the Common Rule? If the marketing of expanded screening results in a decision to substitute nationwide mandatory screening for a nationwide research protocol with an appropriate informed consent process, the nation would seem to be avoiding the protection of human research subjects, with its associated costs. (See chapters 4 and 10–13 for further discussion of these issues.)

The problem is that there has been no national policy calling for a well-funded research arm within state-based newborn screening programs. Such a research arm would abrogate the need to implement mandatory screening prematurely in response to calls for expansion of panels and would develop the necessary evidence base for appropriate implementation. More to the point, government agencies and investigators have not yet clearly defined what it is that we want to know in this realm of public health practice and research. A research protocol indicates to the research subjects that there are unknowns, that the investigators know the questions that need to be answered, and that the investigators have the tools to answer them. It is our obligation in the face of these unknowns to be clear about what the questions are that need to be answered and to implement research protocols with the scientific rigor to ensure that the findings, treatments, and outcomes will be understood.

Some of what the clinical scientific community wants to know about expanded screening is, how many cases? For that, we need to establish a case definition that reflects the natural history so that we know what we are looking for. Some of what we want to know is, what is the effectiveness of early intervention? Again, the need for a case definition looms large so that we can understand the many variables. Finally, some of what we want to know is, is the condition treatable? This involves the development and evaluation of treatments that can only be accomplished with well-designed clinical trials and, to that end, we need to admit to our need for a cohort of well-defined affected infants for enrollment in such trials.

The choice of a consent-based mechanism or de-identification in the recent Massachusetts examples was heavily based on the information being sought. Incidence data for the 19 metabolic disorders could not be collected on de-identified samples because follow-up diagnostic tests were needed to determine the presence or absence of a disorder in infants with positive screening results. Likewise, the predictive values of the CF screening algorithm could not be addressed without diagnostic outcome data. Investigators recognized that data for evaluation of the clinical utility of newborn screening would be compromised or lost if newborn screening testing was de-identified, because any parallel testing system would not be universal and might provide medically relevant information too late to be of use for treatment protocols. Finally, questions about the natural history of a disorder could be addressed only with a consent-based system. Although natural history data on cases identified through screening are limited to information from the timeframe before a positive screening result in a consent-based system, opportunities for gathering such data from family histories are available; in a de-identified system, these opportunities would be lost.

The information we are seeking is of great importance. Of equal significance is the method used to gain this knowledge. Although some people might be impatient to access services that seem to be beneficial or that are beneficial for a select but undefined few, as yet there is no national consensus on how newborn screening as part of the public health service can be the appropriate venue to deny or provide evolving services. Massachusetts demonstrated two viable and successful models for research protocols: one that can inform us about the numbers of individuals at risk for a particular disorder, and one that can, with permission, identify individuals at risk and provide further evaluation and treatment. Notably, one of the protocols (HIV seroprevalence protocol) ended when clinical data changed the circumstances.

State newborn screening programs that work effectively to identify, track, and evaluate outcomes in their populations must be a key component of any national infrastructure that evaluates and implements research proposals for population-based research. State law and policy should protect the integrity of the centralized databases of the newborn screening programs, protect individuals from privacy infringements and coercion into unproven therapy, and provide routes of information about IRB-sanctioned clinical trials. The HIV Seroprevalence in Childbearing Women Study provides an extremely sensitive case study of the ability of state newborn screening programs to generate valuable data while protecting the confidentiality of individuals' private medical information in a state program's gathering of numbers. In Massachusetts alone, during the seven years of the study, more than 600,000 newborns were tested without a single breach of confidentiality or complaint of such a breach (unpublished data). Furthermore, the more recent pilot studies demonstrate the effectiveness of privacy protection and provision of appropriate medical care by the state's newborn screening program for more than 482,904 infants whose specimens were screened with identifiers in place and the results reported to the appropriate health care provider (unpublished data).

Agencies that collect and test specimens under the authority of the state for the provision of a public health service do so with particular stewardship responsibilities. The appropriate use of this authority and the population-based data generated from newborn screening will ensure our ability to be informed about the health of our newborns and our populations with continued public confidence and trust.

ACKNOWLEDGMENTS AND DISCLAIMER

Our sincere thanks to Karen Maschke, Andrea Bonnicksen, Scott Grosse, Jaime Hale, and Mary Ann Baily for their editorial comments and patience. A. Comeau wishes to thank Mary Ann Baily and Tom Murray, of the Hastings Center, for the opportunity to work on the "Ethical Decision-Making for Newborn Genetic Screening" project, and to thank all project participants for their thoughtful and provocative comments. The views and opinions expressed in this chapter do not necessarily state or reflect those of the Massachusetts Department of Public Health.

NOTES

1. The 10 disorders are: phenylketonuria, maple syrup urine disease, homocystinuria, galactosemia, congenital hypothyroidism, congenital toxoplasmosis, congenital adrenal hyperplasia, sickle cell disease, biotinidase deficiency, and medium-chain acyl-Co-A dehydrogenase deficiency.

2. The 20 disorders are: cystic fibrosis, tyrosinemia type I, tyrosinemia type II, 3-methylcrotonyl-CoA carboxylase deficiency, 3-hydroxy 3-methyl glutaryl-CoA lyase deficiency, argininosuccinic aciduria, isovaleric acidemia, hyperammonemia/ornithinemia/citrullinemia, glutaric acidemia type I, glutaric acidemia type II, citrullinemia, methylmalonic aciduria, propionic acidemia, carnitine palmitoyltransferase deficiency, long-chain hydroxyacyl-CoA dehydrogenase deficiency, very long-chain acyl-CoA dehydrogenase deficiency, short-chain acyl-CoA dehydrogenase deficiency, long-chain acyl-CoA dehydrogenase deficiency, β-ketothiolase deficiency, and argininemia. Note that the list approved by metabolic specialists includes long-chain acyl-CoA dehydrogenase deficiency and that recent deliberations have indicated these cases to be very long-chain acyl-CoA dehydrogenase deficiency.

3. The committee members were: Lori Andrews, research attorney, American Bar Foundation; Jeffrey P. Davis, M.D., state epidemiologist, Wisconsin; Martin S. Hirsch, M.D., infectious disease specialist, Massachusetts General Hospital, Boston; Stephen Josephson, Ph.D., University Hygienic Lab, Iowa; Jerome O. Klein, M.D., professor of pediatrics, Boston City Hospital; Kenneth McIntosh, infectious disease specialist, Children's Hospital, Boston; Allen Mitchell, M.D., Sloan Epidemiology Unit, Boston University; Janet L. Mitchell, M.D., Women's Health, Beth Israel, Boston; Nancy E. Mueller, Sc.D., Department of Epidemiology, Harvard School of Public Health, Boston; David J. Sencer, M.D., Management Sciences for Health, Boston; Cladd Stevens, M.D., New York Blood Center, New York City; Ruth Tuomala, M.D., obstetrician/gynecologist, Brigham and Women's Hospital, Boston; Richard Vogt, M.D., Division of Epidemiology, Vermont Department of Public Health; Judith Wilber, Ph.D., Public Health Laboratory, California; Rodney Hoff, Sc.D., George F. Grady, M.D., Marvin Mitchell, M.D., Lynne Mofenson, M.D., Barbara Werner,

Ph.D., and Victor Berardi, State Laboratory Institute, Massachusetts; Anne Willoughby, M.D., National Institute of Child Health and Human Development (NICHD); Antonia C. Novello, M.D., M.P.H., NICHD; John LaMontagne, Ph.D., National Institute of Allergy and Infectious Diseases (NIAID); Timothy Dondero, M.D., Centers for Disease Control and Prevention (CDC); Marguerite Pappaioanou, D.V.M., Ph.D., CDC; Barry Graubard, M.A., biostatistician, NICHD; Peter Glasner, M.D., NIAID.

    4. National Conference of State Legislatures, "Newborn genetic screening privacy laws" (www.ncsl.org/programs/health/screeningprivacy.htm).

    5. This figure is derived from Counseling and Testing Data, Massachusetts Department of Public Health, HIV/AIDS Bureau, Office of Research and Evaluation, showing 26,610 anonymous tests of women, and data from the New England Newborn Screening Program, showing 251,927 women giving birth in those years.

REFERENCES

Accurso, F. J., Sontag, M. K., and Wagener, J. S. 2005. Complications associated with symptomatic diagnosis in infants with cystic fibrosis. *J Pediatr* 147 (3 Suppl): S37–41.

American College of Medical Genetics. 2006. Newborn screening: toward a uniform screening panel and system. *Genet Med* 8 (Suppl 1):1–252S.

Andrews, L. B., Fullarton, J. E., Holtzman, N. A., and Motulsky, A. G. 1994. *Assessing Genetic Risks: Implications for Health and Social Policy.* Washington DC: National Academy of Sciences.

Atkinson, K., Zuckerman, B., Sharfstein, J. M., Levin, D., Blatt, R. J., and Koh, H. K. 2001. A public health response to emerging technology: expansion of the Massachusetts newborn screening program. *Public Health Rep* 116 (2): 122–31.

CDC suspends testing of newborns. 1995. *AIDS Policy Law* 10 (10): 1, 9.

Centers for Disease Control and Prevention. 1997. Newborn screening for cystic fibrosis: a paradigm for public health genetics policy development—proceedings of a 1997 workshop. *MMWR Morb Mortal Wkly Rep* 46 (16): 1–22.

Chatfield, S., Owen, G., Ryley, H. C., Williams, J., Alfaham, M., Goodchild, M. C., and Weller, P. 1991. Neonatal screening for cystic fibrosis in Wales and the West Midlands: clinical assessment after five years of screening. *Arch Dis Child*: 66 (1 Spec No): 29–33.

Comeau, A. M., Parad, R. B., Dorkin, H. L., Dovey, M., Gerstle, R., Haver, K., Lapey, A., O'Sullivan, B. P., Waltz, D. A., Zwerdling, R. G., and Eaton, R. B. 2004. Population-based newborn screening for genetic disorders when multiple mutation DNA testing is incorporated: a cystic fibrosis newborn screening model demonstrating increased sensitivity but more carrier detections. *Pediatrics* 113 (6): 1573–81.

Comeau, A. M., Parad, R., Gerstle, R., O'Sullivan, B. P., Dorkin, H. L., Dovey, M., Haver, K., Martin, T., and Eaton, R. B. 2005. Communications systems and their models: Massachusetts parent compliance with recommended specialty care after positive cystic fibrosis newborn screening result. *J Pediatr* 147 (3 Suppl): S98–100.

Committee for the Study of Inborn Errors of Metabolism, Division of Medical Sciences, Assembly of Life Sciences, National Research Council. 1975. *Genetic Screening: Programs, Principles, and Research*. Washington, DC: National Academy of Sciences.

Connor, E. M., Sperling, R. S., Gelber, R., Kiselev, P., Scott, G., O'Sullivan, M. J., VanDyke, R., Bey, M., Shearer, W., Jacobson, R. L., Jimenez, E., O'Neill, E., Bazin, B., Delfraissy, J.-F., Culnane, M., Coombs, R., Elkins, M., Moye, J., Stratton, P., and Balsley, J. 1994. Reduction of maternal-infant transmission of human immunodeficiency virus type 1 with zidovudine treatment. Pediatric AIDS Clinical Trials Group Protocol 076 Study Group. *N Engl J Med* 331 (18): 1173–80.

Cystic Fibrosis Foundation. 2005. Patient registry: annual data report. www.sgpp-schweiz.ch/downloads_cms/cff_patient_registry_annual_data_report_2005.pdf.

———. 2006. Patient registry: annual data, 1990–1994. www.cff.org/UploadedFiles/living_with_cf/Files/NBSFinalQALH.pdf.

Dao, B. 1994. Bill offered on requiring AIDS report. *New York Times*, March 9.

Farrell, P. M., Shen, G., Splaingard, M., Colby, C. E., Laxova, A., Kosorok, M. O., Rock, M. J., and Mischler, E. H. 1997. Acquisition of *Pseudomonas aeruginosa* in children with cystic fibrosis. *Pediatrics* 100 (5): E2.

Feuchtbaum, L. B., Lorey, F., Faulkner, L. A., Sherwin, J., Currier, R., Bhandal, A., and Cunningham, G. 2006. California's experience implementing a pilot newborn supplemental screening program using tandem mass spectrometry. *Pediatrics* 117 (ACMG Suppl): 261–69.

Fortun, M. 2001. Breaking the code. www.rpi.edu/dept/NewsComm/Magazine/mar01/feature3.html.

Gertz, R. 2004. An analysis of the Icelandic Supreme Court judgment on the Health Sector Database Act. www.law.ed.ac.uk/ahrc/script-ed/issue2/iceland.asp.

Grosse, S. D., Boyle, C. A., Botkin, J. R., Comeau, A. M., Kharrazi, M., Rosenfeld, M., and Wilfond, B. S. 2004. Newborn screening for cystic fibrosis: evaluation of benefits and risks and recommendations for state newborn screening programs. *MMWR Recomm Rep* 53 (RR-13): 1–36.

Grosse, S. D., Boyle, C. A., Kenneson, A., Khoury, M. J., and Wilfond, B. S. 2006. From public health emergency to public health service: the implications of evolving criteria for newborn screening panels. *Pediatrics* 117 (3): 923–29.

Hale J. E., Parad R. B., and Comeau, A. M. 2008. Newborn screening showing decreasing incidence of cystic fibrosis [correspondence]. *N Engl J Med* 358 (9): 973–74.

HIV Seroprevalence in Childbearing Women Advisory Committee. 1987. Approved minutes of Advisory Committee meeting, July 28.

Hoff, R., Berardi, V. P., Weiblen, B. J., Mahoney-Trout, L., Mitchell, M. L., and Grady, G. F. 1988. Seroprevalence of human immunodeficiency virus among childbearing women: estimation by testing samples of blood from newborns. *N Engl J Med* 318 (9): 525–30.

Holtzman, N. A., and Watson, M. S. 1997. *Promoting Safe and Effective Genetic Testing in the United States: Final Report of the Task Force on Genetic Testing*. Bethesda, MD: National Institutes of Health.

Martin, J. A., Brady, E. H., Sutton, P. D., Ventura, S. J., Menacker, F., and Munson, M. L. 2003. Births: final data for 2002. *Natl Vital Stat Rep* 52 (10): 1–116.

Martin, J. A., Hamilton, B. E., Sutton, P. D., Ventura, S. J., Menacker, F., and Munson, M. L. 2004.

Births: final data for 2003. *Natl Vital Stat Rep* 54 (2): 1–116 (available at www.cdc.gov/nchs/data/nvsr/nvsr54/nvsr54_02.pdf).

McCormick, M. C., Davidson, E. C. Jr., and Stoto, M. A. 1999. Preventing perinatal transmission of human immunodeficiency virus in the United States. Committee on Perinatal Transmission of HIV. *Obstet Gynecol* 94 (5 Pt 1): 795–98.

Mofenson, L. M. 2000. Technical report: perinatal human immunodeficiency virus testing and prevention of transmission. Committee on Pediatric Aids. *Pediatrics* 106 (6): E88.

———. 2002. U.S. Public Health Service Task Force recommendations for use of antiretroviral drugs in pregnant HIV-1-infected women for maternal health and interventions to reduce perinatal HIV-1 transmission in the United States. *MMWR Recomm Rep* 51 (RR-18): 1–38.

National Newborn Screening and Genetics Resource Center. 2003. National newborn screening report. http://genes-r-us.uthscsa.edu/resources/newborn/00chapters.html.

Newborn Screening Task Force. 2000. Serving the family from birth to the medical home: a report from the Newborn Screening Task Force convened in Washington DC, May 10–11, 1999. *Pediatrics* 106 (2 Pt 2): 383–427.

Parad, R. B., and Comeau, A. M. 2005. Diagnostic dilemmas resulting from the immunoreactive trypsinogen/DNA cystic fibrosis newborn screening algorithm. *J Pediatr* 147 (3 Suppl): S78–82.

Parad, R. B., Comeau, A. M., Dorkin, H. L., Dovey, M., Gerstle, R., Martin, T., and O'Sullivan, B. P. 2005. Sweat testing infants detected by cystic fibrosis newborn screening. *J Pediatr* 147 (3 Suppl): S69–72.

Rosenstein, B. J., and Cutting, G. R. 1998. The diagnosis of cystic fibrosis: a consensus statement. Cystic Fibrosis Foundation Consensus Panel. *J Pediatr* 132 (4): 589–95.

Wilken, B., and Chalmers, G. 1985. Reduced morbidity in patients with cystic fibrosis detected by neonatal screening. *Lancet* 2 (8468): 1319–21.

Wilson, J. M. G., and Jungner, G. 1968. *Principles and Practice of Screening for Disease*. Geneva: World Health Organization.

Zytkovicz, T. H., Fitzgerald, E. F., Marsden, D., Larson, C. A., Shih, V. E., Johnson, D. M., Strauss, A. W., Comeau, A. M., Eaton, R. B., and Grady, G. F. 2001. Tandem mass spectrometric analysis for amino, organic, and fatty acid disorders in newborn dried blood spots: a two-year summary from the New England Newborn Screening Program. *Clin Chem* 47 (11): 1945–55.

CHAPTER 15

Ethical and Policy Implications of Conducting Carrier Testing and Newborn Screening for the Same Condition

BENJAMIN S. WILFOND, M.D.

While discussion ensues on how new genetic tests will change the practice of medicine *in the future*, adult carrier testing and newborn screening have already been part of the clinical landscape in the United States for decades. These two approaches to genetic testing coexist, but they are characterized by distinct providers, rationales, and approaches.

Carrier testing and newborn screening have been used to detect autosomal recessive diseases such as Tay-Sachs disease, phenylketonuria (PKU), sickle cell disease (SCD), and cystic fibrosis (CF) because there is typically no family history to suggest a particular risk. Carrier testing determines a person's risk for having a child with a rare hereditary condition if he or she were to have a child with another person who also carries the gene. Newborn screening identifies children who may have a medical condition, before clinical symptoms arise. With effective treatments, newborn screening can be used to attenuate morbidity and mortality. Even without effective treatments, newborn screening permits an earlier diagnosis, which may reduce unnecessary clinical evaluations of the child and alert parents to their risk with future children.

Carrier testing and newborn screening can be used for the same condition. Carrier testing for SCD was first used in the 1970s, and newborn screening for SCD became routine in the United States by the late 1980s. Subsequently, there has been only a modest literature on one program's impact on the other, primarily involving studies on the experience of familial carrier testing as a result of newborn screening programs (Laird, Dezateux, and Anionwu 1996; Mischler et al. 1998; Ciske et al. 2001; Wheeler et al. 2001; Parsons, Clarke, and Bradley 2003; Oliver et al. 2004; La Pean and Farrell 2005; Lagoe et al. 2005).

For CF, the American College of Obstetricians and Gynecologists (ACOG) and the American College of Medical Genetics (ACMG) recommended that clinicians offer carrier testing (Mennuti, Thomson, and Press 1999) and the Centers for Disease Control and Prevention (CDC) recommended that states consider newborn screening (Grosse et al. 2004), within a few years of each other. These recommendations are likely to result in the implementation of broad-based programs. As such programs expand, a greater number of people in the United States may be exposed to both carrier testing and newborn screening for CF.

In the United States, carrier testing and newborn screening tend to be considered independent of each other in policy discussions. However, they may be better appreciated as related programs that are used to manage the impact of a genetic condition on the lives of affected individuals and their families over time. Indeed, the National Health Service in the United Kingdom simultaneously addressed newborn screening and carrier testing during pregnancy in policy analyses for both CF and SCD (Murray et al. 1999; Zeuner et al. 1999). The two types of screening—carrier testing and newborn screening—are related because each approach has implications for the other. Each program can influence how the other program operates or how test results are interpreted. The social and clinical context of the information gained through screening is changed by the presence of the other program. Depending on how each program's goals are framed and prioritized, the particular approaches can seem to be at odds with each other, in that the presence of one program might reduce or enhance the effectiveness of the other (Super and Abbott 1998).

In this chapter I argue that, to make good policy, both public and private policymakers must recognize and account for these interactions. The overall policy goal should be to provide information allowing individuals to manage the impact of genetic conditions on their families in ways that respond to diverse family needs and preferences, and in a manner that is both cost-effective and respectful of basic ethical values.

TABLE 15.1
The Different Worlds of Genetic Screening

Characteristic	Newborn Screening	Carrier Testing
Service delivery setting	State health departments	Obstetrics, family practice, genetic services providers
Voluntariness	"Mandatory" programs	Patient choice
Health-related goals	Avoid childhood death and disability	Enhance reproductive decision making
Current delivery challenges	Diminishing impact on health as the range of disease expands	Limited discussion of alternatives presented to some women

A Brief History of Carrier Testing and Newborn Screening
Worlds Apart

Key differences between newborn screening and carrier testing are sum-marized in table 15.1. Newborn screening began with testing for PKU in the early 1960s. By the 1970s, most children in the United States received new-born screening for a handful of conditions, including congenital hypothyroid-ism and galactosemia. A distinguishing characteristic of newborn screening is that it is not primarily offered in the context of routine outpatient medical practice. These tests were originally provided by state health department labo-ratories, using samples collected in hospitals, in part because of concern that pediatricians might be slow to adopt such tests or that parents might refuse such tests. Another key difference between newborn screening and carrier testing involves legislation passed in most states that "mandates" screening (Andrews et al. 1994). This "mandatory" approach was justified by the fact that the conditions screened for required immediate diagnosis and treatment shortly after birth to avoid serious, irreversible harm (Faden, Holtzman, and Chwalow 1982). In practice, almost all babies are screened, but hospitals gen-erally respect the wishes of parents who strongly object to testing. The pri-mary goal of newborn screening has traditionally been direct and profound clinical benefits: avoiding death or serious disability as a result of screening.

More recently, states have added to their screening panels conditions for which there is limited empirical evidence of benefit, or evidence that suggests the benefits are less significant than, for example, the prevention of mental re-tardation through early diagnosis and treatment of PKU (Botkin et al. 2006). Justifications for newborn screening have expanded to include psychological benefits to parents from diagnosis. Diagnosis can reduce uncertainty about the meaning of clinical symptoms, provide parents with the opportunity to prepare for chronic care needs, and allow parents to use the information for family planning decisions(Grosse, Boyle, et al. 2006; see also chapters 4 and 10). The main challenge surrounding this expanded approach is to develop a framework to determine whether the public health expenditures for such benefits are justified.

Carrier testing programs that began in the 1970s for SCD and Tay-Sachs disease followed a different path from newborn screening. While some of these carrier testing programs were community-based, the tests were most commonly offered as part of prenatal care. In contrast to newborn screening, providers' approaches to carrier testing strongly emphasized the role of a patient's choice to undergo or forgo testing. Such decisions are consistent with the commonly stated goal of carrier testing to enhance reproductive decision making based on new information and to offer a broader range of reproductive options. Carrier testing faces the challenge of providing objective information to patients that is easily understood and does not pressure people to choose for or against testing (Asch 1999).

Worlds in Collision

Information from either carrier testing or newborn screening can be used to help make decisions about clinical interventions for the child and to allow parents the opportunity to prepare psychosocially for having a child with special needs. Figure 15.1 demonstrates the complexity of relationships between these programs.

Results from carrier testing and subsequent prenatal testing offer a broader range of options than newborn screening results. Once a couple learns that they have an increased risk of having a child with a particular medical condition, they can decide whether or not to have further children, using gamete donation or preimplantation genetic diagnosis, or can decide to adopt a child.

Abnormal results from either carrier testing or newborn screening provide parents with information about the risk for future pregnancies. This is an interesting convergence because, regardless of which approach was used to generate the information, the results bear similar significance. Information about increased risk for future pregnancies provides the couple with the option of either newborn screening or prenatal diagnosis, regardless of how they learned of the risk initially. Further, such information has implications

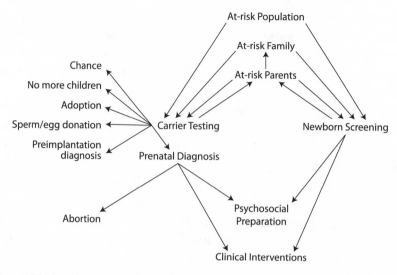

Figure 15.1. The converging worlds of genetic screening.

for family members (such as parents' siblings), who now can consider the options of newborn screening or carrier testing. Couples and their family members will have the same broad range of options to consider, whichever screening approach they chose.

Each program may occasionally provide information commonly associated with the other type of program. Carrier testing programs identify some adults not as carriers but as being affected by the disorder. Newborn screening programs can also directly identify infants as carriers. Testing the siblings of infants diagnosed by newborn screening or testing the children of carrier parents can result in these children also being diagnosed as affected or carriers.

The convergence of these two types of programs raises a broad question: how does the presence and effectiveness of one program influence the other program? To address this question, one must articulate each program's primary goals. Similar programs can have different goals, and a particular program can have multiple goals. However, the normative work to define benefits (goals) is necessary to permit judgments about a program's effectiveness, which then must be balanced with costs and risks. It is also necessary to consider how each program may empirically influence the benefits and risks of the other program. These evaluations can provide some guidance for policy and practice considerations by identifying how one program could be modified to maximize the benefits and reduce the risks of the other program.

An Example: The Implications of Cystic Fibrosis Genotype-Phenotype Relationships for Population Screening

Despite the convergence of population screening programs, few analyses have examined connections between newborn screening and carrier testing (Green et al. 2004; Oliver et al. 2004). This chapter examines these issues through the lens of cystic fibrosis because, in addition to being a contemporary illustration, the complexities of the genotype-phenotype relationships for this disease provide some insight into the challenges faced when addressing the overlap of newborn screening with carrier testing. These challenges may become common themes as more conditions are proposed for both types of program.

The cystic fibrosis transmembrane regulator (CFTR) gene has more than 1500 mutations associated with cystic fibrosis. The CFTR mutations are categorized into five classes (I, II, III, IV, V) that are distinguished by the mechanism by which the mutations affect the functioning of the CFTR protein. Class I, II, and III mutations are clinically associated with pancreatic insufficiency, which can result in poor growth (Mickle and Cutting 2000). Class IV and V mutations are associated with normal pancreatic function. Individuals with CF have mutations on each chromosome of the chromosome 7 pair, but the presence of one mutation that is either class IV or V allows for normal pancreatic function.

The most common CFTR mutation is ΔF508 (class II), which occurs in 7 in 10 "CF chromosomes" (Sugarman et al. 2004). In contrast, RII7H (class IV) occurs in only 1 in 200 "CF chromosomes." The RII7H mutation is found more commonly in the general population (1 in 300 people) than would be expected from its rare occurrence in patients with CF compared with ΔF508 (1 in 45 people). This suggests that RII7H less commonly causes CF when paired with another CF mutation. Part of the explanation is that R117H is disease-causing primarily when it is associated with the variant IVST8 5T. When R117H is associated with other IVST8 variants, either the 7T or 9T variant, CF may not develop at all. Another possibility in this situation is the development of what are sometimes called "CFTR-related diseases," such as congenital bilateral absence of the vas deferens or pancreatitis. Even when R117H is associated with CF, the natural history is often comparatively mild because, in addition to a higher likelihood of normal pancreatic function, individuals with CF who have the R117H mutation have milder lung disease.

These molecular details are important in deciding whether to include R117H in the panel of mutations used in carrier testing or newborn screening. The 2001 ACMG-ACOG guidelines determined which mutations to include based on the criterion of a frequency of at least 0.1 percent of "CF chromosomes" known to be found in people with CF (Watson et al. 2004). Twenty-five mutations met this requirement, including R117H, illustrating that frequency alone may not be an adequate criterion for inclusion in a screening panel. Further attention to the implications of a particular mutation may be necessary to decide whether to include the mutation in a panel.

Some CF newborn screening programs exclusively use a biochemical assay, the immunoreactive trypsinogen (IRT) test, whereas others use a two-tiered approach (IRT and DNA-based testing) (Wilfond and Gollust 2005). The two-tiered approach uses an elevated IRT level (the highest 4% to 6% of values) as a cutoff before performing DNA testing. Infants with a CF mutation either have CF or are carriers. The standard diagnostic test for cystic fibrosis, the "sweat test" (measuring chloride in sweat), is the final determining factor in diagnosing CF.

While carrier testing and newborn screening for CF are independently organized health services in the United States, most states using the IRT-DNA approach employ either the ACMG-ACOG panel or other commercially available panels also marketed for carrier testing (Wilfond and Gollust 2005). Because carrier testing panels include class IV and V mutations, newborn screening programs that use the panel developed for carrier screening will identify some infants with only class IV and V mutations. Most of these infants with CF (having normal pancreatic function) are not at risk for malnutrition. Other infants will have ambiguous sweat test results, making it unclear whether the infant has CF (Comeau et al. 2004). The use of the CF carrier screening DNA panel for newborn screening exemplifies how carrier testing can influence the design and outcome of newborn screening.

Carrier Testing and Newborn Screening: Complementary or Contradictory?
Defining the Goals

Goals for carrier testing and newborn screening can be complex and multifaceted, yet some goals seem more "contradictory" and others more complementary. One goal for CF carrier testing is to provide people with information that allows them to make more informed reproductive choices. Based on this goal, a program is successful whenever people (even a small minority) who want information about their carrier status can obtain and understand such information. Provided no adverse effects outweigh the value of the information, what individuals choose to do with this information is relatively unimportant as long as they understand it.

Reducing the prevalence of the disease represents another goal for carrier testing. As an illustration, much of the Tay-Sachs testing "success" relies on the observation that fewer children are born with Tay-Sachs since carrier testing became available (Kaback 2001). With a goal of reduced prevalence, it is important to maximize the uptake of the testing and provide an environment where acting on the results of testing is socially acceptable. The prevalence of CF will be reduced if carrier couples choose not to have biologically related children, or use preimplantation or prenatal diagnosis to avoid having a biologically related child with CF.

For CF newborn screening, two additional distinct goals exist. One is to improve the health of children with cystic fibrosis. Research studies of CF newborn screening indicate that children with CF diagnosed via newborn screening show improved growth (Farrell et al. 1997). There is also some evidence of improved cognitive development associated with growth (Koscik et al. 2004). Some studies suggest a slight reduction in mortality rates in children with CF below the age of 10 (Lai, Cheng, and Farrell 2005; Grosse, Rosenfeld, et al. 2006). To date, none of the studies reveals a pulmonary benefit from newborn screening. This may be due to the multifactorial nature of the progression of CF lung disease, which reduces the possibility of observing a difference in the small populations studied (generally fewer than 100 individuals in each study) (Wilfond, Parad, and Fost 2005).

The second goal for newborn screening is more family-centered and psychosocial. This goal involves providing information to parents that allows them to (1) avoid the "diagnostic odyssey" that sometimes occurs between the initial appearance of symptoms and the time of diagnosis (Kharrazi and Kharrazi 2005) and (2) use the screening information for further reproductive planning (Mischler et al. 1998). To the extent that newborn screening leads parents of children identified with CF or as CF carriers either to avoid having more children or to use prenatal testing in future pregnancies, followed by termination of affected pregnancies, the birth prevalence of CF will decrease (Scotet et al. 2003; van den Akker-van Marle et al. 2006).

Normative Beliefs Influence Goals

The compatibility of carrier testing and newborn screening programs relates to how particular goals for each program are either implicitly or explicitly endorsed. The endorsement of the particular goals is a decision based on
normative beliefs. These may include subjective beliefs about the nature of the
disease and attitudes about illness in general, as well as beliefs about the value
of information and personal agency in decision making.

Subjective beliefs about CF can influence screening goals. Some people believe that "lung congestion, pneumonia, diarrhea, and poor growth, are all
part of CF, and even with modern medical treatment the average life span is 25
years" (from a CF carrier screening brochure, quoted in Loeben, Marteau, and
Wilfond 1998, p. 1183). Others, however, believe that "the lung and digestive
problems are both treatable, and a baby with CF will need regular medical care
and a good diet."[1] The underlying attitudes and beliefs about CF represented
by these statements can shape which program and goals one would endorse.
Those who believe that CF is best described by the first statement might be
more comfortable with a carrier testing program in which the goal is to reduce
the incidence of CF (Rowley, Loader, and Kaplan 1998). Those believing that
CF is best described in the second statement might be more likely to endorse
a newborn screening program in which the goal is to improve the health of
infants with CF (Farrell and Farrell 2003).

The Compatibility of Programs Is Based on the Goals

Carrier testing and newborn screening can seem contradictory when newborn screening advocates believe strongly that newborn screening will pro-
foundly improve infants' health and when carrier testing advocates believe
strongly that carrier testing can dramatically reduce disease prevalence. In
figure 15.2, the upper left quadrant represents the potential contradictions
between the programs based on these "health impact–related" goals. As the
figure shows, it may be contradictory for a state health department simultaneously to adopt both programs if one program aims to reduce the birth
prevalence of the disease and the other program aims to improve the health of
children with the disease. Of course, public health programs commonly have
simultaneous goals for preventing a disease and treating that disease (e.g.,
heart disease). Yet, what sometimes complicates public health engagement

Goals of Carrier Testing

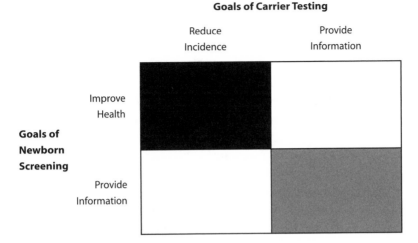

Figure 15.2. The goals of genetic testing through carrier testing and newborn screening can appear complementary (gray) or contradictory (black), or are unrelated (white).

in the prenatal context is that, in at least some cases, disease prevention cannot be disentangled from reducing the births of particular individuals (e.g., infants with CF). However, exceptions exist even in this context. For example, public health recommendations to increase dietary folate during pregnancy to reduce the incidence of neural tube defects do not reduce the births of particular individuals, unlike prenatal screening for neural tube defects.

In other cases, such as for SCD or CF, goals to improve health and reduce prevalence prove more contradictory because each program's success reduces the benefits of the other program. If newborn screening dramatically improves the health of people with CF, it becomes more difficult to justify a carrier testing program whose goal is to prevent the birth of children affected by CF. Alternatively, if a carrier testing program dramatically reduces the incidence of CF, the predictive value of an abnormal newborn screening result will also be reduced, diminishing the value of newborn screening (see figure 15.2, upper right quadrant).

Advocates for either type of screening program may not necessarily believe that the program goals should be related to health impact; they may have more modest goals. Advocates placing a high value on personal decision making could justify either program, if both have a goal of providing information that has a positive psychosocial effect on the family. In this regard, the two programs can be complementary in that both provide information that allows people to address the impact of genetic disease on their families (figure 15.2, lower right quadrant).

Of course, beliefs about the value of information for personal decision making and beliefs about screening goals are not necessarily related. Some people believing in health impact–related goals for one program could still support the other program, as long as they understood its goal of providing information (figure 15.2, lower left and upper right quadrants).

The Impact of Goals on Program Design and Prioritization

It is important to be clear about the primary goals of a screening program because these can be relevant to decisions about the program's specific design. Primary goals can influence how one compares the value of a particular program with the value of the related screening program for the same condition or with the value of other health care programs. Table 15.2 illustrates how goals might influence these issues.

NEWBORN SCREENING. A primary newborn screening goal to improve health might drive the design to maximize the detection of infants with CF. To achieve this goal, the screening panel should include a large number of mutations. However, if the goal is primarily to provide information, the design might balance maximizing diagnosis with minimizing the detection of infants with false positive or ambiguous results by using a smaller, more refined number of mutations. With a primary goal to provide information to affected families, the main risk to families who show false positives is also related to the information provided. Although these benefits

TABLE 15.2
The Impact of Goals on Program Design and Service Delivery Prioritization for Newborn Screening and Carrier Testing for Cystic Fibrosis (CF)

Program Design and Prioritization	Newborn Screening		Carrier Testing	
	Goal: Improved Health	Goal: Information	Goal: Reduced Incidence	Goal: Information
Carrier testing	Give lower priority because the disease is not as severe.	Give priority because it also provides information to families.	Design program to maximize uptake.	Design program with passive approach.
Newborn screening	Design program to maximize detection of infants with CF.	Design program to balance CF detection with detection of false positives.	Give lower priority because the disease is not as common.	Give priority because it also provides information to families.

and risks accrue to different populations, the nature of the benefits and risks is commensurate.

The way in which policymakers view the goals of newborn screening might also influence how they prioritize the value of carrier testing. This is a more nuanced question than that of whether the programs are complementary or contradictory. The point is that lying between these two poles are questions about the relative priority of the programs and how to make decisions about health service utilization as resources become more limited. Alternatively, policymakers may choose to support newborn screening, which is in the public health domain, and ignore carrier testing, which in the United States falls within the clinical domain. Indeed, to date, this has been U.S. policymakers' stance.

Those who believe that newborn screening has medical benefits might not be expected to prioritize carrier testing, because reproductive decision making is a less significant concern for diseases that are not as severe. For example, even if population carrier testing for PKU were feasible, effective treatment for PKU following newborn screening would make the argument in favor of PKU carrier testing for its reproductive benefits less compelling. Alternatively, those who believe that the main value of newborn screening is to provide information may consider carrier testing to be equally important because this testing also has informational value.

CARRIER TESTING.   The goals of carrier testing will also affect the design of these programs. When a program's goal is to reduce the prevalence of the disease, the program must find a way to increase the number of people who are offered carrier testing and to encourage uptake. Significant literature on health behavior provides guidance for designing programs to maximize uptake (Bekker et al. 1993). It is more effective to offer carrier testing to pregnant women than to couples who are not yet pregnant (Clayton et al. 1996) and to provide testing in the context of a routine prenatal visit rather than requiring a separate visit. Finally, physicians simply mentioning carrier testing can increase uptake rates to between 75 and 90 percent (Witt et al. 1996). However, when the goal of carrier testing and prenatal diagnosis is primarily psychosocial, programs can be designed in ways that will predictably limit uptake to individuals who are highly motivated (i.e., a program with a more passive approach). For example, a program that used mail solicitation of an adult population to attend a group counseling session on CF carrier testing resulted in an uptake rate of 15 percent (Tambor et al. 1994).

The goals of carrier testing may also influence how policymakers prioritize newborn screening. Those who support a carrier testing goal to reduce the birth prevalence of the disease may see less need for newborn screening. For example, within suggestions to expand newborn screening to a wider range of diseases, there are no proposals to include Tay-Sachs disease. The main interventions used to reduce morbidity from Tay-Sachs disease (airway management and prolonged mechanical ventilation) are not likely to be more effective following newborn screening rather than symptom-based diagnosis. However, newborn screening for Tay-Sachs would offer parents the typical information benefits of such screening (i.e., avoiding the "diagnostic odyssey") and improve options for reproductive decision making. Thus, despite potential benefits in newborn screening for Tay-Sachs, it is plausible that the lack of proposals for its inclusion in newborn screening panels relates to the greater perceived value of carrier screening.

PRIORITIZATION OF SCREENING. Diverse views about the goals of each type of program might support the simultaneous development of both programs for CF (and for SCD). Alternatively, many view both programs as having goals primarily related to the personal value of the information. One implication of endorsing information-based goals at a policy level might be that both programs are given lower priority than other services for children that produce direct clinical benefits. Primarily information-related goals could negatively affect the cost-utility of each program. For example, for a given cost of newborn screening, a program providing the benefit of improved health in children with CF might be better justified than a program that had little or no impact on children's health but provided valuable information for families. Similarly, for the given cost of carrier screening, a program providing the benefit of reduced prevalence might be considered to have stronger justification than a program having no impact on the incidence of CF even if people found the information personally useful.

Whether informational benefits have sufficient weight to justify costs might depend on resource availability. With more acutely limited resources, programs with either informational or health-related goals would have to be balanced with other specific programs for people with the disease, other health care programs for all children, and, of course, all the other uses of public resources. For example, situations where limited resources exist for providing antibiotics and pancreatic enzymes to individuals with CF might determine whether money would be better spent on starting newborn screening programs or on providing additional enzymes and antibiotics. Resource limitation might even justify decisions not to screen, such as in resource-poor locations where infectious diarrhea is a major cause of childhood mortality.

Interestingly, in the United States, both carrier testing and prenatal diagnosis programs and newborn screening programs have emerged. Although this could be because the primary goals of both types of testing are informational, this does not seem to be the case. The emergence of both types of programs could be due to the goals not being fully articulated. More to the point, different groups with very different interests have promoted the two types of testing. Federal and state officials and disease advocacy organizations promote newborn screening. Clinicians and professional societies (with no direct involvement by state or federal agencies or disease support groups) tend to promote carrier testing. Thus, it is not surprising that each program's policy decisions do not take into account their impact on the other program. However, as the two types of programs move forward, it will become more important for each program to consider the other.

The Interaction between Programs Can Influence the Effectiveness of Each Program

When both types of testing are offered to the same population at the same time, the goals, design, and priorities need to be contextualized to account for the fact that the presence of both programs may have an influence on each program. The examples below illustrate different potential interactions, though many of these hypothesized interactions are contradictory. Empirical research will be necessary to determine how, in fact, carrier testing and newborn screening influence each other.

The Influence of Newborn Screening on Carrier Testing

Some CF newborn screening approaches identify infants as carriers, implying that at least one parent is a carrier. In CF newborn screening programs that use DNA testing, depending on the IRT cutoffs and the number of mutations tested for, 5 to 10 carriers will be identified for each child affected with CF. Only carrier testing of both parents will identify which parent is a carrier

(Rowley, Loader, and Kaplan 1998), and in approximately 1 in 30 tests, both parents will be identified as carriers. Further, the carrier status of any parent identified as a consequence of newborn screening will have implications for that adult's siblings, who may also be carriers and may also consider carrier testing. Newborn screening for CF thus has the potential to increase the up-take of carrier testing in the adult population.

However, newborn screening may also *decrease* the interest in carrier test-ing. First, the mere presence of newborn screening may prompt some adults to decide that rather than having carrier testing, they will defer and have CF newborn screening done on their infants. Second, if newborn screening continues to improve the quality of life for people with CF, there may be less interest in carrier testing because the disease will no longer seem to have as much of a health impact on families. In both examples, the shift in interest in carrier testing could be directly related to changed attitudes in the population or changed attitudes among health care providers who may be less inclined to offer CF carrier testing.

Newborn screening would presumably lessen the cost-effectiveness of rou-tine carrier testing. As more families learned about their carrier status from newborn screening, fewer new carrier couples would be detected through car-rier testing offered in the prenatal setting. Targeted carrier testing of the par-ents, aunts, and uncles of infant CF carriers would identify more carriers per test than population screening and hence would be more cost-effective than routine carrier testing. In this targeted screening approach, approximately 1 in 2 people will be identified as carriers, and those with negative results will have even more certainty that they are not a carrier than they would have with population-based carrier testing. In population-based testing, fewer than 1 in 30 people tested will be identified as carriers, and some carriers will not be identified. Targeted carrier testing would be more cost-effective than popula-tion carrier testing. However, a reduced interest in carrier testing would re-sult in less population benefit (regardless of how the benefit is defined), even though the cost-effectiveness ratio might be improved.

Since the 2004 CDC recommendation that CF newborn screening is "jus-tifiable" (Grosse et al. 2004), the number of states providing such screening using IRT-DNA approaches has increased. Nevertheless, some states choose to use non-DNA-based methodologies. There are no data to systematically explore such decisions, but my direct experience with the decision making in several of these states suggests that reasons and justifications for non-

DNA-based approaches span a broad range, including: (1) carrier identification is undesirable because it adds to the complexity of a newborn screening program; (2) carrier identification is not an explicit goal or even an unintended but welcome benefit; and (3) carrier screening is desirable, but non-DNA approaches are preferable to allow specific issues of newborn screening delivery to be clarified and monitored before considering approaches that would involve the additional complexity of carrier identification. Because the usual non-DNA approaches require repeat testing, they have, for the most part, been restricted to the small number of states where newborn screening programs routinely collect second specimens. If only one specimen is collected, parents would have to take their infants to have a second blood sample taken and analyzed.

The Influence of Carrier Testing on Newborn Screening

Cystic fibrosis carrier testing in the general population might reduce some of the psychosocial concerns that have been raised about CF newborn screening. The main psychosocial concern is worry and distress following a positive test result, as well as confusion about the meaning of a false positive result and carrier status (Farrell and Farrell 2003). However, in the presence of carrier testing programs, there may be an improved understanding of CF for the parents of infants with abnormal newborn screening results. Offering carrier testing during pregnancy alerts parents to the possibility of CF and may give them a basic understanding of their potential carrier status. In this case, discussions with parents after abnormal results from newborn screening for CF will be covering somewhat more familiar information, compared with situations in which parents have no prior familiarity with CF. Almost all parents receive some sort of newborn screening brochure, and they may have some discussion before receiving the newborn screening results, but many parents attend to newborn screening information only when it is clearly relevant to them (after an abnormal result).

Carrier testing might decrease the cost-effectiveness of newborn screening. If, in fact, carrier testing substantially reduces the birth prevalence of CF, the number of infants diagnosed with CF would presumably decrease, even though the cost of newborn screening would not change much. In Canada, it is estimated that the birth prevalence of CF declined from 1 in 2714 to 1 in 3608 in the 10 years after carrier testing became available (Dupuis et al.

2005). Abnormal newborn screening results will proportionally identify more carriers than infants with CF as the incidence of CF decreases.

Conclusion

When carrier testing and newborn screening are offered in the same geographic area, it is important for obstetricians and pediatricians to become more aware of both programs and to incorporate such information when providing education for their patients. For example, in the prenatal setting, discussions about CF should include information on both carrier testing and newborn screening (Grosse et al. 2004). A brochure that discusses CF and includes both approaches, with balanced information, would be useful. In the newborn setting, after a false positive newborn screening result, it is important for families to be referred for consideration of carrier testing. While some newborn screening programs already designate genetic counseling services, in the future it might be feasible to refer parents back to their obstetrician for further discussion about carrier testing (unless it was done earlier).

A comprehensive health care system would presumably develop an integrated carrier testing and newborn screening system. Indeed, the National Haemoglobinopathy Programme in the United Kingdom coordinates both newborn and prenatal carrier screening for SCD and other hemoglobin disorders (Davies et al. 2000), although the U.K. prenatal testing program focuses on β-thalassemia, a condition for which no routine newborn screening test currently exists. Coordinating educational materials for families to include a unified approach to genetic counseling for carriers identified in either the prenatal or the newborn setting might be useful. Clearly, the benefits of such an integrated program would need to be evaluated. Benefit assessments would require specific, measurable outcomes, which would depend on the goals of the programs endorsed by the health system. Just as integrated health systems have become proficient at using "continuous quality improvement" for many services, such approaches could also be used to determine the best way for the programs to achieve their goals.

In the future, as more diseases become candidates for both carrier testing and newborn screening, the development and evaluation of implementation plans should include attention to the programs' goals, assessment of their cost-utility, and creative coordination of related health services.

NOTE

1. Wisconsin Newborn Screening Laboratory, "Newborn screening: parents guide" (www .slh.wisc.edu).

REFERENCES

Andrews, L. B., Fullarton, J. E., Holtzman, N. A., and Motulsky, A. G. 1994. *Assessing Genetic Risks: Implications for Health and Social Policy.* Washington DC: National Academy of Sciences.

Asch, A. 1999. Prenatal diagnosis and selective abortion: a challenge to practice and policy. *Am J Public Health* 89 (11): 1649–57.

Bekker, H., Modell, M., Denniss, G., Silver, A., Mathew, C., Bobrow, M., and Marteau, T. 1993. Uptake of cystic fibrosis testing in primary care: supply push or demand pull? *BMJ* 306 (6892): 1584–86.

Botkin, J. R., Clayton, E. W., Fost, N. C., Burke, W., Murray, T. H., Baily, M. A., Wilfond, B., Berg, A., and Ross, L. F. 2006. Newborn screening technology: proceed with caution. *Pediatrics* 117 (5): 1793–99.

Ciske, D. J., Haavisto, A., Laxova, A., Rock, L. Z., and Farrell, P. M. 2001. Genetic counseling and neonatal screening for cystic fibrosis: an assessment of the communication process. *Pediatrics* 107 (4): 696–705.

Clayton, E. W., Hannig, V. L., Pfotenhauer, J. P., Parker, R. A., Campbell, P. W. III, and Phillips, J. A. III. 1996. Lack of interest by nonpregnant couples in population-based cystic fibrosis carrier screening. *Am J Hum Genet* 58 (3): 617–27.

Comeau, A. M., Parad, R. B., Dorkin, H. L., Dovey, M., Gerstle, R., Haver, K., Lapey, A., O'Sullivan, B. P., Waltz, D. A., Zwerdling, R. G., and Eaton, R. B. 2004. Population-based newborn screening for genetic disorders when multiple mutation DNA testing is incorporated: a cystic fibrosis newborn screening model demonstrating increased sensitivity but more carrier detections. *Pediatrics* 113 (6): 1573–81.

Davies, S. C., Cronin, E., Gill, M., Greengross, P., Hickman, M., and Normand, C. 2000. Screening for sickle cell disease and thalassaemia: a systematic review with supplementary research. *Health Technol Assess* 4 (3): 1–99.

Dupuis, A., Hamilton, D., Cole, D. E., and Corey, M. 2005. Cystic fibrosis birth rates in Canada: a decreasing trend since the onset of genetic testing. *J Pediatr* 147 (3): 312–15.

Faden, R. R., Holtzman, N. A., and Chwalow, A. J. 1982. Parental rights, child welfare, and public health: the case of PKU screening. *Am J Public Health* 72 (12): 1396–1400.

Farrell, M. H., and Farrell, P. M. 2003. Newborn screening for cystic fibrosis: ensuring more good than harm. *J Pediatr* 143 (6): 707–12.

Farrell, P. M., Kosorok, M. R., Laxova, A., Shen, G., Koscik, R. E., Bruns, W. T., Splaingard, M., and Mischler, E. H. 1997. Nutritional benefits of neonatal screening for cystic fibrosis. Wisconsin Cystic Fibrosis Neonatal Screening Study Group. *N Engl J Med* 337 (14): 963–69.

Green, J. M., Hewison, J., Bekker, H. L., Bryant, L. D., and Cuckle, H. S. 2004. Psychosocial aspects of genetic screening of pregnant women and newborns: a systematic review. *Health Technol Assess* 8 (33): iii, ix-x, 1–109.

Grosse, S. D., Boyle, C. A., Botkin, J. R., Comeau, A. M., Kharrazi, M., Rosenfeld, M., and Wilfond, B. S. 2004. Newborn screening for cystic fibrosis: evaluation of benefits and risks and recommendations for state newborn screening programs. *MMWR Recomm Rep* 53 (RR-13): 1–36.

Grosse, S. D., Boyle, C. A., Kenneson, A., Khoury, M. J., and Wilfond, B. S. 2006. From public health emergency to public health service: the implications of evolving criteria for newborn screening panels. *Pediatrics* 117 (3): 923–29.

Grosse, S. D., Rosenfeld, M., Devine, O. J., Lai, H. J., and Farrell, P. M. 2006. Potential impact of newborn screening for cystic fibrosis on child survival: a systematic review and analysis. *J Pediatr* 149 (3): 362–66.

Kaback, M. M. 2001. Screening and prevention in Tay-Sachs disease: origins, update, and impact. In *Tay-Sachs Disease*, ed. R. J. Desnick and M. M. Kaback, pp. 253–65. San Diego: Academic Press.

Kharrazi, M., and Kharrazi, L. D. 2005. Delayed diagnosis of cystic fibrosis and the family perspective. *J Pediatr* 147 (3 Suppl): S21–25.

Koscik, R. L., Farrell, P. M., Kosorok, M. R., Zaremba, K. M., Laxova, A., Lai, H. C., Douglas, J. A., Rock, M. J., and Splaingard, M. L. 2004. Cognitive function of children with cystic fibrosis: deleterious effect of early malnutrition. *Pediatrics* 113 (6): 1549–58.

La Pean, A., and Farrell, M. H. 2005. Initially misleading communication of carrier results after newborn genetic screening. *Pediatrics* 116 (6): 1499–1505.

Lagoe, E., Labella, S., Arnold, G., and Rowley, P. T. 2005. Cystic fibrosis newborn screening: a pilot study to maximize carrier screening. *Genet Test* 9 (3): 255–60.

Lai, H. J., Cheng, Y., and Farrell, P. M. 2005. The survival advantage of patients with cystic fibrosis diagnosed through neonatal screening: evidence from the United States Cystic Fibrosis Foundation registry data. *J Pediatr* 147 (3 Suppl): S57–63.

Laird, L., Dezateux, C., and Anionwu, E. N. 1996. Neonatal screening for sickle cell disorders: what about the carrier infants? *BMJ* 313 (7054): 407–11.

Loeben, G. L., Marteau, T. M., and Wilfond, B. S. 1998. Mixed messages: presentation of information in cystic fibrosis–screening pamphlets. *Am J Hum Genet* 63 (4): 1181–89.

Mennuti, M. T., Thomson, E., and Press, N. 1999. Screening for cystic fibrosis carrier state. *Obstet Gynecol* 93 (3): 456–61.

Mickle, J. E., and Cutting, G. R. 2000. Genotype-phenotype relationships in cystic fibrosis. *Med Clin North Am* 84 (3): 597–607.

Mischler, E. H., Wilfond, B. S., Fost, N., Laxova, A., Reiser, C., Sauer, C. M., Makholm, L. M., Shen, G., Feenan, L., McCarthy, C., and Farrell, P. M. 1998. Cystic fibrosis newborn screening: impact on reproductive behavior and implications for genetic counseling. *Pediatrics* 102 (1 Pt 1): 44–52.

Murray, J., Cuckle, H., Taylor, G., Littlewood, J., and Hewison, J. 1999. Screening for cystic fibrosis. *Health Technol Assess* 3 (8): 1–104.

Oliver, S., Dezateux, C., Kavanagh, J., Lempert, T., and Stewart, R. 2004. Disclosing to parents newborn carrier status identified by routine blood spot screening. *Cochrane Database Syst Rev*, no. 4:CD003859.

Parsons, E. P., Clarke, A. J., and Bradley, D. M. 2003. Implications of carrier identification in newborn screening for cystic fibrosis. *Arch Dis Child Fetal Neonatal Ed* 88 (6): F467–71.

Rowley, P. T., Loader, S., and Kaplan, R. M. 1998. Prenatal screening for cystic fibrosis carriers: an economic evaluation. *Am J Hum Genet* 63 (4): 1160–74.

Scotet, V., Audrezet, M. P., Roussey, M., Rault, G., Blayau, M., De Braekeleer, M., and Ferec, C. 2003. Impact of public health strategies on the birth prevalence of cystic fibrosis in Brittany, France. *Hum Genet* 113 (3): 280–85.

Sugarman, E. A., Rohlfs, E. M., Silverman, L. M., and Allitto, B. A. 2004. CFTR mutation distribution among U.S. Hispanic and African American individuals: evaluation in cystic fibrosis patient and carrier screening populations. *Genet Med* 6 (5): 392–99.

Super, M., and Abbott, J. 1998. Genetic advances in cystic fibrosis: to screen, to treat or both? *Disabil Rehabil* 20 (6–7): 202–8.

Tambor, E. S., Bernhardt, B. A., Chase, G. A., Faden, R. R., Geller, G., Hofman, K. J., and Holtzman, N. A. 1994. Offering cystic fibrosis carrier screening to an HMO population: factors associated with utilization. *Am J Hum Genet* 55 (4): 626–37.

van den Akker-van Marle, M. E., Dankert, H. M., Verkerk, P. H., and Dankert-Roelse, J. E. 2006. Cost-effectiveness of 4 neonatal screening strategies for cystic fibrosis. *Pediatrics* 118 (3): 896–905.

Watson, M. S., Cutting, G. R., Desnick, R. J., Driscoll, D. A., Klinger, K., Mennuti, M., Palomaki, G. E., Popovich, B. W., Pratt, V. M., Rohlfs, E. M., Strom, C. M., Richards, C. S., Witt, D. R., and Grody, W. W. 2004. Cystic fibrosis population carrier screening: 2004 revision of American College of Medical Genetics mutation panel. *Genet Med* 6 (5): 387–91.

Wheeler, P.G., Smith, R., Dorkin, H., Parad, R. B., Comeau, A. M., and Bianchi, D. W. 2001. Genetic counseling after implementation of statewide cystic fibrosis newborn screening: two years' experience in one medical center. *Genet Med* 3 (6): 411–15.

Wilfond, B. S., and Gollust, S. E. 2005. Policy issues for expanding newborn screening programs: the cystic fibrosis newborn screening experience in the United States. *J Pediatr* 146 (5): 668–74.

Wilfond, B. S., Parad, R. B., and Fost, N. 2005. Balancing benefits and risks for cystic fibrosis newborn screening: implications for policy decisions. *J Pediatr* 147 (3 Suppl): S109–13.

Witt, D. R., Schaefer, C., Hallam, P., Wi, S., Blumberg, B., Fishbach, A., Holtzman, J., Kornfeld, S., Lee, R., Nemzer, L., and Palmer, R. 1996. Cystic fibrosis heterozygote screening in 5,161 pregnant women. *Am J Hum Genet* 58 (4): 823–35.

Zeuner, D., Ades, A. E., Karnon, J., Brown, J., Dezateux, C., and Anionwu, E. N. 1999. Antenatal and neonatal haemoglobinopathy screening in the UK: review and economic analysis. *Health Technol Assess* 3 (11): i–v, 1–186.

CHAPTER 16

What Can We Do to Shape the Future of Newborn Screening?

Conclusions and Recommendations

MARY ANN BAILY, PH.D.
THOMAS H. MURRAY, PH.D.

In 2000, a child named Ben Haygood died in rural Mississippi from an undiagnosed rare, inherited disorder known as medium-chain acyl-CoA dehydrogenase deficiency (MCAD). His father became an advocate for expanding that state's newborn screening program to include MCAD and other disorders. Within a few years, the Mississippi legislature had passed the Ben Haygood Comprehensive Newborn Screening Act, the state's test panel had increased from only 5 disorders to 40, and a three-person team had been created in each of nine state districts to manage the cases of children with positive screening results (Bender 2004; see also chapter 6). Most funding for newborn screening programs came from a fee for each newborn screened; to help pay for the expansion, the state doubled the fee to $70. This meant that a substantial share of the resources for expansion came from Mississippi's Medicaid funds, because Medicaid covers more than half of Mississippi births (Johnson 2004). In the first year of expanded screening,[1] 3 cases of MCAD were identified along with 12 cases of other newly included disorders, in a total of 116 newborn screening diagnoses.[2]

At about the same time, according to a *New York Times* article, Mississippi experienced a worrying change in overall infant mortality rate (Eckholm

2007). The state's rate had long been above the national average, but it had been falling. Between 2004 and 2005, however, it increased, especially among blacks. In 2005, 481 infants died, 65 more than in the previous year.

A new governor had taken office in 2004 and promised to keep taxes steady and bring Medicaid costs down. Medicaid eligibility requirements were tightened, and some programs were cut. Were the changes in Medicaid a factor in the increase in infant deaths? Could infant lives have been saved if, instead, the state had increased the availability of Medicaid services and provided state funds to subsidize transportation for low-income rural black women to improve their access to prenatal care? It is hard to know; however, the *Times* article points to the dramatically lower infant mortality rate achieved in one very poor Mississippi county from 1991 to 2005.[3] The county's rate fell sharply after a private charity began providing intensive in-home visits, using local women as counselors, and began busing pregnant black women to prenatal and postnatal classes.

Our goal here is not to single out Mississippi for criticism or to focus on any specific alternative for improving the health of children. Newborn screening, home visits, and prenatal care are all means to the end of helping children. There are many others as well. There could be a systematic effort to identify children with asthma and manage the condition better, especially for poor children who often end up in emergency rooms in asthmatic crises. There could be efforts to reduce smoking by pregnant women, increase the use of car seats for children, or prevent childhood accidents. We do not know which of these programs would produce the greatest benefits for children—but that ignorance is itself a major problem. The problem is heightened when resources available for children's health, such as Medicaid, are decreased or fail to keep up with growing need.

The experience in Mississippi serves to highlight an important ethical issue in child health policy. Although resources for children's health are scarce, too often there is no systematic effort to identify and compare alternative ways to use those precious resources to help children; moreover, the information needed to make an intelligent and informed comparison among such programs is often lacking. This chapter explores this and other ethical and policy issues that arise in debates about public newborn screening programs. We explain the overall conclusion of the Hastings Center's project "Ethical Decision-Making for Newborn Genetic Screening," discuss its implications for newborn screening policy, and make specific recommendations for the future.

As we noted in the Preface, the period during which the project ran—2002 to 2007—was a time of unexpectedly rapid and often controversial change in newborn screening. Project participants were able to reach agreement on the general requirements for ethical newborn screening policy, but they disagreed strongly about the extent to which developments in newborn screening conformed to the requirements. Thus, we emphasize that the opinions about current and future policy expressed here are those of the authors of this chapter and do not necessarily reflect the views of the project members.

Requirements for Ethical Newborn Screening Policy

The conclusion of the Hastings Center's project is that newborn screening policy is ethically acceptable when it is (1) evidence-based, (2) takes into account the opportunity cost of the newborn screening program, (3) distributes the costs and benefits of the program fairly, and (4) appropriately respects human rights. Many would agree that these are sensible requirements for prudent public policy, but some may not immediately see all of them as *ethical* requirements. In particular, the ethical dimensions of the clauses about opportunity cost and evidence may not be clear. In public debates about newborn screening, concern about cost is often seen as opposed to ethics, and some advocates assert that when infant lives are at stake, considering cost at all is morally wrong (Howse and Katz 2000).

In fact, cost itself is an ethical issue in newborn screening policy because, as the experience in Mississippi suggests, the collective resources used for screening programs could always be used in other ways to improve the length and quality of people's lives. The resources used for newborn screening have an opportunity cost, and policymakers have an ethical obligation of *stewardship* to take this opportunity cost into account when they make resource allocation decisions. Policymakers also have an ethical obligation to ensure that the costs and benefits of their allocation decisions are fairly distributed across individuals.

Evidence is an ethical issue because opportunity cost and distributional fairness are ethical issues. Information about the existence, the reliability, the size, and the distribution of the benefits and costs of newborn screening is critical in evaluating the opportunity cost of devoting scarce resources to screening and the extent to which the costs and benefits are fairly distributed. Because gathering evidence consumes resources in itself, policy decisions must often be based on incomplete information. Nevertheless, policymakers have an ethical obligation to use all available evidence and to support systematic, cost-conscious, ongoing efforts to develop additional evidence where necessary.

Evidence and cost are also factors in developing newborn screening policies that respect human rights. The United States has sturdy societal values supporting the rights of individuals to decide what treatments they will have, whether they will participate in research, and what can be done with their personal information and their bodily tissues, such as blood samples. In these matters, parents are normally considered the appropriate people to make decisions on behalf of their children.

Given these values, the mandatory status of public newborn screening has always been ethically controversial. Mandatory screening for phenylketonuria (PKU) was originally sought on the grounds that the urgent need for early diagnosis and the great benefit of the treatment justified omitting informed consent. If mandatory screening requires this kind of justification, then a new condition should be added to the mandatory panel only when there is an established screening test and good evidence that the condition causes serious harm and that the harm can be avoided if the infant is diagnosed and treated immediately after birth. To develop the evidence base for ethical policy decisions, research and data-guided quality improvement activities are essential; however, these activities must be designed to respect individual rights related to participation in research and use of bloodspots.

Even when screening is mandated, parents deserve to receive some information about the screening. To determine how much, the cost of the information process to the program and to parents should be weighed against the value of being informed. Newborn screening programs should maintain the confidentiality of personal health information in program evaluation and research, which may require weighing the value of privacy protection against the cost of security measures and the benefits forgone if security measures make a research or evaluation activity impracticable.

Finally, if society is ethically required to engage in an activity no matter what it costs, the necessary resources must come from somewhere. Because resources ultimately come from people, not from an abstract entity called "society," policymakers must always have an ethical justification for the pattern of individual sacrifice that results when resources are devoted to meeting societal ethical obligations.

Assessment of Current Policies

Does the policy process for newborn screening produce policies that meet these ethical requirements? Unfortunately, the answer is no—not in the past, and not now. To be fair to newborn screening, this is part of the larger picture of disorder and confusion in health policy in general. Below, we take the four clauses in the Hasting Center project's conclusion and discuss each of them with reference to what actually happens in current newborn screening programs.

Newborn Screening Policy Should Be Evidence-Based

Is newborn screening policy based on solid evidence on the nature, size, and distribution of the benefits and costs of newborn screening? Obviously, the information requirements for ethical policy are formidable. For each candidate condition, detailed evidence on the disorder's natural history, its incidence, and the variation in its incidence and expression within the population would be desirable. There should be evidence on the scientific validity, clinical utility, and resource cost of the screening test. There should also be evidence on the effectiveness, resource cost, and availability of treatment. Finally, the positive and negative effects of introducing newborn screening must be measured, aggregated, and compared. This requires evidence on personal values and preferences and how they vary across individuals. Collecting and carefully evaluating all this information is a major challenge.

Currently, the challenge is not being met. The information is far from complete even for conditions that have been included in newborn screening panels for years. Yet, instead of addressing the significant gaps in knowledge about conditions already in the screening panels, states are adding further conditions, many of them only poorly understood.

The nature and extent of the expansion is somewhat unexpected. In a comprehensive report published in 2000, the federally funded Newborn Screening Task Force emphasized the importance of using an evidence-based approach in decisions about the introduction of new tests, and it recommended introducing tests on a pilot basis when evidence was limited (Newborn Screening Task Force 2000). In 2002, the American College of Medical Genetics (ACMG) convened a working group (funded by the Health Resources and Service Administration, HRSA) to evaluate the available evidence on a long list of conditions proposed for newborn screening and to make evidence-based recommendations for a uniform panel of conditions that were suitable for inclusion in state newborn screening programs.

In its final report, the ACMG recommended a uniform panel of 29 primary disorders and an additional 25 secondary disorders that would be detected incidentally while screening for the primary disorders (American College of Medical Genetics 2006). The Advisory Committee on Heritable Disorders and Genetic Diseases in Newborns and Children (the principal national body concerned with newborn screening since June 2004) immediately endorsed the ACMG report in correspondence with the Secretary of Health and Human Services and called for state newborn screening programs to conform to the report's recommendations (Advisory Committee on Heritable Disorders and Genetic Diseases in Newborns and Children 2004; Howell 2005). Other organizations, including the March of Dimes and the American Academy of Pediatrics, also endorsed the recommendations.

The ACMG report acknowledges that there are serious limits to the information available on many of the conditions it recommends for screening. Unfortunately, the information shortfall may be worse even than acknowledged. As discussed in detail in this volume (see chapters 2, 7, and 10), the ACMG's methodology, content, and working process seem to be deeply flawed. Critics have argued that the methodology was highly idiosyncratic and did not conform to established standards for evidence-based reviews. They have also said that the report has insufficient discussion of many important ethical, legal, and social issues that are relevant to such a significant expansion of programs, and have noted that the working group had extensive expertise in metabolic genetics and laboratory medicine but lacked essential expertise in evidence-based medicine, bioethics, primary care, and health economics (Botkin et al. 2006).

The advisory committee responded to criticism of the ACMG methodology by obtaining expert advice on accepted standards and methods for evidence-based medicine. It is developing a new and more rigorous evidence-based process for evaluation of proposals to add new conditions to the uniform panel. The effort to improve a seriously flawed process is commendable; however, the process is unlikely to be in place and ready for evaluating new conditions in the very near future. For now, the committee might be better advised simply to urge states to deal adequately with the management issues in their current programs. Moreover, before an evaluation of additional conditions, the conditions in the current recommended panel should be reevaluated.

In the advisory committee's discussion of the evaluation process, some members of the committee suggested that the criteria used by the U.S. Preventive Services Task Force are too strict for newborn screening programs (Advisory Committee on Heritable Disorders and Genetic Diseases in Newborns and Children 2006). The task force reviews a broad array of health services, including screening tests, to recommend whether they are appropriate for routine use in primary care practice, subject to patient consent. The ACMG is recommending tests for use on every newborn in the country, without full informed consent, and at the expense of public and private third-party payers and individual families, who will incur new costs without consultation. Surely in such circumstances the standard of evidence should be higher, not lower (see chapter 10).

Newborn Screening Policy Should Take Opportunity Cost into Account

Could greater benefits or a fairer distribution of benefits be achieved by reallocating newborn screening resources to another use? In answering this question, all costs should be considered; however, costs are often understated in debates on newborn screening policy. A common error is to consider only the cost of the test itself. Advocates may say, if Baby A had only had a $50 screening test for MCAD, his life could have been saved. Surely a child's life is worth $50! That would indeed be a small price to pay to save an infant's life. But newborn screening programs must test many newborns to identify the few with MCAD. Thus, even if only the cost of testing itself is counted—ignoring, for a moment, the many other activities that must accompany the testing—saving one life costs much more than the price of a single test.

Cost is also understated when advocates claim that the cost of testing all newborns for an additional condition is low because the blood sample is already collected and the infrastructure is in place. For example, if tandem mass spectrometry (MS/MS) is already used for PKU and MCAD, then adding one more metabolic disorder seems to add only a little to the cost. But, again, the real cost is more than the cost of testing. After we factor in the full costs of parental education, follow-up of all positive results to a definitive diagnosis, treatment of affected children, and ongoing data collection and evaluation, adding another disorder to an existing panel can be expensive. Moreover, if the natural history of the condition is poorly understood and effective treatments are lacking, children may receive no benefit, or may even be harmed by unnecessary interventions.

Another way to understate the cost of newborn screening is to count only the net cost of state budget appropriations earmarked for the newborn screening program. In fact, adding a test to a mandatory newborn screening panel automatically imposes costs on private insurance (which is expected to pay for the screening test, follow-up, and treatment for insured infants) and on both the state and federal governments (which, through the Medicaid program, cover more than one-third of births in the United States). Other costs fall directly on families. These include the cost in time and money that families of children who test positive must bear to obtain a definitive diagnosis, and the unnecessary worry and anxiety experienced by the families whose children turn out not to have the disorder, or to have a clinically insignificant form of it.

Finally, the full cost of newborn screening includes the cost of program-related research and quality improvement. The ACMG report concludes that the development and evaluation of evidence before and after introducing a test is an essential part of a national newborn screening system, and makes recommendations for incorporating ongoing research and quality improvement activities into these programs. It does not attempt to estimate the cost of all this work, however, and thus inevitably underestimates the total cost of newborn screening.

Once the full costs of newborn screening are understood, the benefits must be assessed and compared with the benefits that could be achieved from other uses of the resources. The framework for equitable allocation of health care resources outlined in chapter 2 starts from the premise that society has a moral obligation to ensure that every child has access to adequate health care and to distribute the cost of achieving this outcome fairly. The adequate level of care should be determined by considering the relative merits of different health services in the light of the reasons for the special importance of health care. This means that the quantity of resources devoted to newborn screening and treatment for genetic disorders should be established in the context of determining the entire adequate level of health care and the importance of health care relative to other important social goods.

Unfortunately, the policy process is biased against doing this. The U.S. health care system is not really a *system*. It has no institutional structure to take responsibility for stewardship of collective resources and to force consideration of the opportunity cost of decisions about public health programs or additions to standard clinical care. In newborn screening, this system-level problem has been made worse because each state makes its own decisions on newborn screening; furthermore, program financing is plagued by a lack of transparency. Advocacy by health professional groups, makers of screening technologies, and consumer groups such as the March of Dimes and associations supporting parents of children with genetic conditions also affects policy development. These advocates provide important perspectives, but often no one steps up to advocate for the programs that will not be undertaken and the people who will not be helped because health care resources have been directed to newborn screening. (See chapter 2 for additional discussion of the role of advocacy in the policy process.) Consider Mississippi: a state expands newborn screening at the same time that it cuts support for prenatal care for poor women. The advocates for those women, and the children they were carrying, were either silent or ineffective.

Newborn Screening Policy Should Distribute the Costs and Benefits of the Program Fairly

Would changes to newborn screening policies produce a more fair distribution of benefits and costs within the programs? The comprehensive Newborn Screening Task Force report, advocacy groups, and other observers have identified many long-standing fairness issues associated with program structure. These relate primarily to the selection and implementation of tests and the financing and delivery of screening, follow-up, diagnosis, and services for treatment and management (Newborn Screening Task Force 2000).

Given the variation in the composition of test panels across states, being born on one side of a state border instead of the other can mean life or death for a child with a genetic disorder. The incidence of a condition may vary across racial or ethnic groups, and fairness is an issue in decisions about how this variation should influence the selection of a test and whether only the members of specific racial/ethnic groups should be screened. Technical decisions made within newborn screening laboratories can have fairness implications; for example, a laboratory's decisions about the cutoff level that constitutes a positive test result for a disorder can affect different racial/ethnic groups differently. The same is true for decisions about what mutations to include in DNA-based screening.

Currently, the services received by individual families of affected children vary substantially and inequitably both across and within states. Also, the cost of the various elements of newborn screening programs is arbitrarily distributed, largely because of the patchwork nature of health care financing in the United States. This results in excessive burdens on some families and fails to distribute the burden of the total cost of newborn screening, including follow-up diagnosis and care, equitably across the entire nation (Therrell et al. 2007).

As noted in earlier chapters, the traditional public health justification for newborn screening was that a very important benefit to the child would be lost if screening did not occur soon after birth, and the risk to the child posed by screening was minimal at worst. One of the most surprising features of the ACMG report is its departure from this basic principle, which has guided newborn screening from the beginning and was reaffirmed by the highly respected Newborn Screening Task Force (2000) only a few years before the ACMG began its work (Bailey et al. 2006; Grosse et al. 2006). The ACMG's expanded framework for justifying screening allows consideration of benefits to the family and to society. For example, benefits to the family might include the provision of information that could help the family make future reproductive decisions or avoid the so-called diagnostic odyssey. Benefits to society might include the identification of potential research subjects for the study of currently untreatable disorders. Some newborn screening advocates now argue that the decision is not what to include, but what to exclude; in this view, the new default position is to screen for everything possible (see chapter 4).

Both the change and the way it came about are troubling. The ACMG working group adopted the new criteria with little discussion or justification and immediately began using them to select the new uniform panel, which was then released as a fait accompli. As a result, the uniform panel includes conditions that do not urgently need treatment in the newborn period, or for which no proven treatment is available, or for which the benefit of treatment to the infant is much less significant and certain than the benefit of treatment for a condition like PKU. This means that the inequity of the difference in access across states has been exchanged for another kind of inequity. For some of the newly added conditions, it is less obvious that newborn screening for the condition is truly part of an adequate level of care or, if it is, that it should take priority over other ethically urgent health care not readily available to all children at this time.

Moreover, it seems imprudent as well as unfair to expand quickly, without the necessary support services in place for the new disorders and without first addressing the inequities in access to services for the conditions already included in screening panels. The work involved in expanding programs to deal with the long list of conditions in the uniform panel is monumental. It includes educating health care providers and parents about the conditions, resolving many technical issues associated with the new tests, building the infrastructure for follow-up to diagnosis and long-term treatment and management, and providing for continuing research and quality improvement. HRSA is making a significant investment in helping states to do this work, but much more remains to be done. A child harmed because she or he was screened for a condition but the test failed to detect it, or because there was no proper follow-up and treatment, is no better off than a child who is harmed because screening for the disorder was never initiated.

The ACMG report's family benefit justification for screening also raises fairness questions. For example, although some families might benefit from an early diagnosis that lets them avoid a diagnostic odyssey, that benefit should be weighed against the burdens of different kinds of odysseys that other families might have to endure. Families whose healthy children are inaccurately identified as having a condition must endure a period of anxious searching until follow-up tests reassure them that their children are well. Less fortunate families may experience more disturbing long-term outcomes. Suppose parents are told that testing confirms that their child has an abnormal laboratory finding that is sometimes associated with serious illness, but their child never becomes symptomatic. Perhaps the child has a mild or subclinical form that was unknown before newborns were routinely screened for the disorder. (This plausible scenario underscores the need for evidence on the natural history of disorders recommended for newborn screening.) Meanwhile, the family reorganizes its life around medical monitoring and planning for something terrible that never happens. Or a family may be told that a child has a serious disorder with no proven treatment, one that before newborn screening was diagnosed only after death. The family begins a treatment odyssey—searching the internet, visiting specialists, running up debt, medicalizing the child's life—only to have that life end in early death anyway. Or perhaps treatment options exist, but they are terribly burdensome in dollars and parental time and energy—perhaps to the child as well as the parents—and bring, at best, a slight, fleeting improvement in the child's condition. A family with limited resources and no comprehensive health insurance may be forced to choose between embarking on an odyssey of seeking a way to gain access to the services or making the painful decision to forgo them. With the expansion of programs to more conditions, many poorly understood, unhappy medical wanderings such as these have become more likely.

Newborn Screening Policy Should Respect Human Rights

Does newborn screening policy take appropriate account of fundamental and widely respected American values concerning confidentiality, privacy, and informed consent in genetic screening and in research involving human subjects? The mandatory nature of newborn screening seems inconsistent with these values. The standard rationale for mandating public health measures, such as immunization or treatment of infectious disease, is that the measure will avert serious imminent harm to others, but this rationale does not apply to newborn screening. Instead, the justification for a mandate has been that the risk is minimal and the child will lose a vital benefit if screening is not done immediately. Even under these circumstances, not all ethicists think that omitting informed consent is acceptable. Broadening the rationale for screening makes the omission even more questionable. If the rationale is a family benefit, such as information that can inform reproductive decisions or help avoid diagnostic odysseys, or a societal benefit, such as identifying potential research subjects for the study of currently untreatable disorders (Alexander and van Dyck 2006; Wald 2007), then the ethical requirement is clear: parents should be informed and allowed to make their own decisions.

Oddly enough, the new rationale for screening is frequently justified with references to "what parents want" (Alexander and van Dyck 2006; Wald 2007). For example, some argue that parents want to know if the results of MS/MS show that a child has a metabolic abnormality, even if there is no treatment—in fact, even if its clinical significance is unknown. In practice, as we noted in chapter 2, "what parents want" usually means "what some of the parents of children already identified as having a specific genetic condition are advocating for." We should all be deeply sympathetic to parents whose children suffer from diseases whose worst complications could have been prevented by newborn screening. Indeed, in our view, where the evidence that such screening can reliably prevent harm is solid, screening should generally be initiated. The Wilson and Jungner criteria (1968) were an early and largely successful attempt to articulate this standard.

Unfortunately, in more ambiguous cases, there is little hard evidence of what parents typically want. Hearing from parents frightened by a false positive result, or presented with a diagnosis of a condition whose natural history is not clearly understood and for which no reliable and effective treatment is available, would be especially helpful. Moreover, as important as the views of parents are, there are others who should also have a say. When collective resources are being used, taxpayers and those paying insurance premiums also deserve to be heard (Clayton 2006).

Society has not systematically asked individual parents or taxpayers or premium payers what newborn screening policies they think are appropriate. If society decides to ask, framing the question properly will be a challenge. The question should not be, do you want to be able to refuse screening for a specific genetic disorder on behalf of your newborn, given that the program is already in place? Nor should the question be, do you think screening newborns for life-threatening genetic disorders is a good idea? The right question is not a yes-or-no question but a question about alternative paths for pursuing good and valuable ends. For example, we could pose the question in a form that helps people understand that screening has an opportunity cost and that gives them examples of what could be obtained if the resources were used differently (see chapter 2). We could collect information on how respondents' views vary with the specific characteristics of the disorder. Probably most people would agree that screening for PKU is worthwhile; but judgments about the desirability of using scarce resources to screen newborns for conditions that have only minimally effective treatments or whose clinical significance is unclear—especially when those same resources might be devoted to some other worthy activity with proven benefits—are less easy to guess.

Fortunately, there are alternatives to mandatory screening of newborns for all conditions (see chapters 5 and 10). States can establish pilot programs that offer voluntary screening and generate the evidence needed to support an informed policy decision to include the condition in a mandatory universal testing program. States can also make screening for a condition available to all newborns in a public program, but on a voluntary basis with informed consent. Physicians can offer parents the option of newborn screening for the condition in the clinical setting, with informed consent. Attractive and practical alternatives to mandatory screening exist for those disorders for which crucial evidence is lacking. It is vital to understand that these alternatives do not deny a known, life-saving benefit to newborn infants. Instead, under conditions of uncertain benefit, they promote parents' informed choices while simultaneously allowing us to gather crucial evidence.

Finally, in considering the parental role in newborn screening, we err if we focus entirely on the debate between the opposing claims that informed consent is an ethical absolute and that informed consent is too expensive in time and money, and babies will be harmed because some parents will make bad decisions about consent. The reality is that even in a mandatory program, families have to know enough about newborn screening to understand what is at stake and to cooperate appropriately with the enterprise if newborn screening's goal of preventing avoidable harm to the child is to be achieved.

What kind of information is needed? Ideally, expectant parents should be aware that their newborn will be screened for a variety of disorders before leaving the hospital. During pregnancy, there should be basic education designed to convey a few simple messages: "Newborn screening will happen soon after your baby is delivered; your obstetrician recommends it; most babies picked up by screening for a disorder do not have it but those few who do need urgent treatment; you must follow up immediately if notified of a positive result." Obstetricians do not have to provide detailed information about all the individual disorders and their consequences, but they should be able to tell parents where to find more information if they want it. In the hospital, new mothers should be notified that the screening is being done and reminded about how important it is to follow up a positive result, even though most babies turn out to be unaffected. Parents receiving a positive result should receive basic information about the specific condition, and, of course, the parents of a child with a confirmed diagnosis should receive the detailed information and support they need to understand their child's condition and manage its impact on the child and the family.

In our project, we focused especially on the key position of obstetricians in the educational process. As part of the project, the March of Dimes collaborated with the New York State Newborn Screening Program to prepare educational materials for obstetricians, and it also produced an educational video on newborn screening for parents, which can be used by obstetricians to educate their patients. During the project period, HRSA funded the development of educational materials for parents and health professionals. Individual state programs, the March of Dimes, and parent advocacy groups have all engaged in efforts to educate the public, parents, and health professionals. Thus, some progress is being made in this area, even as the rapid expansion of test panels makes the task of informing parents significantly more complex.

There remains the issue of whether and how bloodspots can be stored and used after newborn screening is conducted. Some points are clear. Researchers have realized that newborn bloodspots are a potential treasure trove of human biological material samples. With virtually every child born in the

United States included, the annual set of Guthrie cards constitutes the most complete collection of human biological materials for any population cohort, making them enormously valuable for studies of population prevalence for such things as infectious diseases and allele frequencies for genes of interest. (Questions such as these can in principle be answered by examining samples from which all identifying information has been stripped.) At the same time, with the exception of a few states, parents are not asked for their affirmative consent for newborn screening. In some states, if they object to having their infant's blood drawn, that objection may be honored. But on the whole, the circumstances under which newborn bloodspots are obtained fall short of what we might regard as a thoughtful, thorough, deliberative process of informed consent.

When newborn screening maintained its founding identity as a public health screening program, this casual attitude toward informed consent had some moral justification. The point, after all, was to benefit the infants who were the subject of the screening program. As we have argued, when the test panel is expanded to include conditions that have no scientifically validated treatment or whose natural history is so poorly understood that children may be identified and treated who would never have developed clinical symptoms, newborn screening loses its clear ethical identity as a public health program. Dispensing with parental consent is not so readily justifiable in such circumstances.

The chapters by Maschke and Botkin (chapters 12 and 13) highlight the implications of these developments for research on bloodspots. There is enormous variation among states in how long bloodspots are stored, as well as in the circumstances under which those bloodspots may be shared with researchers. This variation creates inefficiencies and delays in the implementation of quality control projects and of research studies; furthermore, policy variation on matters of informed consent and privacy and confidentiality protections could undermine public trust in the research enterprise.

In chapter 12, Maschke offers several possible strategies for harmonizing policies among states. When the form of bloodspot samples given to researchers renders the samples completely unidentifiable, under the federal rules this is not classified as research with human subjects. That does not, however, let state newborn screening programs completely off the hook. Most programs have not formulated clear policies and procedures governing research with newborn screening bloodspots. We agree with Maschke that programs should have clear policies on the circumstances under which bloodspot samples may be shared with researchers (particularly on whether they are completely anonymized, coded, or identifiable), with whom, and for what purposes. In addition, each state's policy should specify what ethical oversight is appropriate; what form of consent, if any, is required for specific uses; and under what conditions the results of the research should be shared with parents (for samples that are identified or that are coded and then traced back to the source). The job is not finished when policies are formulated. They must be made transparent through some combination of notification to parents at the time of screening or later consent, and they should be posted prominently on the agency's website.

Botkin and Maschke seem to agree that the most readily justifiable uses of bloodspots are those intended to benefit infants who, after all, are the sources of the bloodspots. They may disagree, however, on whether consent may legitimately be waived under an important set of circumstances. In chapter 13, Botkin proposes a hypothetical study that uses bloodspots obtained over five years as a way of evaluating a new addition to the screening menu. If, say, the new screen identifies 20 children per year with that condition, then the five years before initiating the new test would be expected to include the bloodspots of approximately 100 children with the same condition. If those children could be identified retrospectively, researchers could see how well they fared, how many were identified clinically, and how many have not needed any intervention. Such information could be important in ascertaining the value of including such a disorder in the routine newborn screening panel. Botkin argues persuasively that contacting the parents of each child screened in the previous five years could be unreasonably burdensome. (Suppose the condition had a frequency of 1 in 10,000: finding 100 children testing positive would require contacting 1,000,000 parents.) He proposes multiple safeguards before such a study could be conducted. There would have to be evidence that early detection and intervention are beneficial; parents should be able to learn through mass media that this study is under consideration; and efforts should be made to educate and notify pregnant women and parents, with opportunities to opt out offered. The waiver of informed consent holds only until a child has been identified as positive by the retrospective screening. Parents would then be notified and asked to allow confirmatory testing and other follow-up, according to the research protocol. Botkin also urges that notification protocols be carefully designed to minimize adverse psychological impacts on parents and children.

Proposals such as Botkin's will be important to consider as newborn screening programs, researchers, and the public sort out their ethical convictions on research with newborn screening bloodspots. In the meantime, newborn screening programs should speed the development of thoughtful policies on research with the bloodspots in their care, make those policies as transparent as possible, and work with other states' programs to harmonize those policies.

Conclusion

We can and should improve the process through which newborn screening policy decisions are made. We should have a rigorous evaluation of evidence before adding a condition, and we need a systematic, cost-conscious plan for collecting evidence afterward. The evidence review should follow accepted standards and should include the perspectives of experts on evidence-based health policy analysis outside the field of newborn screening. To take adequate account of opportunity cost, we should collect evidence on both costs and benefits, and we should structure the policy process to compare newborn screening with other uses of resources, within and outside health care. To fairly distribute costs and benefits, we need more transparency in the financing of programs, better data on what the distribution of costs and benefits looks like, and more uniformity in access to follow-up and treatment. To respect human rights, programs should insist that benefit to the infant is an essential criterion for making newborn screening mandatory. If the benefit is to anyone other than the infant, or if the benefit to the infant is uncertain, then parental informed consent should be required. Finally, we must clarify obligations with respect to consent for using bloodspots for quality improvement in newborn screening, research related to newborn screening, and research on questions not directly pertaining to newborn screening.

All of these goals would be far easier to achieve in a health care system with certain key elements. All persons should have access to a socially accepted, morally adequate level of health care. The system should have institutional structures to allocate health care resources across the entire spectrum of care, with due regard to opportunity cost and stewardship. It should have an integrated electronic health information system with security measures that protect the confidentiality of personal health information and clear rules that govern data use. It should have a comprehensive program of quality improvement and research, using data accumulated in routine system operation to efficiently generate information that allows patients to better understand their options and allows health care professionals and organizations to provide better care.

Protecting the health of children is a noble goal. Newborn screening has made significant contributions to children's health since its humble beginnings decades ago. New technologies, new voices, and new opportunities have recently challenged the original ethical foundations of newborn screening programs. In this volume we have tried to articulate these challenges, and to show how they can be met honestly and justly.

ACKNOWLEDGMENT

An earlier version of this chapter was previously published as Mary Ann Baily and Thomas H. Murray, "Ethics, Evidence, and Cost in Newborn Screening," *Hastings Center Report* 38 (3): 23–31 (copyright © 2008 by the Hastings Center; used with permission).

NOTES

1. The first full year was June 2003 to May 2004; approximately 42,201 newborns were screened.

2. The other diagnoses were mostly cases of sickle cell disease and congenital hypothyroidism, at 70 and 21, respectively.

3. In this area, the infant mortality rate for blacks is below the national average for whites, which in turn is substantially below the national average for blacks.

REFERENCES

Advisory Committee on Heritable Disorders and Genetic Diseases in Newborns and Children. 2004. Minutes of Meeting 2, September 22–23. ftp://ftp.hrsa.gov/mchb/genetics/Minutes Sept04.pdf.

———. 2006. Establishing an evidence-based process for modifying the uniform newborn screening panel. Minutes of Meeting 9, December 18–19. http://ftp.hrsa.gov/mchb/genetics/dec06/minutes1206.pdf.

Alexander, D., and van Dyck, P. C. 2006. A vision of the future of newborn screening. *Pediatrics* 117 (5 Pt 2): S350–54.

American College of Medical Genetics. 2006. Newborn screening: toward a uniform screening panel and system. *Genet Med* 8 (Suppl 1): 1–252S.

Bailey, D. B. Jr., Beskow, L. M., Davis, A. M., and Skinner, D. 2006. Changing perspectives on the benefits of newborn screening. *Ment Retard Dev Disabil Res Rev* 12 (4): 270–79.

Bender, D. 2004. Mississippi Department of Health PowerPoint presentation at Advisory Committee on Heritable Disorders and Genetic Diseases in Newborns and Children Meeting II, September 23. www.hrsa.gov/heritabledisorderscommittee/presentations/sep04/bender.htm.

Botkin, J. R., Clayton, E. W., Fost, N. C., Burke, W., Murray, T. H., Baily, M. A., Wilfond, B., Berg, A., and Ross, L. F. 2006. Newborn screening technology: proceed with caution. *Pediatrics* 117 (5): 1793–99.

Clayton, E. W. 2006. The concepts of benefit and treatment: current practices and family perspectives. In Minutes of Advisory Committee on Heritable Disorders and Genetic Diseases in Newborns and Children Meeting 9, December 18–19, pp. 39–43. http://ftp.hrsa.gov/mchb/genetics/dec06/minutes1206.pdf.

Eckholm, E. 2007. In turnabout, infant deaths climb in South. *New York Times*, April 22.

Grosse, S. D., Boyle, C. A., Kenneson, A., Khoury, M. J., and Wilfond, B. S. 2006. From public health emergency to public health service: the implications of evolving criteria for newborn screening panels. *Pediatrics* 117 (3): 923–29.

Howell, R. R. 2005. Letters from R. Rodney Howell, M.D., Chairperson of Advisory Committee on Heritable Disorders and Genetic Diseases in Newborns and Children, to Michael O. Leavitt, Secretary of Health and Human Services. June 13. ftp://ftp.hrsa.gov/mchb/genetics/correspondence/ACHDGDNCletterstoSecretary.pdf.

Howse, J. L., and Katz, M. 2000. The importance of newborn screening. *Pediatrics* 106 (3): 595.

Johnson, K. 2004. Johnson Group Consulting PowerPoint presentation at Advisory Committee on Heritable Disorders and Genetic Diseases in Newborns and Children Meeting II, September 23. www.hrsa.gov/heritabledisorderscommittee/presentations/sep04/johnsonpresent.htm.

Newborn Screening Task Force. 2000. Serving the family from birth to the medical home: a report from the Newborn Screening Task Force convened in Washington DC, May 10–11, 1999. *Pediatrics* 106 (2 Pt 2): 383–427.

Therrell, B. L., Williams, D., Johnson, K., Lloyd-Puryear, M. A., Mann, M. Y., and Ramos, L. R. 2007. Financing newborn screening: sources, issues, and future considerations. *J Public Health Manag Pract* 13 (2): 207–13.

Wald, N. 2007. Neonatal screening: old dogma or sound principle? *Pediatrics* 119 (2): 406–7.

Wilson, J. M. G., and Jungner, G. 1968. *Principles and Practice of Screening for Disease.* Geneva: World Health Organization.

Appendix
Descriptions of Five Genetic Disorders

Phenylketonuria (PKU)

Phenylketonuria is a disorder of amino acid metabolism. Affected individuals cannot properly process the amino acid phenylalanine, which accumulates and damages the brain. The effects of PKU are mental retardation, organ damage, unusual posture, and, in women, compromised pregnancy.[1]

Species differ in which amino acids they can synthesize and which must be ingested—the latter are called essential amino acids. Phenylalanine is an essential amino acid for humans; it is obtained from the diet, especially from protein-rich foods such as meat, eggs, dairy, and nuts. It is also found in most wheat products, such as pasta and bread, and in some fruits, such as oranges and cherries (www.pku.com). Symptoms can be prevented by detecting PKU through newborn screening and then placing the child on a strict diet that limits phenylalanine intake. This diet must be followed throughout the individual's entire life to avoid PKU's dire effects (National Institutes of Health 2000).

Classical PKU is an autosomal recessive disorder caused by mutations in both alleles of the gene for phenylalanine hydroxylase (PAH), the enzyme that converts phenylalanine to tyrosine, another amino acid. The mutations on each allele do not have to be the same to cause PKU; as many as 400 disease-causing mutations have been discovered, thus many different combinations are possible (National Institutes of Health 2000). The type(s) and extent of mutations directly contribute to the severity of the disease. Phenotypic expression of a mutated gene presents as either a structurally altered form of the protein (the enzyme PAH) (Friedman et al. 1973) or a complete failure to synthesize it (Ledley et al. 1988). In either case, normal metabolic function is lost, leading to the buildup of phenylalanine levels. The estimated frequency of PKU mutations in newborns in the United States is greater than 1 in 20,000.

As noted above, PKU can result in severe mental retardation unless detected soon after birth and treated with a special dietary formula. In the past, physicians believed that the low-phenylalanine diet was necessary only during the developmental years of childhood and that individuals could go off the diet in adulthood; however, experience has shown that the diet should be adhered to for life. Those who go off the diet complain of an inability to concentrate and behavioral changes, such as depression. Most who resume the diet report cognitive and behavioral improvement (www.pku.com).

Women with PKU must be on a low-phenylalanine diet during pregnancy to protect their babies from serious birth defects that may result from high levels of phenylalanine in the blood. These risks are essentially eliminated if the woman maintains her diet before conception and throughout the pregnancy. Avoiding "birth defects" does not include PKU itself—the gene may be passed on by the mother whether she is on the diet or not. But the effects of maternal PKU on fetal brain development can be severe, whether or not the fetus has PKU (Rouse et al. 1997).

The strict dietary regimen can be difficult to maintain, even with a mature knowledge of the consequences of going off the diet. A major complaint is the expense and unpleasantness of the protein supplement required to make up for the proteins absent from the diet (www.pku.com). Depending on the age of the patient, the cost of the formula may range from $20 to $40 a can, and this may last for only a few days; it also tastes bad (Johnson and Ayer 2007).

Testing Methods

Newborn screening tests for PKU measure the concentration of phenylalanine in the bloodspot. Newborns with a severe deficiency of PAH usually have an increased phenylalanine concentration (relative to tyrosine concentration) in the blood within the first 24 hours after birth. Those with a less severe deficiency may not have an elevated phenylalanine concentration in this timeframe, however, so the test should be performed after the first 24 hours, or a second test should be administered if the first was done too early. Laboratories in the United States use cutoff values for blood phenylalanine levels of 2 to 6 mg/dL (125 to 375 µmol/L) (Kaye 2006). The cutoff value must be deliberated carefully—lower values reduce the risk of false negatives but increase the number of false positives, and vice versa with higher cutoff values (Marsden, Larson, and Levy 2006).

Three main methods are used for screening newborns for PKU in the United States: the Guthrie BIA (bacterial inhibition assay), fluorometric analysis, and tandem mass spectrometry (MS/MS). The Guthrie BIA is inexpensive and reliable, but fluorometric analysis and MS/MS produce fewer false positive results. Preliminary data indicate that MS/MS produces fewer false positive results than the fluorometric method in samples obtained in the first 24 hours of life (Kaye 2006). All states now test for PKU (see table 1.1), and most states now use MS/MS (National Newborn Screening and Genetics Resource Center 2007c). After a positive screening result, confirmation can be obtained by DNA testing if there is a known familial mutation, or by further metabolic testing.

Medium-Chain Acyl-CoA Dehydrogenase Deficiency (MCAD)

Medium-chain acyl-CoA dehydrogenase deficiency is a rare disorder of fatty acid metabolism caused by the lack of an enzyme required to metabolize fat to produce energy. People with MCAD cannot go without food for long. Fasting may cause seemingly well infants and children to experience sudden hypoglycemia, vomiting, lethargy, encephalopathy, respiratory arrest, hepatomegaly, seizure, apnea, cardiac arrest, and/or coma, or sudden death (Wang 2000). Identifying affected children before symptoms appear is vital to preventing such crises.

The primary fuel for the human body is glucose, which is largely obtained from the diet. Each organ uses glucose to generate the energy to carry out cellular functions. If the body runs out of glucose, the normal metabolic fail-safe is for a group of enzymes to begin converting the body's stored fat into energy. People with MCAD are unable to manufacture one of these crucial enzymes, medium-chain acyl-CoA dehydrogenase (National Institutes of Health 2007). As a result, they are unable to use body fats as a source of energy, and some or all of their organ(s) eventually more or less shut down. Coma and death are the most severe consequences of this system collapse.

MCAD is an autosomal recessive disorder caused by mutations in both alleles of the ACADM gene, which produces the dehydrogenase enzyme. The mutations on each allele do not have to be the same to cause MCAD (Andresen et al. 1997); as many as 26 disease-causing mutations have been discovered, which can translate into a large number of possible combinations (Wang 2000). The particular type(s) and extent of mutations directly affect the severity of disease. Phenotypic expression of a mutated gene presents as either a structurally altered form of or a complete lack of medium-chain acyl-CoA dehydrogenase (Andresen et al. 1997). Either situation results in loss of normal metabolic function, leading to the inability to metabolize fats to produce energy. The estimated frequency of MCAD mutations in newborns in the United States is greater than 1 in 25,000.

Treatment includes the avoidance of fasting and the use of a nutritional supplement. It is strongly recommended that children with MCAD should not go without food for more than 12 hours. They should eat high-carbohydrate meals (starches, cereals, pastas, etc.), especially when they are ill. A low-fat diet may be helpful, and a high-fat diet should be avoided. Care must be taken to ensure that infants and children have late-night and early-morning meals to prevent a long period of fasting overnight (www.fodsupport.org/mcad_fam.htm).

There is some uncertainty about how much difference early identification through universal newborn screening would make in the health of children with the genetic mutations associated with MCAD. For example, there is poor genotype-phenotype correlation; some families have healthy children who bear the same homozygous mutant alleles as their severely affected siblings (Korman et al. 2004). Mysteriously, some people with MCAD mutations do not exhibit symptoms until adulthood (Wilhelm 2006). Different combinations of mutations result in different forms of the disease—the most minor of these (still poorly defined) may never be noticeable by the individual or the physician (Zschocke et al. 2001).

Testing Methods

The best method of screening for MCAD is MS/MS, which measures the amount of octanoylcarnitine (C8) and related metabolites in the blood (Chace and Kalas 2005).

C8 is an intermediate product of fatty acid metabolism that is normally further broken down to produce energy when glucose levels are low. Because of the mutation that alters the functioning of medium-chain acyl-CoA dehydrogenase, C8 accumulates in the blood. Healthy newborns typically have very low levels of C8 (<0.3 μmol/L), but newborns with MCAD have higher levels; depending on the mutation(s) and the severity of the phenotype, C8 levels can reach well into double-digit micromolar levels (Chace et al. 1997). C8 concentration should be assessed in relation to other MCAD-associated metabolites; elevated levels of C8 alone can also indicate other metabolic disorders. Each unique disorder demonstrates a specific MS/MS pattern of metabolite levels along with elevated C8 (Chace and Kalas 2005).

Testing of the newborn is the best screening option because C8 levels are significantly higher in the first three days of life than later, making the disease easier to detect (Kaye 2006). Any newborn with a C8 level greater than 1 μmol/L should be definitively diagnosed by urinary and plasma C8 analysis and DNA testing as part of follow-up. MS/MS methods are highly sensitive and specific, with most false positive results being the consequence of setting a rigid cutoff of 0.3 μmol/L (Chace and Kalas 2005). Every state either offers or requires newborn screening for MCAD; all but one require it, although a few have not fully implemented the program (see table 1.1).

Sickle Cell Disease (SCD)

Sickle cell disease is a subgroup of the disorders called hemoglobinopathies, inherited diseases of red blood cells that result in varying degrees of anemia, serious infections, pain episodes, and damage to vital organs. The symptoms are caused by abnormal kinds and/or amounts of hemoglobin (March of Dimes 2008).[2]

Hemoglobin binds oxygen in the lungs and delivers it to body tissues via the bloodstream (Bridges 2002). In SCDs, an abnormal hemoglobin known as HbS can cause some red blood cells to become stiff and abnormally (crescent or sickle) shaped. These red cells can get stuck in tiny blood vessels, causing pain and sometimes organ damage (U.S. Department of Energy 2005). Damage to the spleen makes affected children especially vulnerable to bacterial infection. Sickle cells have a much shorter lifespan than normal red cells, which leads to a dearth of red cells (anemia). Blood transfusions are necessary to restore red cells to functional levels, but this has the side effect of accumulating too much iron in the blood, which can also damage organs (www.sicklecelldisease.org).

Sickle cell disease is an autosomal recessive disease caused by a point mutation in both alleles of the hemoglobin β gene (HBB). The normal gene produces hemoglobin A (HbA) and red cells have a normal shape. Two copies of the mutated gene produce a different version of the hemoglobin, depending on the mutation inherited from each parent, giving the red cell its abnormal shape (U.S. Department of Energy 2005). The type(s) and combination of HBB mutations result in different forms of SCD that differ in severity.

There are three main genetic variants of SCD:

- In sickle cell anemia (Hb S/S), individuals inherit a sickle cell gene from each parent. This disease can cause severe pain, damage to the vital organs, stroke, and sometimes death in childhood. The estimated frequency in newborns in the United States is greater than 1 in 5000, with a higher incidence among African Americans (1 in 500) (U.S. Department of Energy 2005). Young children with sickle cell anemia are especially prone to dangerous bacterial infections such as pneumonia and meningitis. Vigilant medical care and prophylactic treatment with penicillin, beginning in infancy, can dramatically reduce the risk of these adverse effects and the risk of death. Affected babies should receive all regular childhood vaccinations (including *Haemophilus influenzae* type b and pneumococcal vaccines) to help prevent serious bacterial infections. Additional treatments depend on the severity of symptoms, but may include intermittent pain medications and regular blood transfusions (March of Dimes 2008). Until the advent of modern medicine, most children with sickle cell anemia did not live past childhood. Now, about half live past the age of 50 (www.sicklecelldisease.org).
- In S-β-thalassemia (Hb S/A, or Hb S/Th), the child inherits one sickle cell gene and one gene for β-thalassemia, another inherited anemia. The frequency in newborns in the United States is greater than 1 in 50,000. Symptoms are often milder than for Hb S/S, but severity varies among affected children. Routine treatment with penicillin may not be recommended for all affected children.
- In sickle-hemoglobin C disease (Hb S/C), the child inherits one sickle cell gene and one gene for another abnormal type of hemoglobin, HbC. The frequency in newborns in the United States is greater than 1 in 25,000. As with Hb S/A, this form is often milder than Hb S/S, and routine penicillin treatment may not be recommended.

Current newborn screening methods can diagnose the type of disease and identify carriers (individuals with "sickle trait"). Approximately 8 to 10 percent of African Americans are carriers. Sickle trait does not produce symptoms, but this carrier status has implications for reproductive decisions.

Testing Methods

Newborn screening programs look for abnormal hemoglobins in the bloodspot. Abnormal hemoglobins are reported in order of quantity (Kaye 2006). The presence and amount of abnormal hemoglobins are indicative of SCD; the type of abnormal hemoglobin essentially specifies the form of the disease.

The most common screening method is isoelectric focusing (IEF) (Kaye 2006). IEF allows for screening of many samples per test, but it is prone to inconsistency. Another screening method is high-performance liquid chromatography (HPLC), which produces more consistent results than IEF and does not require repeat testing. Though HPLC cannot process as many samples per test as IEF, it may have a higher benefit-to-cost ratio because of its reliability. Both methods may miss or misinterpret rare hemoglobin variants of clinical importance (Henthorn, Almeida, and Davies 2004). All states screen for SCD (see table 1.1), and the majority use IEF (National Newborn Screening and Genetics Resource Center 2007b). Infants with positive screening results should have confirmatory testing of a second blood sample before two months of age. Confirmatory testing is performed by IEF, HPLC, hemoglobin electrophoresis, and/or DNA-based methods. If further confirmation or explanation is needed because the type of disease remains unclear, the parents can be tested to identify their carrier status (Kaye 2006).

Cystic Fibrosis (CF)

In cystic fibrosis, abnormalities in the cystic fibrosis transmembrane regulator (CFTR) protein result in lung and digestive problems and in death at an average age of 36.5 years (www.cff.org). Studies suggest that early diagnosis and treatment improve the growth of babies and children with CF. Treatment varies, depending on the severity of symptoms, but may include a high-calorie diet supplemented with vitamins and medications to improve digestion, respiratory therapy to help clear mucus from the lungs, and medications to improve breathing and prevent lung infection (March of Dimes 2006).

Normal body mucus is smooth and aqueous. It keeps the linings of certain organs moist and prevents them from drying out or becoming infected. In people with CF, mucus is thick and sticky, and it accumulates in lungs and blocks airflow. This environment makes it easy for bacteria to grow and leads to repeated serious lung infections. Over time, these infections can cause severe damage to the lungs. The abnormal mucus also blocks ducts in the pancreas that secrete pancreatic enzymes, which aid in digestion in the small intestine; as a consequence the intestine cannot adequately absorb fats and proteins. This leads to malnourishment and irregular stools. In addition, CF causes individuals to expel excessive amounts of body salts through sweating, which disrupts the body's chemical balance. CF can also cause infertility, mostly in men (National Institutes of Health, National Heart, Lung and Blood Institute 2008).

Cystic fibrosis is an autosomal recessive disorder caused by mutations in both alleles of the CFTR gene (U.S. Department of Energy 2003). The mutations on each allele do not have to be the same to cause CF; more than 1500 disease-causing mutations have been discovered, so a tremendous variety of combinations can occur (Cystic Fibrosis Mutation Database 2007). The type(s) and extent of mutations directly contribute to the severity of the disease (Welsh and Smith 1993).

Cystic fibrosis is one of the most common inherited disorders in the United States, with an estimated frequency in newborns of greater than 1 in 5000. The disorder is relatively common in Caucasians, with an incidence of about 1 in 2500, and has a fairly high incidence among Hispanics, 1 in 13,000 (Centers for Disease Control and Prevention 2007). In the rest of the population, it is relatively rare. As with SCD, follow-up screening identifies carriers of the disorder as well as affected children. One in 29 Caucasians (1 in 31 of the entire U.S. population) are carriers (Cystic Fibrosis

Foundation 2007; March of Dimes 2006). Of the many different CF gene mutations that have been identified, the frequency of each varies significantly in different populations (Centers for Disease Control and Prevention 2007). Testing for the most common CF mutation in the U.S. population, ΔF508, detects 70 percent of mutant alleles, but mostly in the Caucasian population (Kaye 2006).

People with CF can lead active lives, unless they have a severe form of the disease. Their diets need to consist of high-calorie, high-fat meals, which are vital for normal growth and development in children. Adults should stay on the diet throughout life to maintain optimal health. This diet makes up for the underabsorption of nutrients from food and provides the extra energy needed for the laborious breathing experienced by people with CF. In addition, pancreatic supplements must be taken to promote intake of nutrients in the small intestine. People with CF should avoid smoke and polluted air and should take precautions against contact with germs; frequent hand-washing is recommended. With recent advances in medicine, 40 percent of the CF population in the United States is now over the age of 18—a remarkable public health achievement. Those who reach adulthood may live into their forties and beyond (www.cff.org).

Testing Methods

In newborn screening for CF, concentrations of the protein immunoreactive trypsinogen (IRT) are analyzed in the bloodspot; high concentrations are indicative of CF. IRT is an enzyme precursor produced in the pancreas, and in the newborn with CF it leaks into the bloodstream from the damaged pancreas (Sontag et al. 2006). Concentrations of IRT considered a positive result vary by state. Some have a specific numerical cutoff (65 to 100 ng/mL) (National Newborn Screening and Genetics Resource Center 2007a), while others use a more blanket approach by following up on results in the top percentile (top 1% to top 5%).

If the initial IRT screen finds high levels, two methods of follow-up are used: DNA analysis of the dried bloodspot for a set of CF mutations or measurement of IRT concentration in a second bloodspot taken at two to three weeks of age (the latter is called persistent elevation analysis). Follow-up testing is not equivalent to a definitive diagnosis unless two or more mutations are found through DNA testing; persistent elevation testing needs further confirmation. The sensitivity of IRT testing is 95 percent; the specificity exceeds 99 percent after follow-up testing. The gold-standard test for CF diagnosis is the sweat test (measuring chloride level in sweat), which should be performed shortly after follow-up testing. Nutritional complications can arise if the newborn is not diagnosed early (Kaye 2006). Thirty-three states have fully implemented mandated CF screening, and more are in the process of doing so (see table 1.1).

Severe Combined Immunodeficiency Disorder (SCID)

Severe combined immunodeficiency is an extreme condition caused by a defect in the T lymphocytes and/or B lymphocytes, the regulators of the immune system. This defect usually results in the onset of one or more serious infections in the first few months of life. The infections are usually severe or life-threatening, and include pneumonia, meningitis, and bloodstream infections (www.scid.net). Early diagnosis allows for emergency treatment, such as bone marrow transplantation.[3]

Lymphocytes are a type of white blood cell, produced from blood-forming precursors, or stem cells, in the bone marrow. Some lymphocyte precursors move to the thymus gland, where they become T cells. Others remain in the bone marrow, where they mature into B cells and natural pathogen-killer cells. Each type of cell is responsible for a particular immune response. Normally, T cells encourage other immune cells to respond to foreign substances, as well as directly combating certain viral and fungal infections. B cells become antibody-producing cells; the antibodies attack foreign substances (antigens) that mark invading viruses, bacteria, and fungi. "SCID" is a term applied to a group of inherited disorders characterized by defects in both T and B cell responses, hence the term "combined" (National Institutes of Health 2008).

SCID is a genetic condition resulting from a number of different mutations; 10 have been clinically identified, but not all have been genetically mapped (www.scid.net). The most common form of SCID is the X-linked genotype, a mutation of the IL2RG gene. This explains why SCID occurs predominantly in males: males have only one copy of the X chromosome, so the defective IL2RG is the only IL2RG gene that can be expressed. The normal gene makes a protein that is crucial to the production of T lymphocytes (National Institutes of Health 2005). There are also seven (identified) autosomal recessive forms of the disease, with mutations on various chromosomes. One form is ADA (adenosine deaminase) deficiency, a mutation that prevents production of the enzyme that helps cells destroy certain toxic substances. Without ADA, toxins build up and prevent T cells from reaching maturity.

So far, the most significant treatment for SCID is a bone marrow transplant from a relative with identical human leukocyte antigen (HLA). If successful, this enables the recipient to create the protein products essential to proper production and/or maintenance of T and B cells. In the 1980s, a technique was developed that allowed individuals with SCID to receive bone marrow from donors who are not 100 percent HLA matches; this remains the most frequently used treatment for SCID. People with the ADA form of SCID can be treated with enzyme-replacement therapy. Eventually, different forms of SCID may be treated by gene therapy, but attempts at this have resulted in unintended harmful effects (www.scid.net).

The case of the "Bubble Boy" is the most well-known example of SCID. As recounted by B. Ballard, "A mother who had lost a child to SCID was pregnant with another boy. Because having another affected child was a risk, plans were made on how to keep this child healthy until his immune system could be corrected. David was born on September 21, 1971, and was immediately placed into a specially designed isolator crib where the air was specially filtered and all items that went into the crib were sterilized. It was quickly proven that his immune system was indeed defective, but there was hope that his older sister would be a match for a bone marrow transplant. Unfortunately, his sister was not a good match and at that time there were no donor registries. The rest of the family was tested, but no one was a match for David" (www.scid.net). Exasperated after years of waiting for a cure, the boy's doctors and family decided to attempt a bone marrow transplant, using his sister as donor. Unfortunately, the bone marrow contained traces of a virus, and David died two weeks later.

SCID is rare: the incidence among newborns in the United States is not known with any precision, but is estimated at 1 in 100,000. No state currently includes the disorder in its newborn screening program, but efforts are under way to examine SCID for possible future inclusion (Kalman et al. 2004). Screening for SCID raises a number of ethically complex issues. The screening itself is more technically demanding and more expensive than the tests for conditions currently included in newborn screening panels, and the possible treatment options—bone marrow transplantation or gene therapy—are risky, expensive, not available to all children with SCID, and of uncertain effectiveness.

Testing Methods

Currently, no mass screening method is available to warrant the addition of SCID to a state's newborn screening panel. Testing immediately after birth can be done by sequencing DNA, if the family mutation is known, or by counting the number of T and B cells and assessing their function. However, the current tests to confirm SCID must be applied to individual blood samples and take hours to prepare. The high costs associated with this amount of workup make screening prohibitive. To make screening for all newborns affordable, an automated screening method for processing hundreds of samples every day, with minimal hands-on requirements, would need to be developed (National Institutes of Health 2008).

NOTES

1. For general information on PKU, see National Center for Biotechnology Information, National Library of Medicine, National Institutes of Health, "Nutritional and metabolic diseases: phenylketonuria," in *Genes and Disease* (www.ncbi.nlm.nih.gov/books).

2. For general information on SCD, see "Blood and lymph diseases: anemia, sickle cell," in *Genes and Disease* (www.ncbi.nlm.nih.gov/books).

3. For general information on SCID, see "Diseases of the immune system: severe combined immunodeficiency," in *Genes and Disease* (www.ncbi.nlm.nih.gov/books).

REFERENCES

Andresen, B. S., Bross, P., Udvari, S., Kirk, J., Gray, G., Kmoch, S., Chamoles, N., Knudsen, I., Winter, V., Wilcken, B., Yokota, I. Hart, K., Packman, S., Harpey, J. P., Saudubray, J. M., Hale, D. E., Bolund, L., Kolvraa, S., and Gregersen, N. 1997. The molecular basis of medium-chain acyl-CoA dehydrogenase (MCAD) deficiency in compound heterozygous patients: is there correlation between genotype and phenotype? *Hum Mol Genet* 6 (5): 695–707.

Bridges, K. R. 2002. Hemoglobin overview. http://sickle.bwh.harvard/hemoglobin.html.

Centers for Disease Control and Prevention, National Office of Public Health Genomics. 2007.

Cystic fibrosis: clinical validity. www.cdc.gov/genomics/gtesting/ACCE/FBR/CF/CFCliVal _21.htm.

Chace, D. H., Hillman, S. L., Van Hove, J. L., and Naylor, E. W. 1997. Rapid diagnosis of MCAD deficiency: quantitative analysis of octanoylcarnitine and other acylcarnitines in newborn blood spots by tandem mass spectrometry. *Clin Chem* 43 (11): 2106–13.

Chace, D. H., and Kalas, T. A. 2005. A biochemical perspective on the use of tandem mass spectrometry for newborn screening and clinical testing. *Clin Biochem* 38 (4): 296–309.

Cystic Fibrosis Foundation. 2007. Frequently asked questions. www.cff.org/AboutCF/Faqs/ #Who_gets_cystic_fibrosis?

Cystic Fibrosis Mutation Database. 2007. Statistics. www.genet.sickkids.on.ca/cftr/Statistics Page.html#cooliris.

Friedman, P. A., Fisher, D. B., Kang, E. S., and Kaufman, S. 1973. Detection of hepatic phenylalanine 4-hydroxylase in classical phenylketonuria. *Proc Natl Acad Sci USA* 70 (2): 552–56.

Henthorn, J. S., Almeida, A. M., and Davies, S. C. 2004. Neonatal screening for sickle cell disorders. *Br J Haematol* 124 (3): 259–63.

Johnson, A., and Ayer J. 2007. Treatment for disorders identified through newborn screening. www.ncsl.org/programs/health/genetics/nbstreat.htm.

Kalman, L., Lindegren, M. L., Kobrynski, L., Vogt, R., Hannon, H., Howard, J. T., and Buckley, R. 2004. Mutations in genes required for T-cell development: IL7R, CD45, IL2RG, JAK3, RAG1, RAG2, ARTEMIS, and ADA and severe combined immunodeficiency. HuGE review. *Genet Med* 6 (1): 16–26.

Kaye, C. I. 2006. Committee on Genetics: newborn screening fact sheets. *Pediatrics* 118 (2): e934.

Korman, S. H., Gutman, A., Brooks, R., Sinnathamby, T., Gregersen, N., and Andresen, B. S. 2004. Homozygosity for a severe novel medium-chain acyl-CoA dehydrogenase (MCAD) mutation IVS3-1G > C that leads to introduction of a premature termination codon by complete missplicing of the MCAD mRNA and is associated with phenotypic diversity ranging from sudden neonatal death to asymptomatic status. *Mol Genet Metab* 82 (2): 121–29.

Ledley, F. D., Koch, R., Jew, K., Beaudet, A., O'Brien, W. E., Bartos, D. P., and Woo, S. L. 1988. Phenylalanine hydroxylase expression in liver of a fetus with phenylketonuria. *J Pediatr* 113 (3): 463–68.

March of Dimes. 2006. Quick reference: cystic fibrosis. www.marchofdimes.com/professionals/ 14332_1213.asp.

———. 2008. Birth defects & genetics: sickle cell disease. www.marchofdimes.com/pnhec/4439 _1221.asp.

Marsden, D., Larson, C., and Levy, H. L. 2006. Newborn screening for metabolic disorders. *J Pediatr* 148 (5): 577–84.

National Institutes of Health. 2000. Phenylketonuria: screening and management. NIH consensus statement, October 16–18. http://consensus.nih.gov/2000/2000Phenylketonuria113 html.htm.

———. 2005. X-linked severe combined immunodeficiency—genetics home reference. http:// ghr.nlm.nih.gov/condition=xlinkedseverecombinedimmunodeficiency.

———. 2007. Medium-chain acyl-coenzyme A dehydrogenase deficiency—genetics home reference. http://ghr.nlm.nih.gov/condition=mediumchainacylcoenzymeadehydrogenase deficiency.

———. 2008. Genome.gov: learning about severe combined immunodeficiency (SCID). www .genome.gov/13014325.

National Institutes of Health, National Heart, Lung and Blood Institute. 2008. What is cystic fibrosis? www.nhlbi.nih.gov/health/dci/Diseases/cf/cf_what.html.

National Newborn Screening and Genetics Resource Center. 2007a. Cystic fibrosis (CF): laboratory testing in 2007. www2.uthscsa.edu/nnsis/.

———. 2007b. Hemoglobinopathies: laboratory testing in 2007. www2.uthscsa.edu/nnsis/.

———. 2007c. Phenylketonuria (PKU): laboratory testing in 2007. www2.uthscsa.edu/ nnsis/.

Rouse, B., Azen, C., Koch, R., Matalon, R., Hanley, W., de la Cruz, F., Trefz, F., Friedman, E., and Shifrin, H. 1997. Maternal Phenylketonuria Collaborative Study (MPKUCS) offspring: facial anomalies, malformations, and early neurological sequelae. *Am J Med Genet* 69 (1): 89–95.

Sontag, M. K., Corey, M., Hokanson, J. E., Marshall. J. A., Sommer, S. S., Zerbe, G. O., and Accurso, F. J. 2006. Genetic and physiologic correlates of longitudinal immunoreactive trypsinogen decline in infants with cystic fibrosis identified through newborn screening. *J Pediatr* 149 (5): 650–57.

U.S. Department of Energy. 2003. Cystic fibrosis gene. www.ornl.gov/sci/techresources/Human _Genome/posters/chromosome/cftr.shtml.

———. 2005. Sickle cell anemia disease profile. www.ornl.gov/sci/techresources/Human _Genome/posters/chromosome/sca.shtml.

Wang, S. 2000. Fact sheet: MCAD deficiency. www.cdc.gov/genomics/hugenet/file/print/ factsheets/FS_MCAD.pdf.

Welsh, M. J., and Smith, A. E. 1993. Molecular mechanisms of CFTR chloride channel dysfunction in cystic fibrosis. *Cell* 73 (7): 1251–54.

Wilhelm, G. W. 2006. Sudden death in a young woman from medium chain acyl-coenzyme A dehydrogenase (MCAD) deficiency. *J Emerg Med* 30 (3): 291–94.

Zschocke, J., Schulze, A., Lindner, M., Fiesel, S., Olgemöller, K., Hoffmann, G. F., Penzien, J., Ruiter, J. P., Wanders, R. J., and Mayatepek, E. 2001. Molecular and functional characterisation of mild MCAD deficiency. *Hum Genet* 108 (5): 404–8.

Abbreviations and Acronyms

3MCC	3-methylcrotonyl-CoA carboxylase deficiency
AAP	American Academy of Pediatrics
ACMG	American College of Medical Genetics
ACOG	American College of Obstetricians and Gynecologists
AHRQ	Agency for Healthcare Research and Quality
CAH	congenital adrenal hyperplasia
CBA	cost-benefit analysis
CCGP	Communities of Color and Genetics Policy project
CDC	Centers for Disease Control and Prevention
CEA	cost-effectiveness analysis
CF	cystic fibrosis
CFTR	cystic fibrosis transmembrane regulator
CH	congenital hypothyroidism
CK (CPK)	creatine kinase (creatine phosphokinase)
CORN	Council of Regional Networks for Genetic Services
CUA	cost-utility analysis
DHEC	Department of Health and Environmental Control
DMD	Duchenne muscular dystrophy
GA1	glutaric aciduria type 1 or I (glutaric acidemia type 1 or I)
GAC	genetics advisory committee
GAO	U.S. Government Accountability Office (before July 2004, General Accounting Office)
HbS	sickle hemoglobin
Hb S/A	sickle-β-thalassemia (S-β-thalassemia) (also abbreviated as Hb S/β-Th or Hb S/Th)
Hb S/C	sickle-hemoglobin C (sickle-C) disease

Hb S/S	sickle cell anemia
HRSA	Health Resources and Services Administration
ICER	incremental cost-effectiveness ratio
IOM	Institute of Medicine
IRB	institutional review board
IRT	immunoreactive trypsinogen
LCHAD	long-chain L-3-hydroxyacyl-CoA dehydrogenase deficiency (long-chain 3-hydroxyacyl-CoA dehydrogenase deficiency; long chain hydroxyacyl-CoA dehydrogenase deficiency)
MCAD	medium-chain acyl-CoA dehydrogenase deficiency
MCHB	Maternal and Child Health Bureau
MS/MS	tandem mass spectrometry
MSUD	maple syrup urine disease
NARC	National Association of Retarded Children
NBSAC	newborn screening advisory committee
NCC	National Coordinating Center
NICE	National Institute for Health and Clinical Excellence (United Kingdom)
NICHD	National Institute of Child Health and Human Development
NIH	National Institutes of Health
OHRP	Office for Human Research Protections
PCV7	7-valent pneumoccocal conjugate vaccine
PKU	phenylketonuria
PPV	positive predictive value
QALY	quality-adjusted life-year
RC	regional collaborative group (genetics and newborn screening)
RCT	randomized controlled trial
SACGT	Secretary's Advisory Committee on Genetic Testing
SCD	sickle cell disease
SCHIP	State Children's Health Insurance Program
SCID	severe combined immunodeficiency disorder
USPSTF	U.S. Preventive Services Task Force

Index

3-methylcrotonyl-CoA carboxylase deficiency, 131

Advisory Committee on Heritable Disorders and Genetic Diseases in Newborns and Children (Advisory Committee on Heritable Disorders in Newborns and Children), 12, 41, 188, 196, 232, 317
advocates/advocacy: and advisory committees, 150, 155–56; consensus-seeking by, 93; and effectiveness, 94–95; and expansion of testing, 39–40, 131; and fairness, xii, 19–20, 21; group, 92, 93; and mandatory testing, 95–96; measures of success for, 90–91; and parents, 92; personal, 93; perspective of, 89–105; and phenylketonuria testing, 98, 125, 182; and policy, 320; and public level, 92; questions for, 92–97; representation by, 97; role of, 15–16, 21, 125; and tandem mass spectrometry, 127; and test panels, 43, 96; and test selection, 34; and treatment, 93, 96, 102
African Americans, 72, 161–62, 163–64, 167, 169, 172, 184, 215
Agency for Healthcare Research and Quality (AHRQ), 180, 181, 186, 203, 244
American Academy of Pediatrics (AAP), 11, 195, 317; and advisory committees, 140; and funding, 40; Newborn Screening Task Force, xiii–xiv, 11, 32, 41, 181, 186, 206, 244, 245, 248–49, 267, 316, 320; and parental permission, 257
American College of Medical Genetics (ACMG), xiv, 12, 14, 41, 170, 187; and advisory committees, 138; and carrier testing, 293; and cost-effectiveness analysis, 65–66; and funding, 40; recommendations of, xiv, 33–34, 196, 197, 198, 203–6, 207, 208–9, 316–17, 319, 321–22; and research needs, 37
American College of Obstetrics and Gynecology, 293
American Health Decisions, 43
American Medical Association, 190
American Society of Human Genetics, 166
argininemia, 162
Arizona, 59, 65, 79
Ashkenazi Jews, 161
Association of Public Health Laboratories, 40
Association of State and Territorial Health Officials, 244
Australia, 74, 170, 277

benefits: and American College of Medical Genetics report, 204–5, 206; and ethical policy, 314; and fairness, 12–13, 17; of health care, 27; to newborn, 30; and public health, 21–22; variation in, 23–24
bias, 44–45, 66, 226, 259
biotinidase deficiency, 70–71, 78, 128

346   INDEX

blood samples/blood spots, 58; consent for use of, 14; de-identified, 282, 286; and fairness, xi; identifiable, 255, 266; national biobank for, 249–50; and research, 15, 230, 237, 255, 259, 325–27; retention of, 237; retrospective use of, 66, 259; and sickle cell disease testing, 183; testing of, 196–97; use of stored, xiv
BRCA1/2 screening, 170
Burke, Edmund, 146

California, 59, 65, 79, 155, 167, 216
cancer, 131, 199–200
carrier testing, xv, 3, 14, 292–308
Centers for Disease Control and Prevention (CDC), 107, 180–81, 186, 190, 203, 249–50, 293
Children's Bureau, 182, 190
Children's Health Act, 40–41, 232
Children's Hospital of Philadelphia, 249–50
choice, 22, 24, 27, 31, 95, 130, 209
citrullinemia, 161
civic/community orientations, 144, 145
cohort design, 229–30
Communities of Color and Genetics Policy project, 160, 162, 166, 170, 172
community organizations, xiii, 160, 172–73
confidentiality/privacy, ix; and blood samples, 239, 244, 246, 247; and data storage, 14; and ethical policy, 315; and fairness, 17; and justification for testing, 130; and Massachusetts research protocols, 276, 282, 287; protection of, 11; and race/ethnicity, 162; respect for, 323; right to, 13; and state governments, 2
congenital adrenal hyperplasia (CAH), 71–72, 76, 125, 128, 226, 228
congenital hypothyroidism (CH), 63, 68–69, 78, 125, 128, 237, 257, 294
consent, ix; and advisory committees, 152, 155; and carrier testing, 295; and cost, 17; and Duchenne muscular dystrophy, xii, xiii, 111–13, 117; and expanded test panels, 324–25; and fairness, 17; and identifiable blood samples, 266–67; and information provision, 201; and mandatory testing, 13, 14, 199, 200, 323, 325; and Massachusetts research protocols,

276, 278–80, 284, 286; and natural history, 286–87; of parents, 13, 199–200, 255–71, 294; and public health, 270; and race/ethnicity, 167–68; and research, 14, 239–43, 244–45, 246–49, 260–66, 284, 326, 327; waiver of, 261–66, 267, 268–69
consultation, ix, 15–16, 43
cost(s): of adequate health care, 27–28, 29; and cost-effectiveness analysis, 46, 63; defined, 59–60; and diagnosis, 67, 104; direct vs. indirect, 60; and ethical policy, 314, 315; and fairness, 12–13, 17, 20, 31, 318, 321; and false positives, 33; to families, 35; and federal government, 104; and financing, 36; of health care, 25–26; and health outcomes, 60–61; and information, 304–5; and Massachusetts research protocols, 284–85; of Medicaid, 36; and racial/ethnic concerns, 169; and selection of tests, 32, 33; and technology, 33; and test panel expansion, 198; and treatment, 67; understatement of, 318–19; and Wilson and Jungner criteria, 98, 103. See also financing/funding
cost-benefit analysis (CBA), 80, 172; and advocacy, 94; and congenital hypothyroidism, 68; defined, 45–46; and efficacy research, 231; and fairness, xii, 13, 21; method of, 59; and phenylketonuria, 67–68
cost-effectiveness analysis (CEA): and bias, 66; and biotinidase deficiency, 70–71; and carrier testing, 306, 307; and congenital adrenal hyperplasia, 71–72; and congenital hypothyroidism, 68–69; as criterion, 58–81; and cystic fibrosis, 77; defined, 46; and efficacy research, 231; and fairness, xii, 13, 19, 21, 46–52, 81; and health outcomes, 59, 60–61; lack of agreement among, 78; lack of influence of, 79–80; limitations of, 80; and maple syrup urine disease, 69–70; methods of, 59–62; and mortality, 66; and opportunity costs, 58–59; as organizing framework vs. mechanical rule, 47, 51–52; and phenylketonuria, 63, 68, 76, 78; and policy, 209; and quality-adjusted life-year, 47, 67; in